LIBRARIES WITHOUT LIMITS:
CHANGING NEEDS - CHANGING ROLES

EAHIL
sixth
european
conference
of medical and
health libraries

Proceedings of former conferences:

Christine Deschamps, Marc Walckiers (eds.), Medical Libraries: Cooperation and New Technologies. First European Conference of Medical Libraries, Brussels, Belgium, 22–25 October 1986. Amsterdam; New York; Oxford; Tokyo; North-Holland, 1987. (Contemporary topics in information transfer. Vol.5)

David W.C. Stewart, Derek J. Wright (eds.), Health Information for All: A Comman Goal. Proceedings of the Second European Conference of Medical Libraries, Bologna, Italy, November 2–6, 1988. München; London; New York; Paris: Saur, 1989

Suzanne Bakker, Monique C. Cleland (eds.), Information Transfer: New Age – New Ways. Proceedings of the third European Conference of Medical Libraries, Montpellier, France, September 23–26, 1992. Dordrecht; Boston; London: Kluwer, 1993

Tony McSeán, John van Loo, Euphemia Coutinho (eds.), Health Information – New Possibilities. [Proceedings of the fourth European Conference of Medical and Health Libraries, Oslo, Norway, June 28 – July 2, 1994.] Dordrecht; Boston; London: Kluwer, 1995

Suzanne Bakker (ed.), Health Information Management: What Strategies? Proceedings of the fifth European Conference of Medical and Health Libraries, Coimbra, Portugal, September 18–21, 1996. Dordrecht; Boston; London: Kluwer, 1997

LIBRARIES WITHOUT LIMITS: CHANGING NEEDS - CHANGING ROLES

Proceedings of the 6th European Conference of Medical and Health Libraries, Utrecht, 22–27 June 1998

Edited by

Suzanne Bakker

Librarian / Information Specialist,
Central Cancer Library,
The Netherlands Cancer Institute,
Amsterdam, the Netherlands

on behalf of the

EUROPEAN ASSOCIATION FOR
HEALTH INFORMATION AND LIBRARIES

KLUWER ACADEMIC PUBLISHERS
DORDRECHT / BOSTON / LONDON

A C.I.P. Catalogue record for this book is available from the Library of Congress.

ISBN 0-7923-5626-8

Published by Kluwer Academic Publishers,
P.O. Box 17, 3300 AA Dordrecht, The Netherlands.

Sold and distributed in North, Central and South America
by Kluwer Academic Publishers,
101 Philip Drive, Norwell, MA 02061, U.S.A.

In all other countries, sold and distributed
by Kluwer Academic Publishers,
P.O. Box 322, 3300 AH Dordrecht, The Netherlands.

Printed on acid-free paper

Printed in the Netherlands.

CONTENTS

CONFERENCE ORGANIZATION

Local Organizing Committee

Suzanne Bakker
Sieb Bohlken
Loes Donkers
Dinie During-Buis
Joop Dijkman
Paul van Olm
Gertie Veldman

Social Programme Committee

Ingrid Arnold
Sieb Bohlken
Loes Donkers
Marjan Hartog
Inge van Gaal
Gemma Geertshuis
Hans Plettenburg
Gertie Veldman
Leo Vittali
Miebet Wilhelm-de Gouw

International Programme Committee

Suzanne Bakker, the Netherlands Cancer Institute, Amsterdam, NL
Manuela Colombi, Schering-Plough SpA, Milan, Italy
Gaynor Davies, Institute of Cancer Research, London, UK
Gerdien de Jonge, Veterinary Faculty, Utrecht University, NL
Rikie Deurenberg-Vos, Library Medical Science, University of Nijmegen, NL
Joop Dijkman, NIWI, Amsterdam, NL
Patricia Flor, Telemark College, Skien, Norway
Gemma Geertshuis, Medical Faculty, Utrecht University, NL
Arne Jakobsson, Swedish Institute for Health Services, Stockholm, Sweden
Marta Jordà Olives, Agència de Recerca i Docència, Barcelona, Spain
Vincent Maes, Pfizer, Brussels, Belgium
Vanna Pistotti, Instituto 'Maria Negri', Milan, Italy
Manuela Prates Caetano, Faculdade de Ciências Médicas UNL, Lissabon, Portugal
Ingegerd Rabow, Lund University, Lund, Sweden
Friedhelm Rump, Tierärztliche Hochschule, Hannover, Germany
Rüdiger Schneemann, Technische Universität, Berlin, Germany
Ian Snowley, Department of Health, London, UK
Lubimora Soltésová, P.J. Safarik University, Kosice, Slovak Republic
Fons van den Eeckhout, University Library, Universiteit Maastricht, NL
Lívia Vasas, Semmelweis Medical University, Budapest, Hungary
Miebet Wilhelm-de Gouw, Deaconesses' Hospital, Utrecht, NL

AUTHOR ADDRESSES

E. Akre
Norwegian Library Association, Section Medicine & Health, Diakonhjemmet Hospital, Medical Library, Box 23, Vinderen, N-0319 Oslo, Norway

R. Aprea
Istituto Dermopatico dell'Immacolata (IDI - IRCCS), Scientific Library, Via Monti di Creta 104, I-00167 Roma, Italy

H. Brazier
Royal College of Surgeons in Ireland, St Stephen's Green, IR- Dublin 2, Ireland

H. Breul
Pharmacie Centrale des Hôpitaux (PCH-AGAM), 7-17 rue du Fer à Moulin, F-75005 Paris, France

A. Brice
University of Oxford, Health Care Libraries Unit, level 3, John Radcliffe Hospital, Oxford OX3 9DU, England, UK

M. de Cock Buning
Marnixstraat 391',
NL-1016 TB Amsterdam, the Netherlands

L. Cavazza
Soprintendenza per i beni librari e documentari, Regione Emilia-Romagna, Via Farini 28, I-40124 Bologna, Italy

L.A. Colaianni
National Library of Medicine, 8600 Rockville Pike, Bethesda MD 20894, USA

M. Curti
Direzione Scientifica, Policlinico S. Matteo, Piazzale Golgi 2, I-27100 Pavia, Italy

M. da Luz Antunes
Instituto de Clínica Geral da Zona Sul, Largo Prof. Arnaldo Sampaio, Centro de Saũde de Sete Rios, P-1500 Lisboa, Portugal

G.B. de Jonge
University of Utrecht, Faculty of Veterinary Medicine, P.O. Box 80159, NL-3508 TD Utrecht, the Netherlands

M. Della Seta
Istituto Superiore di Sanita', Servizio Documentazione, Viale Regina Elena, 299, I-00161 Rome, Italy

R.L. Faraino
Ehrman Medical Library New York University School of Medicine, 550 First Avenue, New York, N.Y. 10016, USA

D. Flake
Coastal Area Health Education Center Library, P.O. Box 9025, Wilmington, NC 28402, USA

V. Fraser
Department of Health, Room 311A
Skipton House, 80 London Road, London
SE1 6LH, England, UK

G. Gabutti
Biblioteca Direzione Scientifica,
Policlinico S. Matteo, Piazzale Golgi 2, I-27100 Pavia, Italy

B. Gann
Centre for Health Information Quality,
Highcroft, Romsey Road, Winchester
SO22 5DH, UK

L. Ghirardi
ICC, 22 Bd Richard Lenoir, F-75011
Paris, France

S. Godbolt
Regional Library & North Thames
Information Unit, Thames Postgraduate
Medical & Dental Education, University
of London, 33 Millman Street, London
WC1N 3EJ, UK

S. Gove
St Gorge's Hospital Medical School,
University of London, Cranmer Terrace,
London SW17 0RE, England, UK

G. Günther Bjørkenes
Østfold fylkeskommune
Sentraladministrasjonen, P.b. 220, N-1701 Sarpsborg, Norway

L. Haglund
Spri Library and Research Report Bank,
Box 70487, S-107 26 Stockholm, Sweden

A. Hicks
Information Resources, School of Health
and Related Research, University of
Sheffield, Regent Court, 30 Regent Street,
Sheffield S1 4DA, UK

D. Hummel
Amberg Health Sciences Library, 100
Michigan N.E., Grand Rapids, Michigan
49503-2560, USA

J. Hunter
West Suffolk Hospital NHS Trust,
Hardwick Lane, Bury St Edmunds,
IP33 2QZ, UK

M. Jordà-Olives
Unitat d'Informació, Agencia de recerca i
Docència, Hospitals Vall d'Hebron, Pg.
Vall d'Hebron 119-129, E-08035
Barcelona, Spain

R. Kiley
Wellcome Trust, 183 Euston Road,
London NW1 2BE, England, UK

U. Korwitz
German National Library of Medicine,
Joseph-Stelzmann-Str. 9, D-50924 Köln,
Germany

R.E. Lande
University Library of Trondheim,
Høgskoleringen 1, N-7034 Trondheim,
Norway

D. Law
King's College London, University of
London, Strand, London WC2R 2LS,
England, UK

C. Lefebvre
UK Cochrane Centre, Summertown
Pavilion, Middle Way, Oxford OX2 7LG,
England, UK

A. Lusher
Cairns Library, Oxford Radcliffe Hospital
The John Radcliffe Trust, Oxford
OX3 9DU, England, UK

J. MacDougall
Library Association of Ireland, 53 Upper
Mount Street, IR- Dublin 2, Ireland

E. Marinoni
Biblioteca A. Vallisneri, Universita' degli
Studi di Padova, Viale Giuseppe Colombo
3, I-35121 Padova, Italy

C. Massiter
Dept. Information and Library Studies, University of Wales Aberystwyth, Llanbadarn Fawr, Aberystwyth SY23 3AS, Wales, UK

A.A.H.M. Mathijsen
Bilderdijklaan 14, NL-3723 DC Bilthoven, the Netherlands

G. Merlo
University of Torino, Central Medical Library, Corso Dogliotti 14, I-10126 Torino, Italy

G.F. Miranda
Sanofi Winthrop, Research Center Sanofi Midy, Scientific Information Department, Via Piranesi 38, I-20137 Milano, Italy

G. Myers
Witwatersrand Health Sciences Library, PO Box 351, 2050 WITS, Johannesburg, South Africa

M. Nardelli
Zeneca s.P.A., Medical Information Group, Palazzo Volta, Via F. Sforza, I-20080 Basiglio (MI), Italy

R. Nollan
Stollerman Clinical Branch Librarian, University of Tennessee, Memphis, 956 Court Avenue, Box 14A, Memphis, TN 38163, USA

T. Oker-Blom
Veterinary Medicine Library, University of Helsinki, P.O. Box 57, FI-00014 Helsingin yliopisto, Helsinki, Finland

C. Oppenheim
Loughborough University, Department of Information and Library Studies, Lougborough, Leics, LE11 3TU UK

A. Pailley-Katz
Bibliotèque de l'Université Paris 7, Denis Diderot, 2 Place Jussieu, F-75251 Paris Cedex, France

L. Parr
City University Library, Northampton Square, London EC1V OHB, England, UK

F. Pasleau
Bibliothèque de la Faculté de Médecine, Université de Liège, CHU, B-35, B-4000 Sart Tilman, Belgium

P. Pekkarinen
National Library of Health Sciences, Haartmaninkatu 4, FI-00290 Helsinki Helsinki, Finland

V. Pistotti
GIDIF-RBM, Piazza S. Agostino 24, I-20123 Milano, Italy

H. Rabow
Department of Theory of Science and Research, Gothenburg University, S-412 98 Gothenburg, Sweden

K. Reavie
Shiffman Medical Library, Wayne State University, 4325 Brush Street, Detroit Michigan 48201, USA

D. Reinitzer
Veterinärmedizinische Universität Wien, Bibliothek, Veterinärplatz 1, A-1210 Vienna, Austria

M.F. Ribes Cot
Hospital Universitario Marques de Valdecilla Biblioteca Marquesa de Pelayo, Avenida Valdecilla s/n, E-39008 Santander, Spain

H.E. Roosendaal
Elsevier Science, P.O. Box 2400, NL-1000 CK Amsterdam, the Netherlands

T. Roper
Royal College of Veterinary Surgeons Wellcome Library, Belgravia House, 62-64 Horseferry Road, London SW1P 2AF England, UK

R. Rotolo
Biblioteca Polo Didattico di Vialba, Università di Milano, Via G.B. Grassi 74, I-20157 Milano, Italy

A. Rozic-Hristovski
Central Medical Library, Vrazov trg 2, SI-1105 Ljubljana, Slovenia

J.S.M. Savenije
University Library, Utrecht University, Postbus 16007, NL-3500 DA Utrecht, the Netherlands

A. Scheiber
Fachhochschule Magdeburg, Fachbereich Sozial- und Gesundsheitswesen, Maxim Gorkistrasse 31-37, D-39108 Magdeburg, Germany

H. Seger
Bibliothek, Medizinhistorisches Institut und Museum, Universität Zürich, Rämistr. 71, CH-8006 Zürich, Switzerland

L. Smith
Graduate School of Library and Information Science, University of Illinois at Urbana-Champaign, 501 E. Daniel St., Champaign, Illinois 61820, USA

O. Sundin
Boras University College of Health Sciences, Box 55 140, S-504 04 Boras, Sweden

C. Szabo-Balogh
Central Library of the Semmelweis University of Medicine, Úllöi út 26, H-1085 Budapest, Hungary

J. Szabo Szavay
Central Library of the Semmelweis University of Medicine, Üllöi út 26, H-1085 Budapest, Hungary

A. Tomlin
Centre for Evidence Based Mental Health, Department of Psychiatry, University of Oxford, Warneford Hospital, Oxford OX3 7LF, England, UK

N. Tržan-Herman
LEK d.d., R&D, Special Library, Verovskova 57, SI-1526 Ljubljana, Slovenia

J. Tsafrir
Medical Library, Chaim Sheba Medical Center, 52621 Tel Hashomer, Israel

C. Urquhart
Department of Information and Library Studies, University of Wales Aberystwyth, Llanbadarn Campus, Aberystwyth SY23 3AS, Wales, UK

A.M. Uryga
Université Jagiellonne de Cracovie, Bibliothèque Médicale, ul. Medyczna 7, PL-30 688 Krakow (Cracovie), Poland

G.J. van Dieën
Sophia Hospital, Medical Library, P.O. Box 10400, NL-8000 GK Zwolle, the Netherlands

M. van Kuik
National Institute for the Victims of War (ICODO), Maliebaan 83, NL-3581 CG Utrecht, the Netherlands

N.W. van Putte
N.V. Organon (department: SDG InfoCentre), P.O. Box 20, NL-5340 BH Oss, the Netherlands

M. van Wegen
St Lucas Andreas Hospital, Jan Tooropstraat 164, NL-1061 AE Amsterdam, the Netherlands

L. Vasas
Central Library of the Semmelweis University of Medicin, Üllöi út 26, H-1085 Budapest, Hungary

M. Viragos
Central Library, Medical University of Debrecen, P.O. Box 18, H-4012 Debrecen, Hungary

M. Wake
The Library and Information Service, The School of Pharmacy, University of London, 29-39 Brunswick Square, London WC1N 1AX, England, UK

A. Weightman
Herbert Duthie Library, University of Wales College of Medicine, Heath Park, Cardiff CF4 4XN, Wales, UK

A. Weist
Medical Education Centre, Whipps Cross Hospital, Leystone, London E11 1NR, England, UK

C. Wickman
Karolinska Institute Library, Box 200, S-171 77 Stockholm, Sweden

A. Zeccato
Biblioteca Direzione Scientifica, Policlinico S. Matteo, Piazzale Golgi 2, I-27100 Pavia, Italy

PREFACE TO THE PROCEEDINGS OF THE SIXTH CONFERENCE

Suzanne Bakker
CENTRAL CANCER LIBRARY, THE NETHERLANDS CANCER INSTITUTE, AMSTERDAM, THE NETHERLANDS

The Utrecht conference including the continuing education courses, special interest group meetings and preconference symposium took a full week. Being one of the organizers of the conference, I do not consider it appropriate to even try to give an impression of this week.

These proceedings are the scientific account of this conference, published and printed to inform those who were not able to attend and to keep record for those who wish to refer to what has been presented. Not included in these proceedings are the summaries of the continuing education courses that took place on Monday 22 June till Wednesday 24 June; nor an outline of the Editors' Workshop held on Monday 22 June, neither the results of the Special Interest Group discussions during that week. The appendix at the end of this publication contains a list of courses and group meetings in order to give special attention to these initiatives.

The many subjects of importance and interest to the members of the European Association for Health Information and Libraries (EAHIL) are reflected in the contributions in these proceedings. It was noted that the quality of the papers and the presentations had risen since the first conferences. This could be the signal to create permanent special interest groups, next to the pharmaceutical and veterinary groups, in order to discuss matters arising in the fields of academic medical librarianship, clinical lirarianship, database production, nursing and allied health, problem-based learning, and WHO documentation. Electronic mail and discussion lists could add substantially to the exchange of ideas and make international cooperation within the reach of many colleagues. The growth and health of EAHIL will allow for higher quality and further specialization in these and other professional activities.

Will there be EAHIL conferences and workshops after the 8th International Congress on Medical Librarianship in London in 2000? Of course there will! Will there be conference proceedings published after these? Probably not, at least not full-text in print. Scientific communication in many disciplines, also in medicine as well as in medical librarianship, makes extensively use of the Internet. Although the printed version is very handy as a reference tool, the speed of distribution will benefit from electronic alternatives and the problem of archiving can be dealt with by the association.

Information professionals make the difference, i.e. adding value to information services. EAHIL makes the difference and will continue to do so, i.e. adding value, quality and friendship, to the profession.

CHANGING NEEDS - CHANGING ROLES: TAKE CARE OF EVIDENCE

R.B.J.C. van Noort
RIJKSINSTITUUT VOOR VOLKSGEZONDHEID EN MILIEUHYGIENE, BILTHOVEN, NL

Your Royal Highness, Ladies and Gentlemen

The Minister of Health, Welfare and Sport, originally accepted the invitation to open this international congress. She found it particularly unfortunate, however, that she was unable to be present here. As you may know, we just had elections in the Netherlands and are in the process of forming a new cabinet. Our Minister of Health, Mrs. Borst-Eilers, is also the leader of one of the parties and is now therefore closely involved in the formation of the new cabinet. But before Mrs. Borst became Minister, she was a specialist in Internal Medicine and Haematology, Director of a university hospital, Vice-president of the Dutch Health Council and a university professor in "Evidence-Based Medicine". I have the honour to address this congress in her place.

Knowledge sickness in health science

Mrs. Borst told me she has experienced that in the medical and health sciences, excellent information sources and services are available. Not in the least thanks to the US Government, which has even provided free Internet access to the MEDLINE database, the electronic version of the Index Medicus.

However, in spite of the initiatives and the efforts to access knowledge incorporated in documents, there is a serious knowledge sickness in health science. This illness is characterised by insufficiency of *using* available knowledge and relevant information. Solving this knowledge problem by collecting evidence and making evidence available, would establish a more rational and effective medicine. On behalf of my Minister, who is also a doctor herself, I would like to give you her view on this sickness and its therapy. To take care of evidence can be a great challenge, one in which also librarians and information workers have to play important roles.

Medical interventions in the past were made up of treatments like blood-letting, cupping, vomiting techniques, blistering of the skin by compresses, administration of purgatives and drinking of mixtures of herbs, spices and animal extracts. This health care of yesterday was not a random intervention and was really theoretically based. These theories, however, were neither based on clinical observations, nor were they evaluated through experiments or critical observations. In spite of the unsuccessfulness of the treatment procedures in those days, medical interventions were very much in demand because therapists took their time to care for patients: they had a humane, consoling attitude. Also, these therapists did their utmost to stimulate the natural process of healing in the patient.

In 1830, approximately one-and-a-half centuries ago, the first experiments for evaluating medical interventions took place. The movement "Médecine d'Observation" told physicians not to rely on speculation and theory about causes of disease, nor on single experiences. And indeed, their long series of observations showed that care, as opposed to intervention, was far more successful.

After a long period of no more than diagnoses and prognoses and - with good luck - natural healing, the triumphal march in medicine started at the end of 19th century with the development of fundamental laboratory medical sciences, like microbiology and pathology. Causes of disease were discovered and better understood, and this improved knowledge became both the predecessor and condition for the great discoveries of sulpha drugs and antibiotics just before World War II.

Sixty years later we are confronted with overwhelming medical knowledge and technology. The number of diagnostic and therapeutic procedures is immense, and so is the total field of medical practice, with almost 30 different specialisms in clinical medicine. The paradox here is that the explosion of knowledge has become associated with an insufficiency to *use* the available knowledge and relevant information. This applies both to individual physicians and the entire medical profession. In spite of tremendous amounts of medical knowledge, not seldom patients are given inadequate therapies.

The difference with the past is that modern medical interventions *are* logical, based as they are on theoretical predictions, or on what is thought to be a proven causal relation. Because occlusion of carotid arteries is thougt to be a risk for cerebral infarction, surgery has been performed since 1950. Although in 1970, results of a prospective controlled trial showd that an operation was not clearly advantageous, it continued to be popular. Recently, two controlled trials in Europe and the US have given evidence that an operation would only be favourable in an occlusion of more than 70%, and is not in an occlusion of less than 30%. In the latter case, the risk of cardiac or cerebral infarction, and even mortality, is larger. It seems that we rely on "mechanism-based medicine", without realising that it is still not sufficient to *predict* effects of treatments. Rational and effective medicine needs evidence. In spite of the explosion of knowledge, we still know too little of the human organism. A lot of treatments have never been evaluated on effectiveness for distinct groups of patients. This leaves room for non-scientific considerations, such as experience, preference, and influence of the media and industry. I would like to mention two examples of so-called logical treatments which disappeared after being unmasked as totally ineffective. The first is medicinal reducing of eye pressure in glaucoma to reduce the risk of blindness, and the second is placing a duct in the ear-drum of children where there is accumulated moisture.

Evidence based medicine

In the 1980s, the new movement at that time, Evidence Based Medicine, showed us how we could cure the knowledge sickness by collecting evidence and providing it in an accessible and manageable way. Collecting evidence has been done in two ways: by Medical Technology Assessment (MTA) and by Meta-Analysis.

MTA is directed at medical procedures already used in practice but still needing evidence as a base. Meta-Analyses deal with existing and already published investigations.

The Cochrane Collaboration was founded in 1992 to co-ordinate meta analyses and compile databases with systematic reviews. Pregnancy treatments were the first to be systematically reviewed. The results showed that in 1981 seven randomised controlled trials gave evidence of the favourable effect of corticosteroids in cases where there was a risk of a premature birth. However, in 1993 (twelve years later) still only 23% of the women who should have been injected did in fact receive the treatment. This clearly, but very regrettably, illustrates the indolence of health science.

Preceding this conference, yesterday and this afternoon, there have already been course and symposia about Cochrane Library and Evidence Based Medicine. Lectures about MTA and Meta-Analysis will be given by experts from Ireland, Germany, UK and Belgium, about MTA and Meta-Analysis in the Friday afternoon session "Evaluating information: Systematic approach".

Meta-analyses are of course useless if the results do not lead to more rational and effective medical practice. How can a General Practitioner (GP) find the evidence of meta analyses and systematic reviews? He doesn't have enough time to select and read scientific literature. So literature and information have to be brought to the consulting room of the modern doctor. In the Netherlands, over 80% of all GPs uses a computer. Nevertheless professional assistance and even ready-to-use advise is very much needed. Through the Dutch National Information System for GPs it is possible to be linked to Literature Information Systems and find answers in specific cases. Also consultations of librarians and information professionals can be supportive for physicians. In countries, such as Denmark and Great Britain, with isolated practices, out-reach activities of medical libraries are supportive for the GP. Hospital physicians can also get professional assistance - in some local and university hospitals clinical librarians participate in the ward rounds.

Providing specific case-oriented information and literature is one thing. Next to that, it is important to develop practice guidelines and protocols and to make them available to GPs. I would like to mention that the Cochrane Collaboration provides databases with systematic reviews on CD-ROM. An excellent example is the Dutch Poison Control Center, which provides 24-hour assistance service to health workers confronted with cases of acute intoxications. The Center uses an expert information system based on systematic reviews and evaluated literature. In particular medical associations have to publish, propagate and disseminate useful and validated information. In that way the modern doctor has fit-to-use evidence to his or her disposal. I want to underline that a practice guideline should support the doctor and should be patient-oriented, so that the doctor can inform the patient about his or her chances of recovery and can reach decisions together with the patient.

As evidence always applies to groups and not to individuals, guidelines should provide figures and probabilities. Good guidelines quantify uncertainties; they should not be directive - cookery book medicine - or "opinion-based".

Take care

The medical researcher cannot restrict to fit-to-use information or knowledge. He or she should also use dedicated services for current awareness of peer-reviewed relevant information. Next to that, medical investigators should keep up with evidence in their specific research field. In particular, he or she should focus on secondary, bibliographic or referring, information. Literature searches in electronic information sources, such as MEDLINE or EMBASE, can be done through end-user facilities or through professional assistance. In addition, full text, printing-on-demand and alerting services are provided by electronic Journals to an increasing extent. As Internet is not the most user-friendly medium, librarians should preselect useful sites or they should be an intermediary for the client and deliver services in an appropriate format - timely, useful and applicable to the user.

As this conference is devoted to changing roles, it is my suggestion that you should not forget to help your client to adapt to a changing environment in which electronic information is presented. He or she needs your help to get used to the changing information tools. In the Thursday morning and Friday afternoon sessions of this conference you will hear from British, American and Canadian experts about this subject: "Empowering the End-User".

Your Royal Highness, Ladies and Gentlemen. I have come to the end of my speech. I have told you about the development of EBM and explained why it is necessary to care for evidence in medical practice. I have briefly run through the ways GPs and medical investigators can find evidence nowadays. In this digital era one sometimes wonders whether libraries will have a role in the future. I am convinced that if you focus on your clients, give them your time, your attention and your personal interest, like a doctor does with a patient, there will be a continuing need for your excellent services.
Thank you.

Chapter 1: COPYRIGHT

Editorial introduction

The first chapter of these proceedings contains the presentations given at the first plenary session of the conference. Both speakers address the 'problem' of intellectual owners' rights, copyright. Madeleine de Cock Buning is explaining to us the general principles of copyright and the consequences of digitization and the new European Directives. Charles Oppenheim outlines the history of the relationship between publishers and librarians and how the changes in the early 1990s brought tension in this relationship. He points out that the proposed European Directive shifts the law quite significantly in favour of rights holders and against users and librarians. He emphasizes that it is in the scholarly publishing industry's interest to ensure that users get more rights.

The discussion at the end of the session made clear to the attendees that all medical librarians have to take their responsibility and must claim the fair use of electronic documents and databases on behalf of their users, for which licences can be negotiated and agreed upon.

At the closing of the conference the following statement was formulated:

"Medical, Nursing, Health Allied and Health Care Librarians *shall accept only that kind of licence agreements* for (electronic) full-text databases, information sources and data collections *that take into account the non-commercial, educational, scientific and public aspects* of medical and health related information and therefore they *will not accept too many restrictions or unfair limitations in contracts of publishers.*"

It is to the benefit of physicians, scientists, patients and the health care system that (medical) librarians take an active role in negotiating licence agreements.

LIBRARIES WITHOUT LIMITS, LIMITED BY COPYRIGHT?

Madeleine de Cock Buning
INSTITUTE FOR INFORMATION LAW, UNIVERSITY OF AMSTERDAM / DE BRAUW BLACKSTONE WESTBROEK - LAWYERS, AMSTERDAM, NL

Introduction

Copyright law offers statutory regulation of competing interests of right- holders and end-users of information. In a digital era libraries are both consumers and producers of copyright. That gives them a twofold position. On the one hand they are large scale consumers of information and on the other hand they are independent producers of electronic databases. In the Netherlands the famous Lite-ROM case was a result of this new role of libraries as database producers. I will get to that case later on. Without the protection of copyright on these library-produced-databases, the time and effort used to produce the databases could easily be lost. Without permission third parties could commercialize the library-databases.

Most important however remains the role of the library as a user of information. Libraries are, as the recent position paper of EBLIDA puts it, the gateways to information resources. Commercial producers of databases (publishers) currently used by libraries, are asking for rather big licence fees for information that used to be part of the public domain.

In this presentation some general principle of copyright will be introduced in a nutshell. What information is protected? What is the content of the protection? Who is the right owner?

After this introduction the consequences of digitization for copyright will be addressed. New European Directives, such as the Database Directive and the proposal for an harmonisation Directive and the WIPO (World Intellectual Property Organization) copyright treaty shall be addressed.

Copyright in a nutshell

Copyright is the exclusive right of the maker of literary, scientific and artistic works. Different from other intellectual property regimes such as trademarks or patents, for which no formal requirements are made for protection. In order to be protected a work must be created. That is to say it has to be expressed in some form. It also has to be original. In written law no definition of the term originality can be found. The Berne Convention gives no guidance as to what constitutes "originality". Originality is a criterium that emerged in case law. It differs from country to country. In Germany and France a higher standard exists than in Great Britain. At one end of the scale skill and labour must be expended in the work (e.g. not copied) on the other end intellectual and creative effort is required. In any case no qualitative judgement (e.g. whether a novel is to be considered literary art or merely a banal product) is used.

The copyright owner has the right to reproduce, publish or otherwise communicate his work to the public: photocopying, broadcasting, distribution through the Internet et cetera. Also the public lending of a work by a library is an exclusive right that belongs to the copyright owner.[1] Some Member States exempt this right for libraries in their respective copyright laws, libraries are however kept to pay a reasonable renumeration.[2] Scientific libraries are, in Holland at least, again exempted of paying this renumeration.[3] The exploitation rights are also limited in several other ways. These limitations differ from country to country. That is one of the reasons that the European Commission issued a Proposal for a Harmonisation Directive.[3] I will get to that Proposal later.

The initial copyright owner is the person who created the work. Sometimes, the author licences part of his exploitation rights to a publisher. In the field of exact-sciences the author often transfers his rights completely to a publisher.

Consequences of digitization of information

For libraries the consequences of digitization of information are capital. An important function of a library is to serve as a gatekeeper for information to the end-users. This task can be performed much more efficient thanks to digitization. The information demand of a client can be served almost immediately with modern databases that are electronically stored or on-line. Fast searching-software helps the librarians find what the client is looking for.

Database protection

An important and direct consequence of digitization for copyright law is the grow of the economic value of (collections of) information. Is such a collection of information protected?

It must be emphasized that the information as such is not protected. However, the *collection* of facts can be protected. The selection, sequence and organization of a database can be an original work of authorship. So what do you think, is a telephone book protected by copyright law? And what do you think about a dictionary?

In a case called "Van Dale Romme" the Supreme Court of the Netherlands ruled that a collection of facts was protected if the collection is the result of a selection that indicates a personal opinion of the maker.[5]

The Van Dale dictionary could in fact have been protected under a typical Dutch regime called "geschriftenbescherming". This is a thin form of protection without originally requirements which originates in the Dutch history. For example, pricelists, theater programs and time tables were protected in this way. Most famous are the broadcasting tables. Broadcasting time was related to subscribers of the TV-guides. For this reason programming information was considered protected material.

Other European countries that did not have such a historical safety net, were provided on March 11, 1996 with a modern safety net in the European Database Directive.[6] This Directive is aimed at both digital and analogue databases. It introduces a *sui generis* right for non-original databases. The producer of a database is granted an extraction right to protect the information contained in a database. His right lasts 15 years after the first publication of the database. If it is substantially altered another 15 years period of protection follows. Already an up-date of the database can start another 15 years period. If a publisher keeps updating the database, the extraction right lasts forever.

It has to be kept in mind that both the copyright and the *sui generis* protection of the database exists *next to* a possible copyright protection of the content of such a database. In a Dutch case about LiteRom, a database on a CD-ROM containing more than 50.000 book reviews the NBLC (Nederlands Bibliotheek en Lectuur Centrum/Dutch Library Centre) acted as a publisher without asking permission to the authors of the book review. The court ruled in December 1997 that the database contained illegal reproductions of copyrighted material and thus could no longer be used, not even on the spot in the library. The authors of the book reviews (freelance journalists that remained the copyright owners) did not give their consent to electronic publication. For a while Dutch libraries simply ignored this in their view unjust verdict and kept offering the use of the LiteRom to their visitors. Last week the LiteRom case was finally settled. The authors finally excepted the reasonable amount of money that was offered to them.

Last year a Dutch court ruled that also permission of free lance journalist must be acquired before their articles may be digitized and published on the Internet.

The consequence of the Database Directive (that still has to be implemented in some European countries such as the Netherlands) is a general concern for the access to information. Also for medical science the unconditional access to databases is of extreme importance. However, the library can also function as a publisher of a database, as in the production of the before mentioned LiteRom. Than, the library/publisher is of course very well of with some form of copyright or *sui generis* protection.

Proposal for a Harmonisation Directive[4]

Another consequence of the digitization of information is the adoption of the WIPO copyright treaty in December 1996 and the Proposal for a new European Directive.

On November 10, 1997 the EC adopted a Proposal for a Directive on the harmonisation of certain aspects of copyright in the information society. The goal of the proposed Directive is twofold:

1. To present harmonising measures to bring about a coherent and favourable environment for creativity investment in the Internal Market" (Explanatory Memorandum).
2. To implement the WIPO-treaties of December 1996.

In respect of these treaties an important observation can be made: Librarians fought successfully for the deletion of a very important article that was originally proposed by WIPO. In this article the reproduction right was stretched to all forms of reproduction, including the mere technical reproduction that occurs during e.g. browsing and caching. In the final text of the WIPO treaty these acts are no longer explicitly pointed out as restricted acts.

The recent European Proposal for a Directive includes a mandatory exemption for temporary acts of reproduction that are instrumental to the use of a work and that do not have any separate economic significance. If acts of reproduction occur as a part of a technical process, without direct intervention of a person (such is the case in caching and temporary storage in the working memory of a computer) and these acts do not have any economic significance they are exempted. However, certain forms of caching, in particular those which increase the intensity of use, do not fall under this exception. Browsing however, is explicitely allowed in the Proposed Directive's Preamble.

The other issues dealt with in the Proposed Directive are: the right of communication to the public; including making available for access; limitations to the exclusive rights, as well as legal protection of technological measures and rights management information.

If the Directive was adopted unchanged, the main problems for the libraries would be:

1. Member States are not allowed any exceptions for libraries other than those listed in the Directive.
2. All exceptions that are listed are optional (except one), that has as a consequence that harmonisation, the main goal of the Directive, will not come about.Alle member States will remain having their own different regimes.
3. Display on screen is considered as communication to the public. For that libraries cannot show on-site information without obtaining a special licence for such purpose.
4. Legal protection of anti-copying and rights management systems have strong impact on the viability of the exceptions as formulated in the Directive. Circumvention of technical measures should indeed be allowed for activities allowed by the copyright owners or permitted by law.

Concluding remarks

When addressing the question as indicated in the title of this presentation:
"Libraries without limits, limited by copyright"?
the answer will be a typical lawyers answer: **YES** and **NO**.

I START WITH THE NO:

This has to do with the changing role of the modern library. Copyright or *sui generis* protection of databases produced by libraries is not a limitation for libraries but an advantage. First of all, this protection makes it possible to avoid other people misusing or commercializing the library databases. Second, extra funds can be raised when libraries to some extend start exploiting there valuable databases.

AND YES:

..libraries are limited by copyright if the proposed Harmonisation Directive will be adopted unchanged. For this it is instrumental that a strong librarian lobby is formed. As publishers have become professional lobbyist, also libraries should organize and form a tight counter movement. It also makes sense to lobby in a national environment since Member States are left to fill in quit a lot of exemptions. Especially the library reproduction right exemption is left to the Member States; e.g. to reproduce works that are no longer available on the market. Also during licence negotations with publishers about e.g. the making available of information online libraries will strenghten their position by working together. In fact, libraries are getting better and better in putting there position across, if you think of the changes they caused at WIPO in the most important international copyright treaty. I would say, keep up the good work!

Notes

[1] Directive 92/100/EG, Pb L 346/61
[2] Art. 15c paragraph 1 Dutch Copyright Law
[3] Art. 15c paragraph 2 Dutch Copyright Law
[4] Proposal for a European Parliament and Council Directive on the Harmonisation of Certain Aspects of Copyright and Related Rights in the Information Society, COM (97) 628 final
[5] HR 4 January 1991, NJ 1991, 608
[6] 96/9/EG (Pb. L 77/20)

INFORMATION OWNERSHIP, COPYRIGHT AND LICENCES

Charles Oppenheim
DEPT. OF INFORMATION AND LIBRARY STUDIES, LOUGHBOROUGH UNIVERSITY, LEICESTER, UK

Introduction

In this short presentation, I want to look at the tension between librarians and copyright owners - especially publishers - over copyright law.
What I want to demonstrate to you is:
- that a few years ago, there was considerable tension between librarians and copyright owners;
- that in recent years relationships have improved somewhat, although we have a long way to go;
- but that there is a real risk that proposed changes to copyright law will make things far worse.

Some history

Ten years ago, the relationship between publishers and librarians was fairly straightforward. Libraries subscribed to books and journals and placed them on their shelves. Users read or borrowed these items, and in some cases photocopied portions of the material.

Although there was concern about the amount of photocopying going on, in practice the technology of photocopying meant that the problem was self-limiting:
- the quality of photocopies is inferior to the original;
- it is a slow and tedious process to photocopy a large number of pages;
- it is also quite easy to police, as it is obvious when someone is spending hours at the photocopying machine;
- large scale photocopying is also quite expensive.

Ten years ago, there was no relationship between libraries and copyright owners in respect of the digitising of material in print form, or use of electronic information. The only relationships were for licences to use online hosts or CD-ROMs, and the ground rules for what was allowed seem to be well understood and respected.

Although at that time there was much talk about the use of electronic information, and reports had been written on the potential of digitising copyright materials for use in libraries to create an electronic, digital or virtual library, no librarian was seriously developing comprehensive services based on digitised content, and no publisher had been approached on the topic.

Changes in the early 1990s

Librarians began to approach publishers for clearance to digitise. Furthermore, the first use of the word "electrocopying" began to appear. Electrocopying as generally understood refers to the conversion of print material into some digitised form, whether by OCR or by some form of image scanning.

There were good reasons why the publishers should have concerns about these approaches. Once something has been electrocopied, it would be easy for any person with access to this digitised material to send it around the world to thousands or millions of people with a trivial amount of effort. This, of course, would lead to loss of sales of the original materials by the publisher. Furthermore, the copies would be perfect, it would cost the perpetrator virtually nothing to do this copying, and such actions would be difficult if not impossible to police. The contrast with photocopying could not be more marked.

In addition to such straight copying, there is also the risk that something in digitised form would be amended, and yet still have the appearance of the original text. In other words, it appears to have all the authority of the publisher, with all the associated quality control, and yet perhaps have serious errors or misleading statements in it due to the unauthorised changes. Dissemination of such inauthentic copies could lead at best to the loss of reputation for the publisher, and at worst the threat of legal action if the inaccurate information had been relied on, say, for a surgical procedure.

So, because of fears of both loss of revenue and loss of reputation, publishers were eager to keep a lid on the genie of electrocopying. Such approaches as librarians were making were typically rebuffed by publishers, who either had no policy in place, or had a policy of rejecting such approaches.

Librarians encountered scepticism and sometimes outright hostility from the publishers they approached. Thus, around 1992 and 1993, it was clear that publishers and librarians were moving into opposing entrenched positions, with the publishers frequently refusing permission, and librarians becoming more unhappy about the denial of what they regarded as a perfectly legitimate request.

Increasing pressure in the mid 1990s

The pressure increased, partly because of initiatives such as the Digital Library Initiative in the USA and the eLib programme in the UK, and by 1995, publishers found themselves at the receiving end of uncoordinated approaches by a variety of projects requesting similar things. Basically, the project leaders were seeking permission to digitise certain items for the purpose of one of their projects - items whose copyright was owned by the publishers.

At the same time, a number of related issues seemed to be coming up for increasing debate - the nature of fair dealing in the electronic environment, the way charges should be made for permission to digitise, the responsibility for archiving of materials that had been digitised, and the need for some generally accepted standard contractual terms.

In the UK, we decided to do something about the situation. So, since 1996, a series of informal meetings have been held between representatives of the higher education community in the UK and representatives of the UK publishing industry.

What was agreed was that a series of working parties should be set up to explore the details of the issues I have just described. Only informal minutes without attributing comments to specific individuals were kept, people spoke for themselves and not as representatives for their employer or association, and the objective was to find as much common ground as possible. Each working party typically comprised a dozen or so people, about half representing the academic institutions and about half representing the publishers.

It must be said the omens were not that propitious. There has long been tension between copyright owners, creators and users of scholarly materials. Some academics and librarians take an aggressive stance, believing that the publishers with their repeated price rises are the villains of the piece. They argue that publishers will wither away in the electronic environment and to help this trend, they urge that academics should ignore publishers, place their material directly on the Web, and should waive all copyright to that material, relying on netiquette to ensure that their material will not be abused.

Others have argued that librarians should adopt a unified front, refusing to subscribe to materials from publishers notorious for their price rises, and have recommended a series of minimum requirements - basic ground rules - for any deals between a library and a publisher, with the implication that no HEI library should break ranks and accept a deal less favourable than what is agreed.

Despite this somewhat unpromising background to the work, the experiment was a remarkable success. Guidelines on fair dealing in an electronic environment, on the basic charging algorithms that should be employed when granting permissions, the definitions for terms used in contracts and some model clauses for such contracts have all been agreed. Further work is underway to agree what is, or is not allowed under inter-library loan and document supply between libraries in the digital age.

All this work is not going on in isolation. For example, the UK Reproduction Rights Organisation, the Copyright Licensing Agency is working on a one stop shop to provide convenient and simple clearance for any organisation seeking to clear digitising rights, and hopes to launch this service before the end of 1998.

In short, peace - or at least a truce with goodwill - has broken out between the UK user community and the publishers who serve it. This has not gone down well in some quarters, where it is felt that the villains - that is to say, the publishers - should be firmly put in their place. Equally, some publishers will no doubt continue to be aggressive in their approach to the granting of, and the pricing of, permissions to digitise.

Risks and opportunities

The issues raised by electrocopying are a microcosm of broader issues facing the publishing and the user communities. After all, electrocopying is, surely, a temporary issue in the period between publishers offering solely print materials and them offering parallel publishing or solely electronic.

Temporary, electrocopying as an issue may be, but all the tensions, fears and attitudes that were brought out will be seen again when we deal with other thorny issues, such as how to deal with multimedia products.

In my view, the work I have described provides a model of how we can resolve some of these issues. I am sure all parties have learned a lot from their involvement in the Working Parties, in particular in respect of the other sides' concerns and problems they face. Whilst even just three years ago I was very pessimistic about the future of the relationship between libraries and the publishers, I am now cautiously optimistic. Before I tell you why I am only cautiously optimistic, let me tell you a story.

A man was walking along a cliff path when he suddenly slipped and fell. Flinging out his hand, he grabbed hold of a bush. He was left dangling at the end of a hundred foot drop clinging onto the bush.
"Help", he cried, "someone help me".
Suddenly there was a clap of thunder and a deep voice boomed out "This is God. I can help you."
"Please save me from the fall" cried out the man.
God said "Do you believe?"
"Yes" cried the man, "I believe".
"Excellent" said God, "if you believe, just let go of the bush, let yourself fall, and I will save you."
The man thought for a minute. He then cried out "Help, is anyone else there?"

Why did I tell this story? In order to resolve the problems raised by the digital environment, everyone - authors, librarians, users, publishers, bookshops, subscription agents and so on will have to take risks.

I believe there are more opportunities than threats out there, but there can be no doubt that by taking the risks, some will make mistakes, and some will fall by the wayside. We will only have ourselves to blame if, by taking dogmatic attitudes, the good relationship ceases and conflict breaks out. *So why is there a problem?*

So, if everything is fine, why I am only cautiously optimistic? This is because of the proposed changes to the law that the European Union is considering in a draft Directive, and it is this issue I now want to consider for a few minutes.

The EC draft Directive

The European Commission is planning an important new Directive on "the harmonisation of certain aspects of copyright and related rights in the Information Society". The draft Directive was published in its latest form in February 1998.

So what are the features of this draft Directive? It proposes a series of changes to Member States' law so that the changes agreed to the Berne Convention (the international convention controlling much copyright law world-wide) that were agreed late in 1996 can be implemented throughout the EU. It proposes a reproduction right, a communication to the public right, user exceptions, a distribution right, and the legal protection of anti-copying and anti-rights management systems.

The *reproduction right* would give copyright owners the right to authorise or prohibit direct or indirect, temporary or permanent reproduction by any means and in any form, in whole or in part, their work.

The *communication right* would give copyright owners the right to authorise or prohibit communication to the public by any means of their works. Interestingly, the magic words 'in whole or in part" do NOT appear, so the implication is that this right only covers the whole work.

The *distribution right* would give the copyright owner the right to control sale or distribution of his work, but when the owner has sold or distributed the work, the owner cannot control what happens subsequently to that work within the Community - for example, it can be re-sold.

These rights on their own would be draconian, but there are exceptions. These include a mandatory exception to the reproduction right where reproduction is caused by the technology and has no separate economic significance (for example, copying onto a computer's RAM for the purpose of display). Further exceptions that may be incorporated into legislation if the national Government wishes to include photocopying, reproduction of audio visual materials by individuals for private non commercial use, reproduction made by public libraries, museums and other similar establishments, copying for the sole purpose of "illustration for non-commercial teaching or scientific research", whatever that might mean, and so long as the source is indicated, copying for use for visually or hearing impaired people, reporting current events, quotation for criticism or review, and for public security, administrative or judicial procedure.

Any such exceptions shall only apply if the copying does not unreasonably prejudice the righstholders' legitimate interests or conflicts with the normal exploitation of the works by the rightsholder.

The draft Directive also proposes that penalties be introduced against the manufacture, distribution or use of devices to circumvent technological measures to protect copyright; against the removal or alteration of any electronic rights management information; or the distribution or communication of copyright material from which electronic rights management information has been removed in order to induce or facilitate copyright infringement.

Concluding remarks

It is not my intention in this talk to discuss the pros and cons of the proposed Directive. My objective is to point out that the proposals as they currently stand shift the law quite significantly in favour of rights holders and against users and librarians.

It is also to point out that the pressure for these changes has largely come from the audio visual industries, rather than from the publishing industry, although no doubt the latter welcomes the general trend.

The point I want to make is that there is little point in developing a law that is largely ignored by the population because they perceive, for whatever reason, that it is unjust or irrelevant, and that is extremely difficult to enforce, and it is my contention that what is proposed falls into this heading.

I believe the draft Directive as it stands could have a profound negative impact on the relationship, always tense, between publishers and librarians. It could, indeed, lead to the breakdown of the current dialogue between the two parties. This, in consequence, would have catastrophic effects on both the learned publishing industry and the libraries.

The libraries may find themselves under pressure from their patrons to, for example, refuse to buy any products that incorporate Electronic Copyright Management Systems, or that are published by particular publishers that are known to enforce their rights vigorously.

Authors of manuscripts will come under pressure from their employers to either only deal with publishers who are lax about enforcement, or to directly add their materials to the vast amount of data on the Web without going through the traditional channels. Such pressures would lead to publishers receiving fewer manuscripts, and to find themselves increasingly in competition with other publishers that are more relaxed about the law, and with the Web. On the other hand, libraries will find they are having to deal increasingly with material that is difficult to identify, has poor bibliographic control, and is poorly indexed or refereed.

In short, publishers and librarians need each other. They may not always like the fact that they need each other, but they do form a symbiotic relationship. That relationship is under strain, and indeed, in the medium term, it may break completely. New technology may lead to learned publishers, libraries or both vanishing. But right now, and for the immediate future, the relationship seems set to continue. However, the proposed new law being considered by the EU will lead to copyright owners being in a much stronger position than hitherto. If I were a publisher, I would not be rejoicing at this, but worrying. The new law may lead to a complete break with libraries and their patrons, and it is the publishing industry that will suffer.

To sum up, what I am arguing is that it is in the scholarly publishing industry's interest to ensure the draft Directive is watered down to give users more rights. If it joins forces with users in this effort, and if they succeed, then copyright law can stumble along as at present - full of compromises, satisfying no one fully, but everyone willing to work within the rules. But if the law shifts dramatically in favour of the owners, I foresee that everyone - authors, patrons, librarians and scholarly publishers - will be the losers.

Chapter 2: SCIENTIFIC COMMUNICATION

Editorial introduction

In this chapter several aspects of the scientific communication process, of which publishing is an important part, will be dealt with. Hans Roosendaal, physicist by training but now publisher with Elsevier Science Publishers, has presented his view on the process. Recognizing the four functions in scientific communication and publishing, those of certification, registration, archiving and awareness, makes it possible to understand and clarifies the interdependence of scientific authors, publishers, libraries and readers. As his views on this topic are published elsewhere, it is decided not to include these in full text in these proceedings but to refer to the URL.[1]

The presentation of Hampus Rabow draws our attention to the internal, self-correcting system in scientific literature, consisting of peer review, editorial control and public discussion. Notwithstanding this system of quality control occasionally scientific articles are withdrawn after publication. He found that retracted articles still are being cited in order to support arguments in later articles; the fact that the citing author does not refer to the fact of retraction, makes clear that in this respect quality control by authors and referees is not yet optimal, although checking retractions is nowadays very easy if one uses MEDLINE. Maria Nardelli and co-authors argue that it could be the library's added-value to inform users about retractions in the literature, at least to try to make users aware of it.

An important tool for studying scientific communication is citation analysis. Two other papers on this subject were presented during this conference. In his paper Ulrich Korwitz (p. 107) makes a plea for the library to inform the users about the relative value of impact factors and citation analysis, referring to the work of Johann Stegman.[2] Tom Roper (p. 135) reports on the use of citation analysis to understand the communication channels and the relative importance of the scientific journals in a subject field, thereby giving his experience in the field of veterinary sciences.

The paper of Päivi Pekkarinen deals with the cultural and language boundaries that will set limits to the area of understanding in the virtual library. Especially in medical and health information the vernacular terms play a major role in "local" knowledge, understanding and use of the information. In the last paper of this chapter Jean Hunter tells us about her experience in setting up a local, electronic information resource that will help doctors to use and apply up to date clinically effective information. This paper must be read in conjunction with the many papers on evidence based medicine (see chapter 4). End-user support, either by clinical library services (see also Anne Lusher p. 67) or by consultancy (see also Maria da Luz Antunes p. 120) and mediating (see also Veronica Fraser p. 122), are important areas for the medical librarian to contribute to total quality management in patient care (see also Gerhardus J. van Dieën p. 114).

References

[1] <http://www.physics.mcgill.ca/~karttune/crisp97/>

[2] Stegmann J. How to evaluate journal impact factors. Nature 1997;390:550

RETRACTION OF ARTICLES: PEER-REVIEW AND QUALITY CONTROL

Hampus Rabow, Ingegerd Rabow
[1]DEPT. OF THEORY OF SCIENCE AND RESEARCH, GOTHENBURG UNIVERSITY; [2]REFERENCE DEPT., LUND UNIVERSITY LIBRARY UB2, SWEDEN

Introduction

Bibliometric measures such as publication impact factor and total number of citations have in many scientific fields become principal means of evaluating scientific merit. Thus it has become important to study how the system of publication in peer reviewed journals succeeds or fails in maintaining standards of quality control. One particularly interesting indicator of these standards is the response to mistakes in the control system.

Material and method

We have chosen to study articles that after publication were determined to have been based on false data or methodology and therefore officially retracted through a notice in the publishing journal. Our sample consists of all articles published 1986 - 1995 and tagged as retracted in MEDLINE before the end of May 1998 (n=172) We used ISI's SCI ™ to find all citations to these articles (both before and after the appearance of the retraction notice).

Because of the unavailability of reliable data on citation expectancy for different types of articles, we could not do a general comparison of the number of post-retraction citations with the normal case. Through a longitudinal study of the frequency of citations, we were still able to give a general estimate of the impact of retraction upon subsequent citation rates.

A sample of articles citing retracted material was examined for what impact the citation had as support for the scientific argumentation.

We checked whether high impact journals (JCR ™) differed from other journals both in the number of accepted and later retracted articles and in accepting articles citing retracted material.

Results

Retractions were found to be about 8 times as common in journals with very high impact factors (>10) than in MEDLINE average. Retracted articles continued to receive citations in significant amounts well after they had been officially retracted and tagged as such in MEDLINE. Some of the citing articles (n=50) were examined in greater detail. In almost all cases was the citation apparently used to support the arguments. In the 9 articles that could be classified as *review*, there were no indications that the cited work had previously been retracted.

Conclusions

The referee system in high impact factor journals, usually with high rejection rates, does not exclude acceptance of articles later being retracted. Neither does it act upon articles citing previously retracted material. The fact that retracted material is cited as support for scientific arguments has implications both for research - basic and applied - and for citation analysis as a measure of quality.

CHANGING USERS' ATTITUDES TOWARDS INFORMATION

Maria Nardelli, Mariateresa Azzolini, Gabriella Gabutti, Maura Moggia, Fulvia Sirocco
[1]ZENECA S.P.A., MEDICAL INFORMATION GROUP, MILANO; [2]RETIRED LIBRARIAN ISF PHARMACEUTICALS; [3]DIREZIONE SCIENTIFICA POLICLINICO S. MATTEO, PAVIA; [4]ASTRA FARMACEUTIC, MEDICAL INFORMATION AND LIBRARY, MILANO; [5]AZIENDA OSPEDALIERA "OSPEDALE SAN MARTINO", GENOVA, ITALY

Objectives

Invalid literature is undoubtedly a problem involving all scientific fields, but it becomes a more ethical and moral matter when related to the biomedical field. In fact recently was demonstrated that information retrieved to satisfy specific clinical questions can be used by physicians in future patient care decisions.[1] Therefore one of the most important commitments for health information professionals should be to make users well aware of the existence of corrected or retracted articles. Both biomedical documentalists and librarians can play an important role in bringing published errata to users' attention, making them more critical readers and stimulating them to verify constantly the validity of the data contained in the literature they usually consult.

Despite the importance of this matter, health information professionals worldwide still can't refer to a codified method to help them reporting correctly invalid literature. With particular reference to librarians, usually they deal with the problem individually in many different ways, according to the organisation of their libraries and the attitudes of their users. Even scientific publishers show corrected or retracted articles on their biomedical journals in many different ways, making often difficult for the end-users to retrieve this kind of information. It is slightly easier for health information professionals to have access to published errata consulting the most important biomedical databases, such as MEDLINE or EMBASE, that report corrections or retractions through several appropriate keywords. But making a particular reference to librarians, they usually deal with the problem individually in many different ways, according with the organisation of their libraries and the attitudes of their users. However the awareness of both librarians and final users about this problem is rather low.[2]

All the above observations are well explained in the article by Azzolini[3] who intended to emphasise the problem of retracted or corrected scientific literature summarising the international situation and underlining the importance for health information professionals to follow a common procedure in reporting invalid literature.

Materials and methods

In October 1996 we carried out an enquiry, sending a questionnaire to the 140 members of GidifRbm (an Italian Association of Health Information professionals). About 30% of the colleagues answered the questionnaire showing their interest to the problem. Analysing the positive answers, they contacted again these colleagues proposing them to start a common experiment. At the end of February 1997 a meeting was organised between the colleagues accepting the invitation (the authors of this presentation). Aim of the meeting was to start a common experiment devoted to identify a useful and functional method to keep users informed about invalid literature. In the project are involved two public libraries and two libraries of pharmaceutical industries, all members of GidifRbm.

The method we developed consisted of four phases:

1. Exchanging biweekly via fax or e-mail the published errata, retrieved by scanning manually a number of common journals
2. Reporting the errata by writing a short cross-reference under the title of the corrected or retracted paper
3. Creating a database for the retrieved corrected or retracted articles
4. Underlining the importance of comments, which can criticise the referent article question its findings, supplement it with additional data use it as starting point for a discussion of the commenting author's own research or opinion.[4,5] We realised that librarian could do a great service alerting soon users to the existence of comments on a previous article. An article should always be supplied to the user with its own comment .
5. Making our users well aware that obviously we cannot check all the information they need to retrieve, as they still have the responsibility to verify the validity of the data contained in the literature they consult

Our main concern was to find a way to organise a regular exchange of information among the group. We immediately realised that the main difficulty was to find a number of journals which all the four libraries subscribed to. We were able to identify only 4 journals and in the following months we collected only few references. Therefore, while continuing to follow the common experiment, M. Nardelli and G. Gabutti decide to develop another procedure using the data banks and particularly MEDLINE. In fact the NLM began its retraction policy in 1984 and its errata policy in 1987 and links the citations to the published retraction notices, errata or comments; and links the retraction notice with the citation of the original article by inserting the notice "retracted by" and the reference to the retraction notice following the title in the citation to the original article. For appropriate MEDLINE keywords: see Table 1.

PT = Corrected and Republished Article
PT = Duplicate Publication
PT = Integrity
PT = Published Erratum
PT = Retracted Publication
PT = Retraction of Publication
PT = Scientific Integrity Review

Table 1: Appropriate Medline keywords

Results

The Search Strategy performed from 1966 to entry month May 1998 gave the results as presented in Table 2. We think that this result must be deeply considered!

The results can than be crossed with the journals each library subscribes to. We managed the results sorting the references in alphabetical order by source, printing them and showing the printout in the library's notice board, so as to permit internal users to have easy access to the information about invalid literature. Furthermore, the references divided into groups according to the related therapeutic area can be provided regularly to the physicians with different printouts.

#1	475	PT = CORRECTED
#2	665	(CORRECTED and REPUBLISHED) in TI
#3	530	(CORRECTED and PUBLISHED) in TI
#4	**1200**	**#1 or #2 or #3**
#5	217	PT = "DUPLICATE"
#6	828	PT = "ERRATUM"
#7	27614	ERRATUM in TI
#8	27541	(PUBLISHED ERRATUM) IN TI
#9	73	#7 not #8
#10	62	#9 not #4
#11	53	#10 not #6
#12	**28612**	**#5 or #6 or #8 or #11**
#13	15	PT = "INTEGRITY"
#14	264	PT = "RETRACTED"
#15	247	PT = "RETRACTION"
#16	**526**	**#13 or #14 or #15#**
#17	**29808**	#4 or #12 or #16

Table 2: Search strategy used in Medline (1966-1998 April)

Conclusions

Although we started and developed it with great enthusiasm, the first phase of our common experiment clearly shows to have the limit to be based on the librarians good will and so to be lacking in a systematic nature. On the other hand, the method based on the use of informatic tools shows to be really useful and to be able to develop a methodical network of systematically organised information. We adfirm that our experience is a progress in changing user's attitudes towards information.

First: starting to discuss about invalid literature, our small group arose the interest of other Italian colleagues in this important matter and it may have convince them to keep their users informed about this problem.

Second: we are now ready to share our experience with other colleagues, asking for their comments and accepting their criticisms and suggestions in order to improve our method of bringing published errata to user's attention.

References

[1] Marshall JG. The impact of the Hospital Library on Clinical Decision Making: The Rochester study. Bull Med Libr Assoc 1992;80:169-178.

[2] Gabutti G, Carrà C, Zeccato A, Tinelli C, Klersy C, Curti M. The role of the consultant librarian in the Evidence Based Medicine. see page 71

[3] Azzolini MT. [To advise the user: the delicate relationship between libraries and scientific information]. Biblioteche Oggi 1996;14(7):62-64

[4] Colaianni LA. Retraction, comment and errata policies of the US National Library of Medicine. Lancet 1992;340:536-537

[5] Kotzin S, Schuyler PL. NLM's practices for handling errata and retractions. Bull Med Libr Assoc 1989;77:337-342

ON THE ROLE OF VERNACULAR MEDICAL VOCABULARIES IN THE CONTEXT OF THE VIRTUAL MEDICAL/HEALTH LIBRARY

Päivi Pekkarinen
NATIONAL LIBRARY OF HEALTH SCIENCES, HELSINKI, FINLAND

On the virtual medical/health library

The virtual medical/health library in this context is defined as a computer-based, telecommunications-connected, domain-specific information system, providing services as any conventional library does. But its collection of documents, being continuously built and individually configured by the user, expands beyond any single library collection. From a management point of view it is a co-operative of information professionals and information users; it is a continuous interactive process. From a semiotics point of view, which is essential for the context, it can be described as an intertextual process.

As a consequence of the above definition of the virtual medical/health library, the user - whether s/he is a medical or health professional, a student or teacher, or a lay person among the general public – is considered both a reader and a writer of medical/health-related documents.

On the structure: documents and their relations

Regarded as a formal structure, the virtual medical/health library contains documents, their relations and attributes attached to them. Two types of documents may be distinguished by the data they contain: (1) documents as such, consisting of texts and images, as well as multimedia (2) metadocuments consisting of metadata used for the representation and retrieval of the documents. Two types of relations within the context may be differentiated (1) hierarchic: generic and partitive (2) non-hierarchic: associative, including equivalence. Both are manifested on conceptual and expressional levels.

Documents produced by the information user may be regarded as a microstructure, documents supported by the information professional as a macrostructure. The microstructure calls for the local, the macrostructure calls for the global. Both of the structures are implemented by hyperdocuments, comprising nodes and links, and by user interfaces, and are presented as hypernetworks.

On the meaning: signs and significations

Using a semiotics frame of reference, the documents of the virtual medical/health library can be seen as a continuum of texts, a system of signs, and their interrelations, meanings.[1,2] This approach is appropriate for
- implying the dynamic nature of virtual medical library documents, their diffuse and in flux character;
- giving a model for meaning with three basic components: (1) sign (2) user of the sign (3) that to which the sign refers;
- looking at meaning through a linguistic sign, i.e. through the sign giving process, signification;
- focusing on the structure produced by that process, and as a result regarding the user of the linguistic sign, the user of the virtual medical library, as an active producer of new linguistic signs, new meanings.

For the user, the virtual medical library is an opportunity to create meanings in medical/health-related documents, produce microstructures and make them publicly available and accessible through macrostructures.[3]

On vernacular medical vocabularies*

The context of the virtual medical/health library makes it possible to utilise a variety of vocabularies linked together as macrostructures supporting microstructures. Two major domains manifesting in the documents of the virtual medical/health library may be distinguished: expert knowledge domain, that of health professionals, and every day life domain, that of the general public. These lead to two requirements for the macrostructure of the virtual library: the capability to accommodate expert concepts and expressions, terms with precisely defined meanings, as well as popular concepts and expressions, words rather than terms.[4] Due to continuous interaction of these two domains in the context of the virtual medical/health library, the relations between the subject fields within the respective domains are continuously changing, resulting in (1) sharing of vocabularies by different communities (2) a diversity of perspectives, displayed in multiple hierarchies and intricate nets of associations.[5] This can be illustrated by using a semiotics frame of reference: a modification of the classical semantic triangle of Ogden and Richards combined with Bochenski's semantic cube.[6,7]

Tension among tongues

There is tension among tongues, rivalry among resources: which of the local words will become global terms; autonomy grows among asymmetry.

The electronic media that bind the world together are essentially carriers of words. While the English language is now the operating standard for global communication, the English language, as the global tongue, is taking over the world.[8,9] In fact, this trend is reflected in the impact of the U.S National Library of Medicine's Medical Subject Headings (MeSH) vocabulary: since the early 1960s MeSH has gradually developed into a de facto international standard for information organization and retrieval in medicine and related areas. Yet, the Unified Medical Language System (UMLS), a long term development project of NLM, implies a 'counter' trend by welcoming vernacular versions of MeSH as parts of its metathesaurus.[10] In the 1990s a growing movement for vernacular versions of MeSH has emerged: not only French, German, Portuguese, Spanish and Russian versions have come into being but a version in Czech and in Slovak, as well as Hungarian, Finnish and Swedish versions are in progress, being structured on respective local needs and resources for communication.

Towards health literacy

Changes in information technology and changes in information ideology, the interdepence of the strategies of Health for All and Information for All have resulted in changes in the clientele of medical libraries and have created an increasing demand for vernacular medical/health-related vocabularies.[11] They have become essential to make an "informed opinion and active participation on the part of the public" into "an informed public debate";[12] they have become essential to health literacy.

Consequently it is suggested that the primary tool for health literacy in the context of the co-operative and interactive process of the virtual medical/health library is an information-user-interface-interlinked metathesaurus [cf. UMLS]. Characteristic of the thesaurus is transparency: the information professional-built relations between terms and concepts are continuously evaluated by the information user on the basis of their meanings; how well the information professional-built perspectives correspond to those employed by the information user to structure his/her thinking in medical and health matters.

Ideally the virtual medical/health library as a continuum of documents, texts, provides the information users, i.e. the readers/writers, with a concurrent access to all medical/health-related documents from the ancient times to the present day - to documents, such as ancient records of symptomatology, e.g. Mesopotamian clay tablets, Egyptian medical papyri, Hippocratic medical writings, as well as to documents, such as modern descriptions of illnesses, e.g. the international classification of diseases. Innumerable interrelations of the documents and texts empower the readers to reveal and to create new meanings in the old as well as in the new texts through the linguistic sign giving process, through microstructures and macrostructures, through local and global vocabularies, instruct and inspire them in health literacy. Vernacular medical vocabularies in the organization, structure and function of the virtual medical/health library add to the awareness building and knowledge empowering of medical and health information users.

References

[1] Fiske J. Introduction to communication studies. 2nd ed. London, Routledge, 1990

[2] Sebeok TA. Handbook of semiotics. Bloomington, Indiana University Press, 1990

[3] Pekkarinen P. On 'new' Ranganathanian laws for structuring the content of the virtual library. In: Knowledge organization for information retrieval: proceedings of the Sixth International Study Conference on Classification Research, University College London, 1997. The Hague, FID, 1997:144-146

[4] Multilingual glossary of technical and popular terms in nine European languages / Heymans Institute of Pharmacology, University of Gent and Mercator College, Department of Applied Linguistics. Gent, 1995 <http://allserv.rug.ac.be/~rvdstich/eugloss/information.html>

[5] Vickery B. Issues in knowledge organization. In: Knowledge organization for information retrieval: proceedings of the Sixth International Study Conference on Classification Research, University College London, 1997. The Hague, FID, 1997:180-182

[6] Ogden CK, Richards IA. The meaning of meaning. 4th ed. London, Kegan Paul, 1936:11 / ARK 1985:11
[7] Bochenski IM. Die zeitgenössischen Denkmethoden. 3. Aufl. Bern, Francke, 1965:40
[8] Crystal D. The language that took over the world. The Guardian 22.2.1997
[9] The coming global tongue. The Economist 1996;Dec 21st:45-48
[10] UMLS knowledge sources. 9th ed. Bethesda, MD: U.S. National Library of Medicine, 1998 <http:www.nlm.nih.gov/research/umls/UMLSDOC.HTML>
[11] Pekkarinen P. On 'FinMeSH' for empowering users of Finnish medical and health information. In: EAHIL '97 Workshop on Managing Information in the New Electronic Age, Budapest, 1997: proceedings. Debrecen, Hungarian Association of Medical Libraries, 1997:114-121
[12] WHO Conference on European Health Care Reforms, Ljubljana, Slovenia, June 1996: proceedings of the conference. Copenhagen, World Health Organization, Regional Office for Europe, 1998

* 'Vocabulary' refers to
(1) a medium of speech, reading and writing ≈ collection of words
(2) to a medium of information organization and retrieval ≈ collections of terms and rules for using them

ELECTRONIC PINK BOOK - BUSINESS CASE

Joan Hunter
WEST SUFFOLK HOSPITAL NHS TRUST, BURY ST EDMONDS, UK

Executive Overview

The original Pink Book (1991) was produced in hard copy form and was intended to provide a communication link between the West Suffolk Hospitals NHS Trust and General Practioners. Unfortunatley it was not revised and became out of date.

The revised Pink Book has been produced in electronic form using industry standard software, so that it can be updated more regularly. It is hoped that it will be able to continue to supply up to date clinically effective information to GPs in an easily accessible form and provide a protocol and guideline resource to facilitate clinical risk management within the Trust. Currently 80% of GPs in West Suffolk have the Pink Book on their computer systems; it has also been widely distributed throughout West Suffolk Healthcare Services.

It is intended that the Pink Book will contain the following information:
- Details about current members of staff in the West Suffolk Hospitals Trust, Mid Anglia Community Trust and primary care
- Current clinical effectiveness initiatives
- Current clinical guidelines in use within the West of Suffolk
- Areas of expertise in WSH, MAHCT, GP practices and primary care
- Latest drug guidelines issued by the Trust's Formulary Review Group
- Pre and post operative and discharge information and procedures issued by Trust wards and clinical areas
- Examples of good practice from published sources such as Effective Healthcare, MEDLINE and Bandolier
- Local Postgraduate medical education programmes
- GP surgery locations, times and availability

Strategic Context

West Suffolk Hospitals Trust aims to provide healthcare to the people of West Suffolk which is:
- effective, accessible and focused on the patients
- of the highest possible quality

- in the best possible environment
- clinically effective while representing the best value for money
- able to improve health to reduce illness, injury and disability
- in collaboration with other providers, purchasers and related organisations to ensure the provision of seamless services
- associated with the provision of excellent teaching and training for health professionals and support for research and development.

The new White Paper 'The New NHS' states that *"the new National Institute for Clinical Excellence will be set up to produce and disseminate clinical guidelines based on relevant evidence of clinical and cost effectiveness".* (p 58) The Pink Book has been designed not only to support local guideline initiatives but also in its development version to give links via the Internet to national guidelines.
Also the government will spread best practice and drive clinical and cost effectiveness in a number of ways:

- By ensuring through the R&D program the provision and disseminatin of high quality scientific evidence on the cost effectiveness and quality of care.
- By developing a program of new evidence based national service frameworks settting out the patterns and levels of service which should eb provded for patients with certain conditions
- By establishing a new commission for health improvement
- To support and oversee the quality of clinical governance and of clinical services
- By working with the professions to strengthen the existing systems of professional self regulation (p 56)

Aims of the Pink Book

The Pink Book directly assists in fulfilling both the above local and national strategic requirements and specifically aims to improve communication between primary and secondary care and to further develop partnerships between healthcare providers in Suffolk and its environs.

The Pink Book is directly linked with clinical effectiveness and evidence based practice, not only via the guidelines contained in it but also via the links with the library and information service, finding the evidence, and links to relevant sites on the Internet. The Pink Book organisers recognise the importance of patient information material and have included leaflets in order to boost health improvement at the primary care level.

The Pink Book provides relevant, accurate and up to date information at the point of patient care, both in the Acute Hospital and at primary care level as well as being the focus of information about healthcare in the west of Suffolk.

Benefits of the Pink Book

The Pink Book evolved from the Trust's clinical effectiveness strategy and clinical staff are benefitting from the protocols and guidelines which have been developed since the concept of the EPB came into existence:

- Give GPs the necessary information to refer patients to appropriate consultants thereby producing efficiency savings at the WSH

- Assists GPs in deciding when and if to refer patients thereby reducing unnecessary referrals.
- To act as a protocol and guideline resource to facilitate Clinical Risk Management, and ensure clarity of clinical policy
- Give doctors in training ready access to local protocols
- Reduction in calls to the switchboard from GP surgeries with queries
- Centralisation of clinical and management information which obviates the necessity for large and diffuse paper based documents, which have a tendency to either get lost or mislaid in busy wards, clinics and departments.

Patient leaflets for instant GP/patient healthcare information provision
- Instant telephone and fax information – time saving

WHERE WE ARE NOW

- A technically excellent version 1 has now been distributed to 80% of GP practices and throughout West Suffolk and Mid Anglia and various other relevant healthcare organisations
- The technical editor is being funded by a grant from Suffolk Health Authority till the end of September 1998 from GP funding.
- The technical editor is updating and expanding the first version of the Pink Book and also preparing it for conversion to HTML in order that it can be accessed via Web technology.
- Evaluation questionnaires have gone out to all users to assess the effectiveness, usefulness of the PB and also to identify areas which need upgrading.

Future Developments

The contributors to the Pink Book come from both clinical and management areas. It is vital for the continued usefulness of the PB that information contained therein is kept up to date on a regular basis particularly in the area of clinical guidelines, procedures and protocols which must be kept up to date so that care provided in the Trust is based on the most recent evidence.

The Trust is therefore asked to fund the appointment of a permanent editor, who, under the auspices of the Clinical Effectiveness Co-ordinator, will undertake the maintenance of the information, liaison with contributors to the PB, and continued evaluation of its contents and resulting development.

The post of Clinical Effectiveness Co-ordinator has to become more substansive and IT hardware and network links at point of patient care must be improved.

Formal recognition and commitment of the Trust to the PB is very important, as well as the backing of marketing the concept of the PB, to raise awareness of its potential outside the confines of West Suffolk. This will raise funds for development, in particular consultation fees for any technical problems or developments that may arise on an ad hoc basis. This requires the trust to recognise that there may be financial/staffing resource considerations, as members of the PB committee will need to involve themselves in marketing promotions from time to time.

Action: Ensure that developments are well advertised and written up in the professional press by developing a marketing strategy.

Risk analysis

If no money is forthcoming for support of the PB, the PB cannot be updated in the long run and the work presently being done on linking the healthcare organisation of Suffolk will no longer be able to be sustained.

The short term contract of the Clinical Effectiveness Co-ordinator who has spent about 70% of her time in promoting and developing the PB poses a major problem. Her contract is due to expire in March 1999 and is funded at present by Audit funds. The importance of clinical effectiveness in the trust's strategy cannot be underestimated and the key role that is played by the CE Coordinator could present serious problems if this post was terminated in 1999.

The present state of IT hardware and network links on the wards within the hospital could prevent the PB being used to its full potential. The PB is now a nationally recognised project and has been given an award by the British Association of Medical Managers and is also part of the Anglia and Oxford Virtual Institute Project. Should the project fail through any of the above risks – *"yer all going to have egg on yer faces maties"*.

Chapter 3: CONSUMER AND PUBLIC HEALTH INFORMATION

Editorial summary

The excellent paper of Bob Gann and Veronica Fraser makes clear that the rapid changes in the National Health System in the UK offer great opportunities for Library and Information Services. The New NHS includes strategies for information management, information technology and public information. In this chapter the emphasis is on public and consumer information; in chapter 6 we will find the paper of Veronica Fraser (p. 122) that explains the consequences of the New NHS for medical library services.

These developments in the NHS will turn out to have a larger and wider impact on medical librarianship and health care than in the UK only. So far as consumer health information concerned, these changes will certainly be followed in other European countries and medical librarians on the continent could benefit of the UK experience and examples. This is already proofed by the presentation from Ireland by Jennifer MacDougall.

According to the research reported by Jennifer MacDougall the information provision to the public in Ireland can and must be improved. The reference framework set out in this paper fits nicely with the practical examples from the USA here represented by reports of the projects of Diane Hummel (Michigan) and Donna

Flake and John Rader (North Carolina). Their papers are not only informative but also a good stimulus to try to follow these examples.

The importance of the Internet and good quality Web-sites for consumer and health information for the public is emphasized by the presentations of Robert Kiley and Sally Hernando (UK) and by the poster presented by Nada Trzan-Herman and Anuška Senčar (Ljubljana, Slovenia). The latter presentation, not included in these proceedings, discusses the information sources available on the Internet for high incidence diseases. Their investigation showed that the number of sites is not so much related to the number of deaths worldwide; more sites are found for diseases that prevail in the developed countries. It is stated that also the pharmaceutical industry has a role to play in offering reliable information for the public on the Internet.

HEALTH INFORMATION IN ACTION: NEW NHS - NEW LIS

Bob Gann, Veronica Fraser
[1]Centre for Health Information Quality, Winchester; [2]NHS Library Adviser, London, UK

Introduction

Since the election of the new Labour government a year ago, there has been an atmosphere of change and innovation in the British National Health Service. Many of these innovations have enormous implications for library and information services (LIS). In this paper we will be examining the policy framework for these changes, in particular the reforming white paper *The New NHS.*[1] We will give an early preview of strategies currently being developed: the new Information Management & Technology (IMT) Strategy and Public Information Strategy. We will describe some practical information service developments. And we will conclude by identifying implications and opportunities for library & information services. For our new Prime Minister Tony Blair everything is new. The election was won on the slogan New Labour: New Britain. We will be proposing another - "New NHS: New LIS".

The new NHS

The British National Health Service was founded 50 years ago, the proudest achievement of the post war Labour government. After 18 years in opposition a new Labour government was elected on 1 May 1997. The National Health Service was inevitably a priority for the new administration. By the end of 1997, the government had produced a policy white paper *The New NHS: Modern, Dependable,* which aimed at building a "modern & dependable health service for the twenty first century". There was a strong emphasis on quality assurance throughout the NHS - "A service with quality at its heart". And a recognition of the importance of the information base for all health care partners - "Knowledgeable patients advised by knowledgeable professionals" and the underlying technology - "Supported by accurate and up to date information and information technology".

Partnerships

The previous Conservative government had introduced an "internal market" to the NHS where different health care providers competed for contracts from health authorities. Information systems in the NHS were focused on contracting data to the detriment of other, knowledge based applications. Although continuing with the purchaser-provider split in health care, *The New NHS* introduces a statutory duty of partnership rather than competition. Health authorities and trusts are encouraged to work more closely together, and in partnership with local authority social services, other public sector organisations including transport and environment agencies, education, the voluntary sector and private health care organisations.

INFORMATION MANAGEMENT & TECHNOLOGY STRATEGY

Information technology in the NHS has had a very poor reputation over the past ten years. Privatisation of NHS computer services, scandals around computer procurement, and failure to take advantage of new technologies created a climate of defeatism and cynicism. Reform of the IM&T strategy was therefore an early priority. Replacement of the internal market enables the new IM&T strategy to concentrate more explicitly on the core purposes of the NHS, in particular:

- Providing access to convenient services
- Ensuring seamless multi-agency care
- Informing and educating professionals on best practice
- Informing and empowering patients and the public

The strategy has now been completed and will be published very soon. Key components will include national development of the electronic record, capturing the total experience of the patient through the health (and increasingly social care) system. After a slow start, the NHS's own intranet *NHSnet* will provide for quicker test results, online appointment bookings etc. Particularly relevant to librarians will be the establishment of an electronic clinical knowledge base. The "evidence trolley" of key clinical knowledge available in real time at the bedside or primary care consultation will be as important a resource as the medicine trolley. We can expect to see increasing integration of text based information & data sources. And for the first time, an NHS IT strategy will recognise NHS responsibility for "providing knowledge about health, illness and best treatment practice to the public through the Internet and emerging public access media".

PUBLIC INFORMATION STRATEGY

For several years now, policy on information for the public has been split across a number of NHS departments - public health, information management and technology, communications and public affairs, patient partnership, library services. Recognising the importance which Health Ministers attach to this work, there has now been established a Public Information Strategy group to bring these initiatives together. The group is headed by an NHS Executive Director (deputy Chief Executive level) and includes the authors of this paper. The strategy is currently under development as a complement to the IM&T Strategy with the following priority themes:

- Intergovernmental scoping of initiatives within the Department of Health and other government departments
- Ways of developing key access points and gateways to health information
- Establishing a national mechanism for quality control and accreditation of consumer health information
- Ensuring that the government's social exclusion agenda is reflected in information policy (so that the fault lines of social exclusion are not reflected in those of information exclusion)

- Making the most of the enormous advances in telecommunications - in particular establishment of the NHS Direct service
- Evaluation of the effectiveness of mechanisms for communicating information to the public
- Development of a public communication strategy which engages fully and constructively with the mass media.

NHS Direct

Having mapped out the policy context, we will now move on to some of the practical information service developments which will be implemented between now and 2000. Perhaps the most radical and far reaching is NHS Direct, providing 24 hour telephone based access to nursing advice and health information for all. The government intends to invest £50 million in NHS Direct - but the expectation is that the service will be "resource neutral" with £50million saved in increased self care & reduced inappropriate calls on general practitioners and accident and emergency services, particularly out of hours. Pilot services are currently being funded to cover about 10 million people with NHS Direct going national in 2000. All services will use algorithm software for symptom advice with the potential to build in other information pathways for referral to community agencies, self help groups etc. Although the initial focus of NHS Direct is on nurse triage for current symptoms it is likely that it will develop into national telephone access for a wide range of consumer health information services and helplines - wherever possible without need to redial. Taking the model of tele-banking, NHS Direct also has the potential in time to become the single NHS telephone number through which contact can be made with any health care service, appointments can be booked, test results given, complaints recorded and public views sought.

Healthy Living Centres

One of the lasting innovations of the previous government was the National Lottery. Later this year funding from £300 million of National Lottery funding will be made available for a network of Healthy Living Centres. These will be community based centres - or could be a network of local health promoting initiatives. Healthy Living Centres will provide facilities for leisure and fitness, as well as a meeting place for self help or community groups. There is considerable potential for Healthy Living Centres to have an important information role - with touch screen information kiosks and libraries of health information. Public libraries will be important partners in Healthy Living Centre consortia. The Public Health Minister, Tessa Jowell, spoke during National Libraries last year of the potential for Healthy Living Centres to combat information exclusion. Despite the rapid spread of the Internet, most Internet access in the UK remains in the workplace and in education. Those excluded from employment or education run the risk of being doubly disadvantaged. Public access to the Internet within Healthy Living Centres could some way towards combatting this.

Health Action Zones

The Labour government seems more inclined than its predecessor to recognise and make moves to combat inequalities in health. Fifteen Health Action Zones (HAZs) have recently been established as a focus for partnership efforts to tackle health inequalities. Despite some initial lack of clarity about how they were to work (not for nothing were they called Hazies) multi-agency approaches to health are now taking shape: housing, transport, employment, education etc. working together in innovative ways. Working with other agencies, Health Authorities are drawing up 3 year Health Improvement Plans. There are clear targets for improvement in national priority areas (such as coronary heart disease and cancer) as well as locally defined priorities reflecting the needs of the local population. If HAZs are to work, there will be a particular need for multi-agency information sharing.

National Institute for Clinical Excellence

In recent years a number of initiatives have been charged with reviewing the evidence base of health care (including the UK Cochrane Centre, NHS Centre for Reviews and Dissemination, guidelines from the Royal Colleges etc.) The *New NHS* white paper announced the intention to establish a National Centre for Clinical Excellence. Although there is little sign of action on this front so far, the National Institute will coordinate production of clinical guidelines based on relevant evidence on clinical & cost effectiveness. It will bring together work of current initiatives and produce information in range of formats to range of audiences - including consumers - in a similar way to the Agency for Health Care Policy and Research (AHCPR) in the United States.

Our healthier nation

Earlier this year the New NHS white paper was joined by a green paper (a consultative document) on public health called *Our Healthier Nation.*[2] *Our Healthier Nation* identifies 3 settings for public health and health promotion: healthy schools, healthy workplaces, and healthy neighbourhoods. Tony Blair has identified his top priorities as Education, Education and Education. Recognising the importance of creating the next healthy generation, there are proposals to facilitate access to high quality health resources for schools through a gateway site *Wired for Health* linked to the National Grid for Learning. Following a series of public health scares in the UK (in particular on food safety) the green paper places a particular priority on clear and unambiguous communication of risks to health, including responsible reporting in the media. And the new Health Action Zones & Healthy Living Centres, and national targets for health improvement, are important mechanisms for achieving better public health.

Health information quality

As we have already noted, the New NHS will have quality at its heart. This concern with quality also extends to information for patients. The need for a national resource centre was identified two years ago, and set out in the NHS Patient Partnership

Strategy and the white paper on primary care: *"The Centre will act as a source of expertise & knowledge for the NHS & patient organisations aimed at improving provision of good quality, evidence based patient information"*
The Help for Health Trust won the contract to develop the Centre for Health Information Quality from April 1997. The work of the Centre includes:

- Promotion of quality tools, checklists & guidelines
- Appraisal of consumer health information material in print and other media
- Databases of contacts, references, reviewed material
- Newsletters & topic bulletin
- Training programme
- Web Site *www.centreforhiq.demon.co.uk*

As part of the Public Information Strategy we are developing proposals for the Centre to be involved in the development of a UK version of the US government *Healthfinder* site.

New NHS: New LIS

So what about library and information services in the New NHS? How can we make the most of this remarkably fertile information environment? Of course we have our traditional bedrock skills in organising & retrieving information and the skills developed over recent years: teaching information skills and expert searching. In the past five years or so we have established an emerging role in areas including critical appraisal and consumer health information and many of us are now creating information sources eg. websites. Library and information work has always been a partnership profession based on networking and sharing resources. In tune with the times there is a role in facilitating, negotiating, brokerage. Health care information professionals in the 21st century, the New NHS and health care systems throughout Europe will be knowledge managers.

References

[1] The New NHS: Modern, Dependable. Cm3807 Department of Health, 1997
[2] Our Healthier Nation: a Contract for Health. Cm3852 Department of Health, 1998
[3] Primary Care: Delivering the Future. Cm3512 Department of Health, 1996

CONSUMER HEALTH INFORMATION - DEVELOPMENTS IN THE USA

Donna Flake, John Rader
LIBRARY COASTAL AHEC; DEPT. OF WELLNESS SERVICES, NEW HANOVER REGIONAL MEDICAL CENTER; WILMINGTON, NORTH CAROLINA, USA

Introduction

Health professionals are seeking ways to improve the health status of our communities. In ever growing numbers, consumers have started to take responsibility for their own health status by paying attention to nutrition, exercise, and general wellness. We are seeing consumer health information in ever growing quantities.

The United States government and particularly the National Library of Medicine is making consumer health information more available to all its citizens than ever before. One example is that in 1997, MEDLINE became available free of charge on the Internet. This Internet free MEDLINE is known as PubMed. Before this event, the National Library of Medicine had always charged for access to MEDLINE.

The Medical Library Association has also shifted its emphasis from medical libraries being for only the health professional, to medical libraries and medical librarians serving and supporting consumers as well as health professionals. Rachel Anderson, past president of MLA, addressed the importance of MEDLINE to the general public when she said, "Patients and their families are regularly turning to health sciences librarians to find reliable health information."

One of the 23 major sections of the Medical Library Association is Consumer and Patient Health Information Section. This section's membership is growing dramatically and it has a web site. It also publishes a newsletter and provides lively and well attended sessions at MLA devoted to consumer health.

Health professionals are broadly endorsing consumers right to know about health. As an example, pioneering heart surgeon and Chair of the National Library of Medicine's Board, Dr. Michael E. DeBakey, said, "Even with our modern advances in health care, I still consider good information to be the best medicine."

Other examples of the growing interest in consumer health information in the US are that most pharmacies now sell videotapes on various health conditions created by the former Surgeon General of the United States. Also, the number of consumer health Internet sites is growing rapidly.

The consumer health library

Moving from consumer health trends in the US to one local area - in Wilmington, North Carolina, there is an excellent new consumer health library. The library is a comprehensive and coordinated source of consumer health information in this community.

Actually, the vision and dream of creating this library was based on an European model. In the mid 1980's, I (Donna Flake) had the privilege of working at the Wessex Medical Library in Southampton. Thankfully, Southampton also housed another library - Help for Health. This library was directed by an enthusiastic knowledgeable and visionary consumer health librarian, Bob Gann. Bob and Help for Health provided the inspiration for the development of this consumer health library in North Carolina. (Of course, Bob now works for the British National Health Service and oversees consumer health libraries throughout Britain.)

I (Donna Flake) have been the Library Director of the Coastal Area Health Education Center (a medium sized medical library) for six years. The mission of our library is to serve local health professionals. Because of this, we purchase a very small number of consumer health resources In spite of this, over 1,500 consumers visit our library each year. Our library cannot meet their needs. The public library offers some consumer health information, but it lacks the currency, depth, and breadth of information most people seek. Other agencies in our city of 100,000 citizens offer almost no health information. I saw this lack of consumer health information in our city as a problem to be solved.

Other people in our city were also concerned. The Director of Wellness Services (John Rader) at our medical center, the former Head Reference Librarian at our Public Library (Dan Horne), and I (Donna Flake) established a small group of people to look for solutions to the problem of a lack of consumer health information. We formed a committee of University faculty, health educators from the health department and citizens and developed a proposal to establish a consumer health library.

Our proposal asked for $276,000 budget for the first two years of operation, a librarian and library technical assistant, a building measuring 2,000 square feet, and all the furniture, books, videotapes, magazines, computers and computer program necessary to have an excellent library.

Our committee decided to ask the largest hospital in our city to fund the library. I (Donna Flake) met with the President of New Hanover Regional Medical Center and asked for funding and support. The hospital thoroughly supported the library, and placed the library administratively within the hospital (under John Rader's Wellness Division). The hospital provided the library with:

*$500,000 for the first two years
*one librarian
*one library technical assistant
*2,200 square foot building
*All the money from a celebrity golf tournament (about $150,000)

Furthermore, the hospital funded a trip to California for John Rader, Dan Horne, and Donna Flake to examine and study the most outstanding consumer health libraries in the U.S. (We selected these 3 libraries based on the opinions of Bob Gann and Alan Rees (Alan is the most prominent consumer health librarian in the U.S.).

We visited the Planetree Health and Resource Center in San Jose, California, the Planetree Health Library in San Francisco, and The Health Library in Palo Alto.

Planetree Health and Resource Center in San Jose, California, is located in an ornate Victorian house. Candace Ford is the librarian and creator of the library. Here we learned the value of creating a healing atmosphere with live plants, artwork, and comfortable furniture with pillows.

The second California library we visited was the Planetree Health Library in San Francisco. This was the largest Consumer Health Library we visited. Here we learned that it is possible to sell information packets to consumers for a fee. This fee helps to financially sustain this library. Also, the library operates a small book store of consumer health books which brings in $10,000 per year.

The third Consumer Health Library visited was The Health Library in Palo Alto, California. We hope to model our library after this one. The library is located in the upscale Stanford Shopping Center, owned by Stanford University. This library served an amazing 19,000 last year. This library benefits greatly by having 100 volunteers.

After visiting these libraries, we returned to Wilmington, NC and began the process of planning and building. We plan to open our library in September 1998. It is located in a shopping center across the street from the medical center. It is open 5 days a week, has 10 volunteers, two public computers with Internet, MEDLINE and Health Reference Center, contains 2,000 circulating books and an extensive clipping file.

We are proud that our medical center has responded so positively to our proposal to build the library. We want to tell you about our medical center, our areas of responsibility within it, and our community. New Hanover Regional Medical Center is a 638 bed regional medical center located in a very rural area of North Carolina. The medical center serves a seven county area which is approximately 2/3 the size of the Netherlands. The population of our seven county area is 400,000. Conversely, the Netherlands has a population of 15,452,903.

North Carolina

"The Old South" is a name often given to the southeastern portion of the United States. Images of plantations and "Gone With the Wind" might come to mind. North Carolina is in this region where most people get little exercise and eat a high fat diet. Here in the Netherlands more people use the excellent bike paths and often cycle to work. Conversely, most cities in the US are designed not for walkers or cyclists but for drivers of cars. As an example of poor health habits in North Carolina, food historically eaten here include fried chicken, potatoes in butter, greens cooked with animal fat, corn meal fried in oil, and pecan pie. This results in an unhealthy population, and North Carolina is one of the unhealthiest in America. The 50 states of the United States are ranked from the best to the worst in terms of the prevalence of deaths.

North Carolina ranks 8th from the worst in cardiovascular disease deaths.
North Carolina ranks 2nd from the worst in stroke deaths.
North Carolina ranks 15th from the worst in coronary heart disease deaths.
North Carolina ranks 12th from the worst in diabetes.
There are fewer physically active adults in North Carolina than any other state in America.

Wellness services

The poor statistics for our area of the country provide a challenge for me (John Rader) and my staff at NHRMC. I am the Director of the Wellness Services Department within the medical center. Six sub-departments comprise the Wellness Services Department. They are:

1. The Coastal Consumer Health Library
2. The Coastal Diabetes Center
3. The Community Charge on Cancer
4. The Diabetes Peer Educators Program
5. Wellness Services
6. Life Wise

All of these subdivisions of Wellness are located across the street from the primary medical center. Each one has the primary mission of reaching out to the community. Most of the activities of the Wellness Services Department are to provide educational programs, health fairs, referral information, and preventative services to all of those in need. We charge for very few of our programs. The Coastal Consumer Health Library will be the glue that binds service departments together. All the employees of our Wellness Services Department will encourage all of their contacts to use the Coastal Consumer Health Library. Because the consumer health library is adjacent to the Wellness Services Department, clients can be referred back and forth between the library and Wellness Services. Also, the Wellness Services Department contains lecture rooms which the Consumer Health Library can use for educational classes. In addition, the Coastal Consumer Health Library is located near a number of physicians offices and is very convenient for the patient to stop at the Coastal Consumer Health Library after a visit to the physician.

We are pleased to be here to tell you about our innovative Wellness program and its Consumer Health Library.

THE INTERNET AND CONSUMER HEALTH INFORMATION: IMPLICATIONS FOR SOCIAL EQUALITY AND THE ROLE OF THE LIBRARIAN

Robert Kiley, Sally Hernando
WELLCOME TRUST, LONDON

Introduction

Speaking at the launch of PubMed[1] - the free MEDLINE service developed by the National Library of Medicine - Vice President Al Gore stated that this service (and the supporting HealthFinder[2] site) would enable all Americans to access 'timely and accurate medical information' via the Internet. Evidence that the Internet is being used by health consumers can be seen in the survey conducted by FIND/SVP which showed that 43% of all Internet users searched the Internet for health information[3].

However, is it realistic to expect that all but a tiny minority of health care consumers can use these resources effectively? And, by legitimising the use of electronic networks for delivery of health information, do we risk creating an even wider gap in quality of care available to the world's rich and poor?

This paper will investigate these issues, and look at some of the ways in which librarians, both internationally and in the UK, are helping consumers to make sense of the vast amount of electronic information which is now, as least nominally, only a keystroke away.

Using the Internet effectively - results of a survey

To identify *how* consumers are using the Internet to find health information, a questionnaire was mailed to a number of health-based Usenet Newsgroups and discussion lists[4]. Though the value of such a survey has some limitations - all respondents are self-selected, motivated, English speaking and Internet-aware - the 42 responses provided a useful snapshot of how the Internet was being used. Specifically, the survey revealed that:

- 95% of all respondents use the Internet once-a-week or more for health information;
- most respondents used non-subject specific search engines (e.g. AltaVista) and only 5% used specialised tools like Medical Matrix[5];
- 82% of respondents discussed their findings with a health professional;
- 57% thought that their doctor was supportive of them using the Internet for health information;
- only 16% had ever acted on the information they found on the Internet without consulting a health professional.

Respondents were very positive about the Internet as an information resource, because it helped them to study different treatment options and to be better informed about their own health. For librarians - and those involved in teaching health consumers to search the Internet - the key conclusion is that much greater attention must be paid to promoting the quality-assured, subject specific search tools such as OMNI[6], Medical Matrix[5] and HealthFinder[2].

Information Rich - Information Poor - the role of the librarian

Though poor search skills may result in consumers finding irrelevant, inaccurate, and possibly dangerous information, a more immediate problem is simply that access to the Internet is restricted to the privileged few. Figures from NUA for example, indicate that though around 120 million people have direct access to the Internet, this is less than 2.5% of the world's population[7]. Even in the UK, only 1 in 25 households have access to the Internet[8].

Librarians however, steeped in the principle that information should be available to everyone and free at the point of use, can be key players in democratising access to the Internet. One example of a library initiative in this field - which could be used as a model of good practice - is the Ohio Public Library Information Network (OPLIN).

PROVIDING ACCESS: THE OHIO PUBLIC LIBRARY INFORMATION NETWORK EXPERIENCE

OPLIN was created to ensure that "all citizens have equal access to information, regardless of locations or format and regardless of the location of the user". This ambitious objective was achieved by setting up a direct connection to the state's telecommunications network in each of Ohio's 250 public libraries.

In addition to proving access to the Internet, OPLIN has negotiated contracts with a number of commercial providers to allow any member of public - calling from within the OPLIN network - to access high quality consumer health resources such as HealthSource Plus, and Health Reference Center. For further details see: http://www.oplin.lib.oh.us

PROVIDING THE EXPERTISE -IDENTIFYING RESOURCES AND DELIVERING TRAINING

In addition to providing access to the Internet, librarians are key players in identifying, and bringing together, high quality Web resources. One premier Internet product that librarians and information specialists play a significant part in compiling and keeping up-to-date is Healthfinder.

Developed by the Department of Health and Human Services, Healthfinder has been established to help lead consumers to "selected online publications, clearinghouses, databases, web sites, and support and self-help groups, as well as the government agencies and not-for-profit organisations that produce reliable information for the public". The success of this service can be gauged by the fact that in the first 12 months Healthfinder attracted 1.7 million visitors to its site. For further details see: <http://www.healthfinder.gov/>

Teaching consumers how to search the Internet, and evaluate the information they find, is another skill librarians can bring to this process. To ensure that this done effectively, it is important that to all librarians have the appropriate skill and knowledge to deliver this training. To meet this need the Director's of OPLIN initiated a state-wide training program. Believed to be the largest public library training program in Ohio history, training was provided to 2,666 public library staff from 250 institutions. This training is now being cascaded down to the users of the Ohio public library service.

DEVELOPING PARTNERSHIPS - THE NETWELLNESS EXPERIENCE

Providing good library access to the Internet also requires librarians to develop partnerships with other key agencies, such as telecommunications providers and electronic publishers. One good example of what can be achieved through partnership is the Netwellness project. Developed by the University of Cincinnati Medical Center, Netwellness is a Web-based consumer health information service that aims to provide consumers with the most current and accurate health information. To achieve this partnerships were established with companies such as TriState Online - an Internet Service Provider - and Cincinnati Bell Telephone the local telecommunications provider. In all, over 40 partners joined the NetWellness project and as a result of this, residents in 29 counties in three midwestern states now have free and easy access to consumer health information on the Internet. For further details see: <http://www.netwellness.org/>

LIBRARY INITIATIVES IN CONSUMER HEALTH THE UK EXPERIENCE

Though co-operation between different library sectors is not so evident in the UK, there are nevertheless examples of good practice both in terms of providing gateways to quality resources and providing free Internet access.

The OMNI gateway[6] provides both consumers and health professionals with a searchable and browseable database of Internet resources that meet a defined quality criteria. And, though the OMNI service is not aimed predominantly at consumers, a search for 'patient education' identifies around 500 quality Internet sites that would be suitable for health consumers. (These consumer sites represent 15% of the total resources catalogued by OMNI.)

Initiatives that focus on providing access for consumers include the Family Resource Centre[9] at the Great Ormond Street Hospital for Sick Children and the "Health Information 1st" service developed at Lister Hospital[10].

INITIATIVES AT THE WELLCOME TRUST

The Wellcome Trust, the world's largest biomedical research charity, has an information centre which is available to members of the public. In addition to providing a free telephone and e-mail enquiry service, study and research facilities are available to all users. Research facilities include *free* access to the Internet and a wide range of health databases and multimedia resources.

To help consumers make effective use of the Internet a number workshops have been organised - which we intend to repeat - and a series of free printed guides are available. Moreover, qualified library staff are always available to provide practical, hands-on advice and guidance.

Conclusion

The Information Society is, after many false starts, becoming a reality. However, to ensure that *all* citizens can enjoy the benefits of this, librarians must recognise the key role they can play in this process.

As this paper has demonstrated librarians are the ones who can provide the access, the training and ongoing support, and the skill to search the Internet and provide pointers to high quality Web sites. Moreover, the culture of sharing and collaborating - which is so prevalent amongst librarians - is perhaps our greatest asset, and one which me must develop and promote. Librarians have all the necessary skills to deliver effective electronic services to health consumers. It is time to act.

References

[1] PubMed <URL: http://www.ncbi.nlm.nih.goc/PubMed> [Accessed 27 May 1998]

[2] HealthFinder <URL:http://www.healthfinder.gov/> [Accessed 28 May 1998]

[3] FIND/SVP <URL: http://www.cyberdialogue.com/isg/features/cas/casindex.html> [Accessed 28 May 1998]

[4] Newsgroups and discussion lists contacted were: alt.migraine;, alt.eating-disorders, alt.cancer.prostate, sci.med.aids, alt.arthritis, alt.multiple-sclerosis, lupus-l, and allegry-l

[5] Medical Matrix: <URL:http://www.medmatrix.org/index.asp> [Accessed 28 May 1998]

[6] OMNI <URL:http://omni.ac.uk> [Accessed.28 May 1998]

[7] NUA <URL:http://www.nua.ie/surveys/how_many_online/index.html> [Accessed 28 May 1998]

[8] OPCS Internet access in the UK - 1997

[9] Family Resource Centre <URL: http://www.ich.ucl.ac.uk/dnqcs/html/resource/inform/webpage.html> [Accessed 28 May 1998]

[10] Health Information 1st <URL: http://www.nthames-health.tpmde.ac.uk/hifirst/ index.htm/>index.html> [Accessed 28 May 1998]

ACCESS TO CONSUMER HEALTH INFORMATION: A DEVELOPMENT MODEL[1]

Jennifer MacDougall
LIBRARY ASSOCIATION OF IRELAND, DUBLIN, IRELAND

Best practice in CHI

Following the 1995 research report *Information for Health*[2], which investigated access to healthcare information in Ireland, the report *Well Read*[1] looks in detail at a number of examples of best practice and initiatives worldwide. The research also involved detailed consultations with over 70 Irish health organisations, study visits to 12 CHI services in the UK, a case study in Wexford, and extensive literature searching and document collection. A review of international best practice and the development of a pilot database of CHI sources were also undertaken.

The development and extent of the UK NHS Health Information Service has been well documented and provides many examples of best practice which serve as models for other countries. Apart from individual services like the Help for Health Trust, the Health Information Service National Support Unit provides support, networking, advice and training and other services and constitutes another example of best practice.[3,4]

There are many examples in Europe and the USA of (cross-sector) cooperaton and networking between public library, university and hospital libraries which provide a flexibility of access for the consumer. Information for patients in GPs' or doctors' surgeries is increasing in the UK, for example in Hertfordshire developed by Health Information First at the Lister Hospital in cooperation with the County Library authority.[1] Over 50% of hospital libraries in the USA and Canada provide a service for the public, while others allow public access with restrictions.

The importance of quality issues in relation to CHI are also examined in the report including evidence based consumer health information. It is the consumers of healthcare and their families who are most affected by the effectiveness or not of treatments and interventions.[5,6] Patients need access to evidence based information in order to make truely informed choices and take part in decision making.[7] Research shows that this can produce more successful health outcomes.[5,8] It is essential that CHI services include good quality accessible information on clinical effectiveness.

Readability and recall are essential qualities for patient information in order to ensure compliance with treatment regimes and medication. Research shows that the incomprehensibility of patient information is an international problem, and that many health professionals seriously underestimate the levels of illiteracy among their patients. Availability and accessibility of a wide range of CHI is important. It has been shown that patients need more information than is usually provided by health professionals, especially by consultants. Nurses and paramedical staff report that patients often want more information following consultations.[9] Patient involvement in the planning and evaluation of information materials will directly improve the effectiveness of information and, therefore, patient satisfaction.[10-12]

The evaluation and monitoring of CHI services is vital to ensure continued effectiveness and quality of service provision. In the UK Trent Healthline has developed *Quality principles for health information services* which provides valuable guidelines for developing a quality service adaptable to different situations.[13] The Centre for Health Information Quality at the Help for Health Trust has been set up to improve the quality of health information for the public by empowering those responsible for producing information with expert advice and examples of best practice.[14]

There are still relatively few training opportunities or resources for CHI staff who collectively have a wide range of experience and skills. Specific skills required include communication, health service structure and organisation, health information sources including CD-ROMs and the Internet, management, IT training, marketing, design and production of information materials and the implementation of monitoring, evaluation and quality systems.[15] The skills base of all health sciences librarians should be extended with specialist CHI training and continuing education opportunities.

Ireland has no formal consumer health information service although there are a range of specialist information services of varying size and sophistication. Examples of best practice include the Irish Cancer Society with its free telephone help-line manned by trained oncology nurses, and a wide range of other cancer-related services nationwide. There is also the National Children's Resource Centre run by Barnardo's which provides a comprehensive information, counselling and training service relevant to the health and welfare of children in Ireland.

The Irish experience - recent initiatives

In recent years the Irish government, the 8 health boards and other bodies have developed a number of initiatives which have served to encourage a more open and accessible face of government and health management, as well as a move towards more public participation in policy and planning. Examples which illustrate an increased awareness of the need for better CHI:

The Charter of Rights for Hospital Patients (1992) was a welcome first step towards recognition of the consumer in healthcare, but much remains to be done. The Charter is not reinforced by legislation and requires broadening to specialist areas, revising and updating.[16]

The Department of Health's strategy document *Shaping a healthier future* highlights the importance of ensuring that services are consumer oriented and "that detailed and accurate information is available when required."[17]

A Plan for Women's Health was developed from an extensive consultation process with women from all over Ireland, with help from the National Women's Council. The resulting document revealed that there was a lack of information on all aspects of health services and issues affecting not only women's health but that of their families.[18]

Research in Ireland

A number of independent studies and recently published reports point to deficiencies in consumer healthcare information provision like problems of access, availability and appropriateness of information on health. There is increasing public demand for information on health, while the provision of CHI is ad hoc, access to CHI is inadequate and there is a lack of awareness of health information - what is available and how to get it, and CHI aimed at groups with special needs is lacking.[2,19]

WEXFORD CASE STUDY

A small case study conducted in the Wexford area, a county town south of Dublin, to assess health information needs showed that:

- the majority of people (67%) go first to their doctor or GP for information on health;
- other sources included friends or family, the public library, the local pharmacy, and the hospital or community care clinic;
- the types of information of most interest were:
  - diseases, conditions and treatments (indicated by 45% of respondents)
  - maintaining and improving health (39%)
  - alternative therapies (19%);
- the type of health information service of most use to respondents would be
  - a free and confidential telephone service (25%)
  - information centre in the hospital/clinic (19%)
  - a drop-in information shop in the town centre (18%).

It is significant that alternative therapies were overall of more interest than health services and patients' rights and entitlements, reflecting the enormous increase in public interest in this area. The survey revealed a need for confidentiality and ease of access to CHI such as could be provided by a free help-line. There was a clear indication that health information should be available from "neutral" sources in addition to the traditional medical environment.

INFORMATION PROVIDERS

Developments in the health boards in recent years include the improvement of customer services, information on women's health, disability, and health promotion. Library and information services are at different stages of development in the health boards but the number of librarian's posts have been greatly increased following recommendations in the report *Information for Health*.[2]

A common problem in the health boards, however, is a lack of coordination and consistency in terms of information provision. Different departments, hospitals and clinics are producing information leaflets for example, without cooperation or collaboration with other sections or departments, and without the aid of any overall health board policy or guidelines. Current staffing and resourcing levels of library and information services are inadequate to meet the increasing demand. Information libraries and services targeted at the public need to be developed in all health boards.

The publication of the Department of Health and Children's *Information guide to our health services* in 1996, compiled by the Department's Library and Information Unit, was an important step in improving healthcare information for the public in Ireland and provides an example of good practice for the health boards. It is also available on the Department's web site.[20]

The Library and Information Unit receives many requests for health information from the public in addition to its main role as resource for the Minister and the staff of the Department. A Working Party has been set up recently by the librarian to look into the provision and quality of public information on health services in Ireland.

Healthcare staff and paramedical professionals are, of course, primary information providers and the first source of information for many patients and their carers. Nurses and GPs receive constant requests for more information from patients and their relatives who have limited access to doctors and specialists. Public health nurses visit patients in isolated rural areas who have no other access to information. Information support for health staff is, however, often neglected and/or insufficent to provide the increasingly wide ranging and sophisticated information needs of patients. Relatively few primary care professionals have regular computer access to information.

Statutory and national bodies are important providers of CHI, for example, Citizens Information Centres, the Consumers Association of Ireland, the National Rehabilitation Board, the Health and Safety Authority, and the Irish Nutrition and Dietetic Institute.

Generally there is very little consumer health information held in Irish medical and health sciences libraries or medical school libraries, and very few encourage access by the public.[19] Notwithstanding the increasing demands by patients for information *"we often send people away disappointed because the level of information we can supply is too complex and aimed at the health professional"* (Health Science librarian).

Many librarians report frequent requests from hospital staff, especially nurses, public health nurses and GPs for information to give to their patients.

The voluntary sector is a major provider of CHI in many areas from large national organisations to small self-help groups. Examples of best practice in Ireland include the Irish Cancer Society and the Irish Heart Foundation.

In many ways the public library is the ideal location for CHI services. Libraries are widely spread with branches in many small towns, they have long opening hours and are more accessible to many people than hospitals or health board headquarters. Public libraries also provide an anonymous, and comfortable environment which is very important to many people.

There is a need for public libraries to foster and maintain links with local community and state bodies which produce and distribute CHI materials. It is important that libraries take a proactive approach to collecting and disseminating information on health. Cooperation between the public libraries, the health boards and health sciences libraries on information provision is one important area for development.

Conclusions and recommendations

Consumer health information is a fast growing area, illustrated by an enormous expansion in publications for the lay person, the growth of large numbers of voluntary organisations and self-help groups, and far-reaching developments in health informatics, interactive CD-ROMs and computer networking. On the Internet health information forms one of the larger components. Many research studies have shown that more information is needed by patients and their carers than is currently provided by health professionals; also that an informed public produces a more efficient use of health services, improved compliance with treatment regimes and greater patient satisfaction. Increased access and availability of information on all aspects of healthcare services, conditions and related issues are required in Ireland, with an urgent need for a coordinated approach both regionally and locally within the health boards and hospitals, and nationally by government, voluntary and statutory bodies. Coordination and development of CHI is necessary to ensure comprehensive cost effective CHI services for the public, as well as to provide essential support for healthcare professionals in their role as information providers.

It is important that recognition is also made of the multidisciplinary skills needed to provide effective comprehensive CHI services for the public. Information as well as management and administrative skills are essential in exploiting the vast area of information resources to achieve the most cost-effective services, improve customer satisfaction and increase health gain for people in Ireland. It is essential that an inclusive approach is used involving a partnership of health professionals, health management, information and administrative staff.

A coherent framework should be developed at national level within which targeted information can be provided and disseminated on a national, regional and local basis. A National CHI Strategy for Ireland, drawn up by a panel representing key stakeholders would highlight the issues involved, provide a strategic plan and develop policy guidelines for national and regional initiatives. In addition, a National CHI Resource Centre would establish a focus for the development of CHI. This centre would provide support for CHI services nationwide in terms of a clearing house, examples of best practice, training, and guidelines on service development.

Regional CHI strategies would facilitate the coordination of services and initiatives by the health boards, ensure value for money, and provide guidelines for future developments. One individual in each health board should be designated as having responsibility for CHI overall.

The challenge in developing services is to reconcile local needs and sensitivity with economies of scale and expertise. Local information gathering (especially on services and self-help groups) is extremely important and must be kept up to date. The role of the health boards, hospitals, and public libraries is paramount here. Local information should be available in a number of locations including hospital libraries, clinics, public libraries, pharmacies, shopping centres, sports facilities, and other community "wellness" centres. This local access should be supported by a National CHI Resource Centre as already mentioned, to provide coordination and resources.

Public libraries should be enabled to play a much more proactive role in the improvement of CHI in Ireland with increased resources to exploit their network of branches and professional expertise. Mutually beneficial cooperative partnerships developed between health boards and public library authorities, as well as health sciences libraries, would facilitate wider access to CHI for the public.

References

[1] This paper is based on: MacDougall J. Well read: developing consumer health information in Ireland. Dublin: Library Association of Ireland, 1998

[2] MacDougall J. Information for health. Access to healthcare information services in Ireland. Dublin: Library Association of Ireland, 1995

[3] Gann R. New developments in the NHS Health Information Service. Assignation 1996;14(1):9-11

[4] Gann R. Information resources for Health Information Services. Winchester: NHS HIS Central Support Unit, Help for Health Trust, 1996

[5] Coulter A. Partnerships with patients: the pros and cons of shared decision making. J Health Serv Res Policy 1997;2:112-121

[6] Kai J. Parents' difficulties and information needs in coping with acute illness in pre-school children: a qualitative study. Brit Med J 1996;313:987-990

[7] Coulter A. Assembling the evidence: patient focused outcomes research. Health Libr Rev 1994;11:263-268

[8] Caldwell A. The influence of preference for information on preoperative stress and coping in surgical outpatients. Appl Nurs Res 1991;4:177-183

[9] Barlow J, et al. How are written patient-education materials used in out-patient clinics? Health Educ J 1996;55:275-284
[10] Lowry M. Knowledge that reduces anxiety. Professional Nurse 1995;(Febr):318-320
[11] North G, et al. Guidelines for producing patient information literature. Nursing Standard 1996;10(47):46-48
[12] Edmondson M. Patient information. In: P.Penn et al. Principles of day surgery nursing. Oxford: Blackwell Science, 1996
[13] Chapman J. Quality principles for health information services. Nottingham: NHS Executive Trent Regional Health Authority, 1995
[14] Centre for Health Information Quality. Hi Quality Matters (newsletter), 1998 http://www.centreforhiq.demon.co.uk]
[15] Gann R. Consumer health information services. In: Brittain J, Abbott W (eds) Information management and technology in healthcare. A guide to education and training. London: Taylor Graham, 1993:284-291
[16] Department of Health. A charter of rights for hospital patients. Dublin: Stationery Office, 1992
[17] Department of Health. Shaping a healthier future. A strategy for effective healthcare in the 1990s. Dublin: Stationery Office, 1994
[18] Department of Health. A plan for women's health 1997-1999. Dublin: Stationery Office, 1997
[19] Cullen J. An evaluation of consumer health information provision in the Republic of Ireland. Thesis. Dublin: LIS, Univ College Dublin, 1995
[20] Department of Health. Information guide to our health services. Dublin: Department of Health, 1996 <http://www.doh.ie/>

CONSUMER HEALTH INFORMATION: A REGIONAL SYSTEMS APPROACH

Diane Hummel
Cook Institute for Health Research and Education, Grand Rapids, Michigan, USA

First initiatives

Healthy Kent 2000 and the Cook Institute's Consumer Health Library began in 1992 as independent regional initiatives to improve the health of West Michigan residents.

Discussions for a Consumer Health Library began at Spectrum Health as a dialogue among physicians, nurses, educators, and community members, in response to two task statements:

- Spectrum Health's mission statement to:
  "Improve the health of the community by serving each individual and family with superior quality personal care."
- JCAHO's revision in 1992 Accreditation Manual which mandates informed consent by the patient and the 1994 revision in sec. IM.9 which provides: "The extent of knowledge-based information services, resources, and systems (for example, professional library and health information services) is related to ... the needs of ... patients and their families" and further states: "Accessible knowledge-based information resources includes... information in multiple formats for patient education (brochures, articles, pamphlets, audiovisual materials, and models)."

Research and consultation

Research into the consumer health information movement in the U.S. established that such services enhance the decision making partnerships among patients, health care practitioners, and institutions to manage individual health care issues. The essential conclusion was that the better informed the consumer, the better the health care choice.

After consultation with architects and designers, Spectrum determined to establish an outreach Consumer Health Library in the Devos Women's and Children's Ambulatory Care Center on the campus to maximize the community's access to health information using state-of-the-art technologies, as well as traditional video and print formats.

Infrastructure

To build an information service that reflected the specific health care issues of residents, it was necessary to create local infrastructure, benchmark regional needs, and select appropriate resources. Healthy Kent 2000 was selected as best data source to provide a definitive picture of health care issues in West Michigan and direction to select appropriate, priority resources to build a Consumer Health Library that provided health information services to the region.

The Kent County Health Department had convened the Healthy Kent 2000 Community Health Committee to enact a local community health plan to reflect the national health agenda, defined by the United States Department of Health and Human Services initiative, Healthy People 2000.

Health assessment

In 1992 the local committee began a year-long, three-phased community health assessment that included:

- A Community Health Profile which used data from state and local databases and registries to synthesize statistics concerning the prevalence and distribution of disease, morbidity and mortality, as well as key demographic and health status data.
- A Behavioral Risk Factor Survey which collected data from 600 Kent County adults through a random, anonymous telephone survey. The survey questions identified healthy and health-risk behaviors, and the results identified Kent County's most prevalent health risk factors.
- Community-based Focus Groups which were used as a qualitative research method to permit the collection of data as it relates to health beliefs, attitudes and perceptions. Six target populations (Caucasian, African American, Hispanic, Native American, Asian/Pacific Islander, and Disabled Individuals) provided an overview of the subjective perspective of Kent County's individual and community health.

Statewide access

MichiCard was selected as the best tool to provide local infrastructure to circulate traditional video and print items within the West Michigan region. Michicard began in 1988 when the Library of Michigan Board of Trustees Task Force on Interdependency and Funding recommended the adoption of a statewide library card to provide walk-in and flexible borrowing arrangements for Michigan citizens to access voluntarily participating libraries. This State Library initiative provided the Consumer Health Library with a gateway to distribute its unique resources to the West Michigan region.

Chapter 4: EVIDENCE BASED MEDICINE

Editorial comment

As a preconference event, Jenni Tsafrir and Barbara Aronson together with Carol Lefebvre organized a well appreciated symposium on evidence-based medicine (EBM). The strong movement of EBM is spreading around the world, not the least by the work and energy that is put into the Cochrane Collaboration and coordinated by the growing number of Cochrane Centres in different countries.

It is sometimes said that *"The concept of a "clinical librarian" who attends ward rounds and provides information on demand for the busy clinicians, is more or less idealized and Utopian, and most libraries suffer from manpower shortages which do not allow them to send off a specialist librarian on such missions.*" That nevertheless clinical librarianship is a viable service is proofed by the experience of several colleagues (see e.g. the paper of Anne Lusher on p. 67) as well as the North American Clinical Librarian SIG and discussion list <clinlib-l@harthosp.org> with Elizabeth Killingsworth as moderator <ekilling@stfranciscare.org>. Also the discussion in the EAHIL Clinical Librarians Special Interest Group meeting in Utrecht pointed out that clinical librarian's services are very efficient and, although labour intensive, nevertheless cost effective service to the benefit of patient care and supportive for evidence based clinical practice.

"Evidence-based" is a subject found extensively in the medical as well as in the medical libraries' and medical informatics' literature. Not surprising that this subject was included in the programme of the Utrecht conference. The urge for physicians to make evidence based decisions in daily patient care and hospital procedures, will offer a chance and a challenge to medical librarians to reorganize and to change library services (≈ document delivery) into information & knowledge management services (≈ providing the answers).

The articles in this chapter of the proceedings will give more examples of how to provide evidence services, on the 'many faces of' evidence and the impact this change of practice in medicine and related fields has on library services in general and the position (and image!) of the medical librarians.

Other papers in these proceedings with relevancy for EBM are found in chapter 10 (Massiter and Urquhart p. 188; Brice and Tomlin p. 203). The papers of Keir Reavie (Chpt. 8 p. 164) and of Urquhart and Davies (Chpt. 9 p. 173) underline the interdependence of teaching and the introduction of evidence-based practice.

EVIDENCE-BASED MEDICINE: PERSPECTIVES AND ROLES OF THE HEALTH LIBRARY

Jenni Tsafrir, Barbara Aronson
[1]CHAIM SHEBA MEDICAL CENTER, TEL HASHOMER AND SACKLER SCHOOL OF MEDICINE, TEL AVIV UNIVERSITY, ISRAEL [2]WORLD HEALTH ORGANISATION, GENEVA, SWITZERLAND

A different perspective

The Evidence-Based Medicine movement, as launched at the beginning of this decade, has proved to be a most controversial and extensively debated approach to the provision of medical care, in terms of the volume of literature published about it within such a short period of time, the range of interpretations placed on it, and the opinions expressed. The criticisms and attacks are sometimes personal, on the supposedly patronizing, ivory tower attitude of the proponents as self-appointed "guardians of the truth", or on the policy-makers and managers who support them, who allegedly think only in financial terms and disregard patient values and preferences or the expertise of individual physicians. Sometimes the concept itself is attacked, either on the grounds that medicine has always been evidence-based and it is presumptuous to present EBM as a new discipline; or on the philosophical or logical grounds that in medicine the term "evidence" is incorrect and misplaced;[1] or on methodological grounds, on the basis that the results of Randomized Controlled Trials (RCTs), meta-analyses and systematic reviews are irrelevant when applied to individual patients. It is claimed that "infostat" medicine i.e. based on "information and statistics" (or "practising medicine by numbers") abrogates clinical responsibility, because it ignores what happens to the individual patient once the guidelines and rules have been applied.

Sometimes the objections are aimed at the application of EBM as a cost-containment tool by managers and policy-makers, or "health care purchasers", to the detriment of patient-specific considerations or their preferences. Conversely, EBM is sometimes attacked for being too clinically- and patient-oriented, and ignoring the population-health ethic which aims for cost-effectiveness and efficiency in the allocation of scarce health-care resources.

As recently as this year an article in an Otolaryngology journal was entitled: "Can we be faithful to the Hippocratic Oath in the Era of Managed Care?". The author uses the term "managed" reservedly in conjunction with "care", preferring the more accurate "managed cost", and urges physicians to challenge each other to remain true to the fundamental principles of the oath they took on graduating from medical school.[2]

Background of EBM

Historically, clinical epidemiology can be traced back to the dawn of medicine, since scientific evidence or information and the communication of such information have always been linked to practice, as have the conflicts between research and statistical results on the one hand and their application to medical practice on the other. EBM as we know it is, first and foremost, a response to the tremendous expansion in size and scope of scientific information. This response takes the form of:
- specialization and standardization of the form in which medical information is published;
- development of new tools for indexing, abstracting and evaluating source materials;
- computerized clinical decision support systems, and problem-based learning which integrates specialized up-to-date information into practice, applied to individual patients or groups.

The well-established discipline of clinical epidemiology gave rise in the early 1990s to evidence-based medicine or evidence-based health practice, as an approach aimed to translate the information obtained from clinical epidemiology into daily practice. The alleged transformation from a clinically-led Clinical Epidemiology approach to the managerially-led approach of EBM, seen as a Quality Assurance tool "capable of regulating not just medical practice, but the whole of the health service"[3] was at the base of much of the harsh criticism aimed at EBM.

The practice guidelines which are based on the best evidence available, with the aim of reducing variation in practice patterns, outcomes and costs of care, should ideally be flexible enough to tailor to individual patients, while being broad enough to cover the majority of patients. These guidelines are more likely to be accepted by clinicians if they focus on the process of care rather than on costs.

The classic definition of EBM shows that most of the criticism is biased or unfounded. According to Sackett et al.[4] Evidence-Based Medicine is:
"the conscientious, explicit, and judicious use of current best evidence in making decisions about the care of individual patients", by "integrating individual clinical expertise with the best available external clinical evidence from systematic research". It is not self-evidently practised, as witnessed by the striking variations in clinical behaviour in different centres, even within one country. It is not a "*cost-cutter*" - the most efficacious interventions for individual patients may raise rather than lower costs. It is not *restricted to the evidence from RCTs or Meta-analyses;* it involves tracking down the best external evidence with which to answer clinical questions, including cross-sectional studies of patients with the relevant disorder, and follow-up studies. RCTs are clearly most relevant for therapeutic questions, although some conditions do not require RCTs, or cannot wait for trials to be conducted, or do not lend themselves (for ethical or practical reasons) to RCTs, such as most surgical procedures.

This detailing of what is and what isn't EBM, from the pen of its founders, seems to refute one by one, each of the arguments against it. The translation of these principles into practice has also been precisely outlined in a number of papers, and re-iterated by Sackett in 1997.[5] Because patient care creates the need for clinically important information about diagnosis, prognosis, therapy, and other clinical and health care issues, it is necessary to:
1) convert these information needs into answerable questions;
2) track down, with maximum efficiency, the best evidence with which to answer them;

3) critically appraise that evidence for its validity (closeness to the truth) and usefulness (clinical applicability);
4) integrate this appraisal with clinical expertise and apply it in practice; and
5) evaluate performance.

If these precepts are adhered to, then "the final integration in the mind of the physician, between the theoretical basis and the empirical observations is not in probabilistic (or statistical) terms, but in explanatory patient-oriented terms."[6]

The problems arise, of course, in the application of these principles - the extent to which they are understood, interpreted and applied, and by whom. This part of the clinical decision-making process has been referred to as "heuristics", or ad hoc rules of thumb.[7] Although it is assumed that medical decisions are driven by established scientific fact, even a cursory review of practice patterns and the variation thus revealed, shows that they are not. This is because there are not nearly enough randomized trials or epidemiological studies to guide all clinical decisions, mainly because of ethical or cost considerations. However, since physicians clearly do decide, and generally do so with ease and confidence, it is assumed that they must have some mechanism for making such decisions, derived from "personal theories, assumptions, experience, traditions and lore."

All these concepts have been expressed slightly differently in an approach rejoicing in the catchy acronym POEM, standing for "Patient Oriented Evidence that Matters",[8] which concentrates slightly more narrowly on the importance of the evidence to the patient, with the question: "Does the information focus on an outcome that my patients care about?"

Clearly, Evidence-Based Medicine should apply to decisions that have to be made for populations as well as for individual patients - e.g. public health decisions, preventive medicine, screening, purchasing, all of which involve resources and different types of values from those exercised in the practitioner-patient relationship, although these decisions undoubtedly ultimately affect the care of patients.

Another definition aims to clarify this concept. "Evidence Based Health Care takes place when decisions that affect the care of patients are taken with due weight accorded to all valid, relevant information." This definition evolved out of the premise that "decisions that affect the care of patients" are taken by managers and health policy makers as well as by clinicians. "*Due weight'* acknowledges that many factors other than the results of RCTs may have to be weighed in taking a decision, and that no single sort of evidence should necessarily be the determining factor. "All", although seemingly Utopian, implies that there should at least be an *active search* for all the valid, relevant information, where this presupposes an assessment of the accuracy and applicability of any type of information before using it in coming to the decision, giving "due weight" to each type.

Evidence: information based

Using evidence as the basis for practice is, on the one hand, regarded as something health practitioners have always done and, on the other, as a revolutionary concept challenging current practice.[9] Both notions are in fact true, "if we view the evolution of the concepts behind evidence-based practice as a response to technological advances" These advances include:
- improved quality and range of databases;
- the availability of such databases through CD-ROMs and the Internet;
- improved, user-friendly search techniques;

- aids to systematic ways of appraising a wide range of literature;
- use of Internet services, such as lists, discussion groups, bulletin boards, etc.

Technologically, this has enabled practitioners to use not just the evidence they come across in routine reading, but much more in depth and systematic collective information, which can be targeted at a specific, perhaps immediate need. "What we are seeing, in fact, is the effect of the information technology revolution on medicine",[10] and much of what is being carried out now in Cochrane Centres around the world would not have been possible without improved access to the published literature and better communication between research centres. We see thus, that the focal point in the evolution of the concept of EBM is in fact, *information*.

EBM is based on:

- judicious and efficient information gathering;
- critical appraisal of written materials
- finding appropriate answers for different types of questions
- information as an educational tool

This is obviously the aspect which most interests us as librarians and information specialists, for just as the practice of EBM may be context-oriented, so is the information-gathering process.

The needs and methods of librarians in an academic or research setting may be quite different from those in a hospital or public health or National Health setting. The main issues in question are:

1) Where does the information come from?
2) What does it consist of? Factual information, statistical, anecdotal, guidelines?
3) For whom is it intended and for what purpose?
   - patients; primary care or secondary care setting
   - funding decisions
   - policy making and management
4) How is it processed, interpreted and applied?
5) By whom is it processed? (Clinicians or other health care workers, managers, policy-makers, economists, librarians, statisticians, etc).

Librarians have been heavily involved in promoting EBM approaches in many settings, the best known of which are probably the Cochrane Collaboration, the NHS Centre for Review and Dissemination in York, the Health Information Research Unit at McMaster in Canada, the Information Resources Unit at the University of Sheffield, and a number of lesser known but no less important examples from Germany, France, Italy and Spain.

The concept of a "clinical librarian" who attends ward rounds and provides information on demand for the busy clinicians, is more or less idealized and Utopian, and most libraries suffer from manpower shortages which do not allow them to send off a specialist librarian on such missions. Under these circumstances, it is fortunate indeed that the technological revolution has come to our aid, and that much of the information our clinicians need is electronically-accessible.

Opportunities of EBM

A number of articles in the Health Libraries Literature (e.g. the Special Issue of the Health Libraries Review in 1994) as well as in the Medical Literature, have described EBHC as "an opportunity" or "a new challenge" for health service or health care facilities libraries. As recently as April 1998, in the EAHIL Newsletter, an important article tied us into this "new wave" of EBHC. Miranda and Ginestet in an article on

Knowledge Management,[11] concluded that "our know-how and experience in collecting, selecting, organising and distributing information could help information professionals contribute to the organisation of a knowledge base".

"EBM has its basis in the systemization of a search process of the relevant information in order to apply it to specific clinical cases"[12] and "in order for the retrieved information to guarantee relevance and scientific accuracy several searching techniques must be used, to enable the retrieval of the most specific information relative to the case". It is therefore important to know how each information resource has been designed and constructed, and to be acquainted with the whole range of available resources, including unpublished literature, non-English language literature, etc.

Another evidence-gathering skill required in the context of EBHC is the ability to interpret the question in the situation in which it is presented by the particular health professional. There are different types of "evidence-based requests". We have to understand whether a question is for immediate patient care, for research, for clinical guidelines, for cost-containment considerations - in other words, selection and evaluation of the information for relevance to the particular question and conditions, and whether for professionals in management and policy situations or for clinicians, who will tend to focus on the practicalities of patient care, such as applicability to their patients, patient preferences, adverse effects, etc.

Clearly, these are the specialized skills which a librarian or information specialist can contribute to the information-gathering needs of the clinicians - the added value which they can contribute. Moreover, in addition to information-gathering skills, the health services librarian has to understand the information he/she is handling - the language, the medical terminology, the research methodology, current medical technologies and marketing approaches. And over and above all these, the librarian is expected to play an educational role, in assisting the health professionals to use available resources effectively in their information-gathering.

EBM in practice

Can EBM work in practice? No, if you consider that in a recent review it was found that "physicians are more likely to turn to other physicians to meet their information needs than to other sources, including the published literature".[13] Furthermore, "in seeking information, physicians are also looking for guidance, support and approval". What are the possible obstacles to the implementation of EBM?

- inaccessibility of evidence at the "point of care", at the moment when it is needed
- much of the evidence from studies supposedly answering all the criteria is "confusing, conflicting, inapplicable or unavailable".[14] There is a need for a "guide to interpreting discordant Systematic Reviews";[15] there are examples of discordance between Meta-analyses and large-scale RCTs on specific management issues, and review articles sometimes reach different conclusions based on the same source literature,[16] while articles on the limitations of Meta-analyses abound in the literature.
- physicians tend to believe that clinical guidelines in particular and EBM in general, are being used more for cost-containment and less for improving quality of care.[17]
- it is difficult to bring about changes in behaviour, especially when the newest evidence clashes with beliefs and established procedures or guidelines. In such cases, an appeal can frequently be made to opinion leaders, or "influential others" who are more receptive to innovation, and can "sell" the idea to their colleagues.

SO, can EBM work in practice? Yes, if one considers that new technologies have enabled unprecedented dissemination of expert-based, critically-appraised resources through an ever-increasing array of points of access, to complement and supplement the knowledge accumulated by physicians and other health care workers through practice, experience and education, basic or continuing.

The very availability and greater accessibility of reliable up-to-date information will encourage more and more practitioners, whether in primary or secondary care, to seek out this information, and by acquiring the appropriate judgmental skills, to appraise this information and apply it in their patient care activities. The interpretation of this information and its application to cost-management and population-based decisions, is the one area most open to abuse of the principles of EBHC, and will have to be subjected to constant criticism in order to prevent it undermining the very positive benefits inherent in the application of the optimal scientific evidence to patient care.

We, as Librarians and Information Specialists, may not want to presume to judge the values or merits of EBM in practice, as we are not directly involved in patient care, but as it seems to be here to stay, then wherever our clients or readers wish to implement it, we have to be there for them, if only to ensure efficient and intelligent information-seeking and appraisal, although we believe that our added value contribution can do much more than this.

References

[1] Shahar E. A Popperian perspectiave of the term 'evidence-based medicine'. J Eval Clin Pract 1997;3:109-116

[2] Healy JB. Can we be faithful to the Hippocratic Oath in the era of managed care? Arch Otolaryngol Head Neck Surg 1998;124:497-8

[3] Charlton BG, Miles A. The rise and fall of Evidence Based Medicine. Q J Med 1998;91:371-4

[4] Sackett DL, Rosenberg WC, Muir Gray JA, Haynes RB, Richardson WS. Evidence-based medicine: what it is and what it isn't. BMJ 1996;312:71-2

[5] Sackett DL. Evidence-based Medicine. Semin Perinatol 1997;21:3-5

[6] Vandenbroucke JP. Evidence-based medicine and 'médecine d'observation'. J Clin Epidem 1996;49:1335-8

[7] McDonald CJ. Medical heuristics: the silent adjudicators of clinical practice. Ann Int Med 1996;124:56-62

[8] Slawson DC, Shaughnessy AF. Obtaining useful information from expert based sources. BMJ 1997;314:947-9

[9] Batstone G. Practising by the evidence: the role of pathology. J Clin Pathol 1997;50:447-9

[10] Marshall T. Scientific knowledge in medicine: a new clinical epistemology? J Eval Clin Pract 1997;3:133-8

[11] Miranda GF, Ginestet J. Knowledge management: a changing scene for information professionals. EAHIL Newsletter 1998;(43):16

[12] Castillo-Martin MR. Literature information applied to clinical practice: the clinical librarian. EAHIL Newsletter 1998;(43):13-15

[13] Smith R. What clnical information do doctors need? BMJ 1996;313:1062-8

[14] Hayward RS. Clinical practice guidelines on trial. Can Med Assoc J 1997;156:1725-7

[15] Jadad AR, Cook DJ, Browman GP. A guide to interpreting discordant systematic reviews. Can Med Assoc J 1997;156:1725-7

[16] Barnes DE, Bero LA. Why review articles on the health effects of passive smoking reach different conclusions. JAMA 1998;279:1566-7

[17] Inouye J, Kristopatis R, Stone E, Pelter M, Sandhu M, Weingarten S. Physicians' changing attitudes toward guidelines. J Gen Intern Med 1998;13:324-6

GETTING EVIDENCE TO THE BEDSIDE: THE ROLE OF THE CLINICAL LIBRARIAN

Anne Lusher
CAIRNS LIBRARY, JOHN RADCLIFFE HOSPITAL, OXFORD, UK

Clinical librarianship

The role of the clinical librarian, as developed by Lamb in 1971, was to provide highly specific, patient-centred information to clinicians in support of patient care.[1] The clinical librarian would usually attend bedside rounds or clinical meetings where individual patients were discussed, questions on care were raised and specific information sought. The objectives of the clinical librarian were to conduct literature searches for clinical problems and continuing educational requirements, and to provide same-day or next-day access to quality-filtered information in the form of articles or reference material.[2]

Following the introduction of end-user searching, more recent papers have examined the additional role of the clinical librarian as advisor and teacher to enable clinicians to search effectively for themselves.[3-4]

Evidence-based medicine

Increasing emphasis is now being placed on the practice of Evidence-based Medicine (EBM), which calls for the integration of clinical expertise with the best available external evidence.[5] The evidence sought should be rapidly retrieved, directly relevant to the clinical problem raised and critically appraised for validity and applicability, for implementation into clinical practice. An opportunity arose for the Cairns Library to explore the role of clinical librarian within a clinical team encouraged to practice evidence-based medicine in an acute general medicine setting. The Oxford Consortium for Getting Evidence to the Bedside, a collaborative group from the Centre for Evidence-Based Medicine, Oxford, is investigating strategies for optimising access to evidence-based resources at the point of need, i.e. ward or unit.

Pilot project

One of the Consortium's pilot projects involves the attachment of a clinical librarian to a medical team comprising medical students, house officers, a senior house officer, registrars, a clinical epidemiologist and a consultant, initially for 2 months, in September 1997 and in April 1998.

The primary objective of the clinical librarian was observatory, to identify the information-seeking behaviour of a busy clinical team in order to determine how best to support the team in patient-centred, self-directed, problem-based learning at the bedside.

The secondary objective was participatory, to assist the clinical team to practice evidence-based medicine on clinical service. To do so, clinicians are encouraged to follow five steps: (1) formulate a clinical question arising from a patient-centred problem, (2) find the best evidence to answer the question effficiently and effectively, (3) critically appraise the evidence for its validity and relevance, (4) act upon the evidence by applying it in patient care decisions and (5) evaluate the outcome.[6]

The clinical librarian attended war-based post-take rounds, team rounds and student teaching rounds where the presentation, evaluation, clinical course and management of patients were discussed, clinical problems identified, clinical questions formulated and evidence sought immediately.

The post-take rounds were usually of 3-5 hours duration. Every patient who was seen had been referred to the general medicine service by local general practitioners or by the Accident and Emergency Service during the previous 8-16 hour shift. For each patient admitted, a team member presented the patient's history and findings as a result of the initial clinical examination. The patient was examined. Questions were raised and evidence for clinical decision-making was sought.

The team rounds were of 1-2 hours duration and held in a seminar room adjacent to the wards. The evaluation and management of each patient on the service was reviewed verbally and additional questions on patient care issues were often generated.

The student teaching rounds were of 1.5-2 hours duration and held in the seminar room adjacent to the wards. The students gave concise case presentations of patients recently admitted to the clinical service, went to the bedside for demonstration and teaching of clinical skills and returned to the seminar room for discussion and filling of 'educational prescriptions'. These consisted of a three-part clinical question based on a specific patient problem the students had raised.[7]

MATERIAL AND METHODS

The evidence-based resources used by the team to retrieve information were made available on a number of computer terminals in key clinical areas (linked to the Internet, medical texts and various biomedical databases) and on an 'evidence cart' (containing summary critical appraisals, CD-based MEDLINE, Best Evidence, projector and printing facilities). The cart was later replaced by hand-held touch-screen radio-linked computers (containing a subset of the above including access to laboratory reports, web-based MEDLINE and full-text journals).

RESULTS

The clinical team's information needs were identified as (1) immediate and to be in an easy assimilated form, particularly on the post-take and team rounds, where appropriate management decisions needed to be made rapidly or multiple clinical problems needed to be identified accurately; (2) specific, centred on the patients admitted to the clinical service, usually to determine the appropriate diagnostic test to perform or therapeutic intervention to make and (3) evaluative to determine if the evidence found for the management of one patient might be applicable to others with the result that a clinical service team policy might be devised to ensure appropriate patient care in the future.

In order to fulfil the needs for immediacy and specificity, the clinical librarian's interventions in support of the clinical team usually needed to be performed in the clinical setting. This support comprised (1) searching bibliographic databases (usually MEDLINE) and secondary sources of critically appraised evidence (usually Best Evidence and the Cochrane Libray) to answer clinical questions arising from individual patient-centred problems, (2) advising how to retrieve specific, patient-related evidence using advanced subject search strategies allied to search filters for therapy, diagnosis, aetiology and prognosis studies in order to optimise specificity without sacrificing sensitivity, (3) providing rapid access to the full text of articles and other reference material identified as useful.

Discussion and conclusion

Participation by the clinical librarian in the practice of evidence-based medicine in the setting is highly challenging. Despite a highly motivated EBM-oriented clinical team, some clinical questions raised were left unanswered. This occurred particularly if the evidence sought was not retrieved from the easily assimilated secondary literature sources (usually Criticaly Appraised Topics (CATs), summary data, or Best Evidence). Searching the primary literature on bibliographic databases was found by the team to be slower and more demanding of search skills. The information retrieved required the full article to be obtained and then appraised for its validity and applicability to clinical practice. This finding confirmed the assessment of clinician's information needs made by Smith, that questions generated in a clinical setting do go unanswered, even though many could be answered, usually by electronic sources.[8] This route was felt to be time consuming. He concluded that "the ideal information source will be directly relevant, contain valid information, and be accessed with a minimum amount of work."[8]

Even if the clinical librarian had at all times been able to understand the clinical issues raised in the questions generated (which was not always the case) and had conducted comprehensive searches of the primary literature on behalf of the team, the team had little time to appraise the validity and applicability of the article selected. The service demands on clinical teams allow for little reading time to assimilate information for clinical problem-solving. Self-reports at several UK hospitals have recorded average patient-centred reading times per week for medical students, house officers, senior house officers, registrars and younger and older consultants of 90, zero, 20, 60, 45 and 30 minutes respectively.[8] This finding suggests the need for a further extension of the clinical librarian role to include critical appraisal of the primary literature and presentation of the evidence in a readily assimilated form.

The challenging experience of two separate months attached to a clinical team has helped to define the multiple skills which the clinical librarian needs to acquire in order to support the clinical team effectively in the practice of evidence-based medicine. To be truly proactive in a clinical setting, the clinical librarian must (1) acquire and sustain a clinical knowledge base in order to understand the clinical issues of the questions generated, (2) conduct complex searches swiftly on a variety of resources that optimise specificity without sacrificing sensitivity in order to retrieve evidence that is trustworthy and directly applicable to the patient-centred problem, (3) assist the clinical team members to enhance their searching skills to retrieve evidence efficiently and effectively for themselves, (4) appraise the articles selected, (5) present the evidence in a readily assimilated form to enable the clinical team to integrate their clinical expertise with the best available external evidence. The clinical librarian role is thus multiple and requires specific training in the tenets of evidence-based medicine and a commitment to lifelong learning.[9]

The pilot study in Oxford is set to continue into a fully developed research project to explore the multiple roles now identified, the training issues required and to evaluate the impact of the clinical librarian on clinical decision-making, quality of patient care, the clinican's trust in the information provided and the effect on health care costs.

References

[1] Lamb G. A decade of clinical librarianship. Clin Libr Q 1982;1:2-4

[2] Cimple K. Clinical medical librarianship: a review of the literature. Bull Med Libr Assoc 1985;73:21-28

[3] Halsted DD, Ward DH, Neeley DM. The evolving role of clinical medical librarians. Bull Med Libr Assoc 1989;77:299-301

[4] Horak EB. Clinical librarianship in an era of end users. Med Ref Serv Q 1987;6(2):65-69

[5] Sackett DL, Rosenberg WMC, Gray JAM, Haynes RB, Richardson WS. Evidence-based medicine: what it is and what it isn't. BMJ 1996;312:71-72

[6] Sackett DL, Richardson WS, Rosenberg WMC, Haynes RB. Evidence-based medicine: how to practice and teach EBM. London: Churchill-Livingstone, 1997. p. 3.

[7] *opus cit.*, pp. 31-35

[8] Smith R. What clinical information do doctors need? BMJ 1996;313:1062-1068

[9] Giuse NB. Advancing the practice of clinical medical librarianship. Bull Med Libr Assoc 1997;85:437-438

THE CONSULTANT LIBRARIAN AND EVIDENCE BASED MEDICINE

Gabriella Gabutti, Cesare Carrà, Andrea Zeccato, Carmine Tinelli, Catherine Klersy, Moreno Curti
[1 2 3 6]LIBRARY AND [4 5]EPIDEMIOLOGY SERVICE, POLICLINICO S. MATTEO, PAVIA, ITALY

Background

Evidence Based Medicine (EBM) is a term coined at McMaster Medical School (Canada) in the early eighties to identify a process of critical learning, aimed at solving clinical problems. This process consists of four phases:
- Clinical problem formulation in terms of a clear question;
- Systematic identification of the literature able to answer this question, through a computerised search;
- Critical evaluation of the retrieved literature;
- Use in clinical practice of the evidence found.

In order to assess the link between this process and the librarian's role, we conceived a MEDLINE search strategy joining with 'OR' the exploded terms 'Information Science', 'Information System' and 'Librarians'; the obtained result was joined with 'AND' to 'Evidence Based Medicine'. Starting 1980, the search retrieved 23 papers: surprisingly, none of them dealt with the ability required to the consultant librarian; they all concerned training and activity of physicians and researchers.

Despite the lack of literature, it's evident that the role of the consultant librarian in phases 1-3 is essential.

Study

Aim of this study is to assess the role and the abilities to be acquired by or professional qualification of the librarian for the phases of EBM, namely:
1 Clear formulation of questions based on the patients' clinical problem (strictly related to the type of patient, the treatment performed, the clinical outcome, etc.);
2 Retrieval of the most specific bibliographic references (optimal recall/precision);
3 Critical appraisal of bibliographic references;
4 Purchasing the full-text paper in the shortest time.

At that purpose 2 questionnaires were set up. The first was aimed to the librarians of 116 public and private biomedical libraries in Italy, to perform a survey of the services offered for EBM and to identify the characteristics, limits and potentialities of the librarians themselves. The second was administered to doctors, whose papers in 1997, reported on MEDLINE, dealt with application of EBM to the study of a clinical case.

Results

Data resulting from both questionnaires were analysed to show the relationship between demand and supply and to check whether doctors' requests are met by actual offers of services.

116 questionnaires were sent to physicians and 35 returned (30%).
95 questionnaires were sent to librarians and 26 returned (27%).

On the average *responding libraries* have 5 persons as staff, an opening time of 39,5 hours/week, are connected to national and foreign libraries for the retrieval of full text articles; 69% of the libraries has an internal network and the 61% has an Internet connection.

Responding physicians have an average age rather low (41,5 years) and belong to 15 different specialities, with a prevalence of Gynaecologists, Nursing researchers and Internists.

Conclusions

1 Both categories know which tools must be used to perform a bibliographic research, but beyond the common use of MEDLINE, physicians use more specialist databanks (e.g. TRIPS) while librarians use more traditional ones.
2 Both categories must improve the ability of critical appraisal; the majority (77%) doesn't know or doesn't use methods aimed at pointing to and eliminating erroneous literature; the use of JAMA or BMJ guidelines for evaluating medicine is low in physicians (34%).
3 Surely there is a gap between the physicians' demands and the librarian's knowledges, especially for the use of foreign languages. The bibliographic research made up by the physician without the co-operation of the librarian is always longer; furthermore, it's impossible for physicians to obtain all the full-text articles needed without using the documentation retrieval organised services.

In EBM the role of the librarian will always be more important and irreplaceable, above all if the librarian himself tries to improve his/her own knowledges and abilities, and specifies his/her preparation and training with a continuous refresh about languages, terms, bibliographic and electronic tools at his/her disposal.

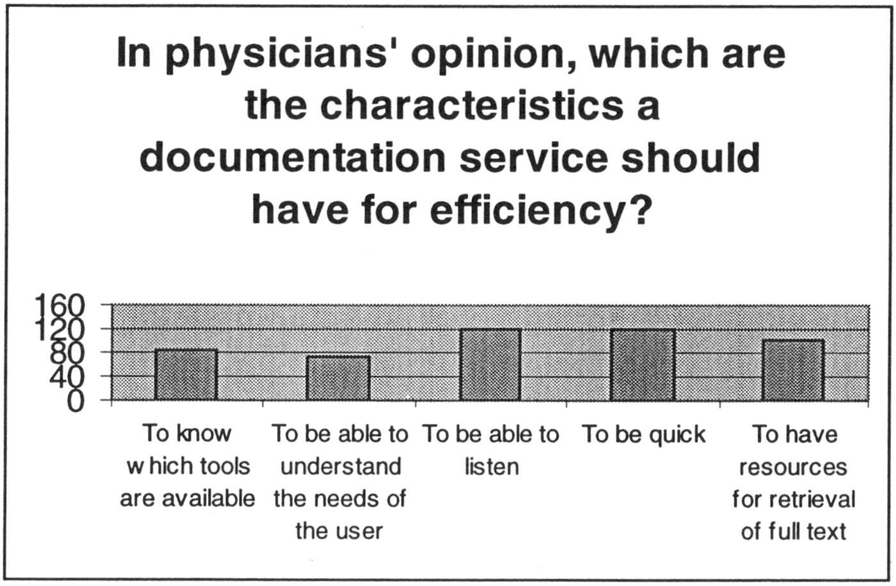

TABLE 1

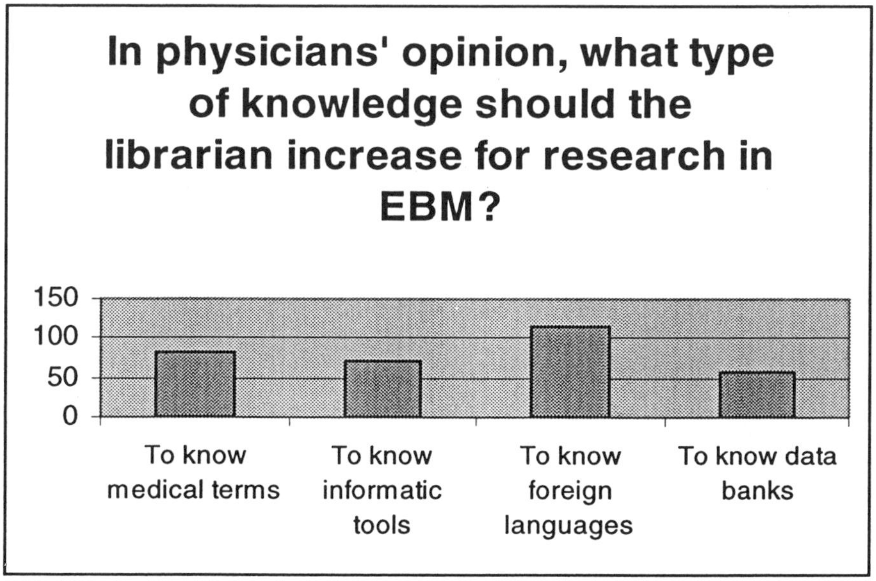

TABLE 2

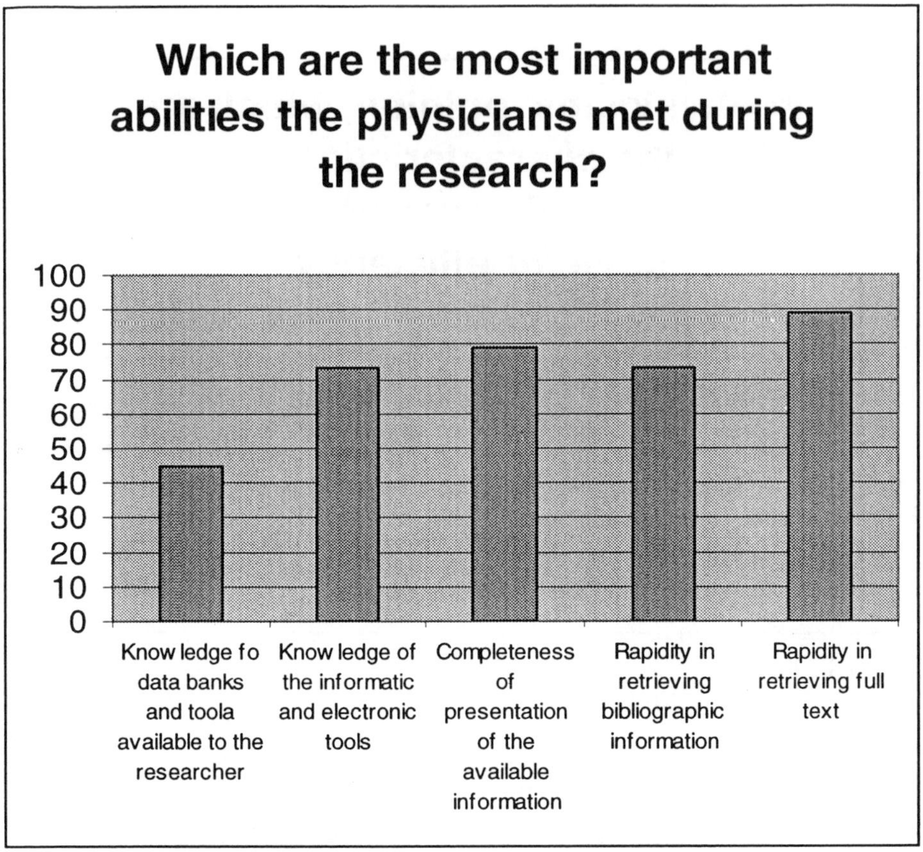
Which are the most important abilities the physicians met during the research?
100
90
80
70
60
50
40
30
20
10
0
Know ledge fo data banks and toola available to the researcher
Know ledge of the informatic and electronic tools
Completeness of presentation of the available information
Rapidity in retrieving bibliographic information
Rapidity in retrieving full text

TABLE 3

ZEBRAS AND HORSES: CAN THE MEDICAL LITERATURE BE USED TO ANWER CLINICAL QUESTIONS

Richard Nollan
STOLLERMAN CLINICAL BRANCH LIBRARY, UNIVERSITY OF TENNESSEE, MEMPHIS, TENNESSEE, USA

Summary

Clinicians are aware of the fact that they cannot know everything they need to know, and that medical information is growing by quantum leaps. So it is important to identify resources, which can fill information gaps as they arise. Literature databases, such as MEDLINE, provide access to information that clinicians need, but do clinicians use the literature to answer their questions? This evidence-based literature review examines the clinical use of computerized literature databases.

Three studies indicate that very few physicians use computerized databases.[1-3] Is this a problem? Perhaps physicians intuitively employ a cost/benefit model (as one study suggests), thereby selecting the best information resources and ignoring those that are too expensive or difficult to use.

Two studies demonstrate a significant gap between what is available in the literature and what clinicians know,[4,5] while one study (representing many more) reports on the underuse of established therapies, making it readily apparent that physicians are not keeping up with the literature.[6] What would be the outcome if clinicians were to increase their use of the literature?

One study shows that 46% of questions asked in a clinical setting found a "clear answer."[7] Another study draws a statistical correlation between MEDLINE searches and patients' length-of-stay and cost.[8]

If the benefits of using the literature are apparent, why do so few clinicians avail themselves of it? The size of the literature is enormous, and finding an answer can be compared to looking for a needle in a haystack. The quality of the literature is variable, not only in terms of publication types, but also in terms of methodologies. Consensus is not always available, and it isn't always clear that the information found is relevant to a clinician's needs.

Finding timely, pertinent information in an easy-to-access format, evaluating that information, and then applying it to the patient is one of the biggest challenge the clinician faces.

References

[1] Covell DG, Uman GC, Manning PR. Information needs in office practice: are they being met? Ann Intern Med 1985;103:596-9

[2] Williamson JW, German PS, Weiss R, Skinner EA, Bowes F. Health science information management and continuing education of physicians. Ann Intern Med 1989;110:151-60

[3] Connelly DP, Rich EC, Curley SP, Kelly JT. Kowledge resource preferences of family physicians. J Fam Pract 1990;30:353-9

[4] Stross JK, Harlan WR. The Dissemination of New Medical Information. JAMA 1979;241:2622-4

[5] Williamson JW, German PS, Weiss R, Skinner EA, Bowes F. Health science information management and continuing education of physicians. Ann Intern Med 1989;110:151-60

[6] Anderson FA, Wheeler B, Goldbert RJ, Hosmer DW, Forcier A, Patwardhan NA. Physician practices in the prevention of venous thromboembolism. Ann Intern Med 1991;115:591-5

[7] Gorman P, Ash J, Wykoff L. Can primary care physicians' questions be answered using the medical journal literature? Bull Med libr Assoc 1994;82:140-6

[8] Klein MS, Ross FV, Adams DL, Gilbert CM. Effect of online literature searching on length of stay and patient care costs. Acad Med 1994;69:489-905

THE WELSH PROTOCOL ENHANCEMENT PROJECT

Alison Weightman, Jacqueline Barker, John Lancaster
HERBERT DUTHIE LIBRARY, UNIVERSITY OF WALES COLLEGE OF MEDICINE, CARDIFF, WALES, UK

Summary

The Protocols for Investment in Health Gain were commissioned by the Welsh Office, and published in the early 1990s, to identify areas of health care where further investment could lead to improvements in the health of the people of Wales. The documents also highlighted current practices which were of questionable value.

This poster presentation did summarise the results of a three year project, coordinated within the UWCM Library, which began in 1995 to 'enhance' the original documents by providing clear, updated, statements in each subject area with a precise indication of the strength of the evidence and its sources for each statement. The publications represent a systematic summary of the evidence found through formal literature searching across a broad range of sources and act as signposts to the best available evidence in a particular area. The evidence has been critically appraised using internationally accepted methods, under the direction of a public health physician, and reviewed by a team of experts who are directly involved in patient care. Detailed attention has also been given to the dissemination and appraisal of the enhanced Protocols in text and electronic formats. The resultant documents are intended for use in a wide variety of settings - to assist in the planning and purchasing of health care, to inform clinical practice, in the development of the undergraduate curriculum where appropriate, for continuing education and audit and to identify potential areas for further research.

SYSTEMATIC REVIEWS DEPEND ON SYSTEMATIC LITERATURE SEARCHES

Hugh Brazier
ROYAL COLLEGE OF SURGEONS IN IRELAND, DUBLIN, IRELAND

Introduction

Well designed systematic reviews and meta-analyses make important contributions to medical knowledge, and for many years the production of such reviews has been recognised as a key component in evidence-based medicine. Writing a systematic review is a scientific activity which must be judged by the same standards as those applied to other scientific research. The validity of the review depends on rigorous and explicitly stated methods, including the literature search methods used to identify studies for inclusion.

Eleven years ago Mulrow[1] examined a sample of fifty medical review articles and found that the source of the information was specified in only one review. In an editorial in the same issue of Annals of Internal Medicine, Huth[2] recommended that a review should describe the method of the literature search "clearly and unequivocally", specifying the indexes searched, the search terms used and any constraints including language and years of coverage. Eleven years on, there are many papers and books on the systematic review process,[3,4] and most of them stress the need for a clear research design and an explicit statement of methods.

How well do authors of reviews follow these guidelines? How well do they carry out their literature searches, and how clearly do they document the methods used?

Methods

I searched MEDLINE (1966 - June 1998) for papers including the words 'systematic review' or 'meta-analysis' in their titles, limiting the search to those papers published up to the end of 1997 in seven journals: Annals of Internal Medicine, Archives of Internal Medicine, BMJ, CMAJ, JAMA, The Lancet or the New England Journal of Medicine.

Papers were included only if they were themselves reviews, as opposed to papers about the review process. The sample was further limited to those systematic reviews or meta-analyses which set out first to identify and then to review the literature, showing some evidence in their methods sections of having searched for studies to include in the review. Reviews which took as their starting point an already known set of data (for example from a series of co-ordinated trials) were excluded.

Each of the reviews which satisfied the inclusion criteria was read, with particular attention paid to the abstract, introduction, methods and discussion sections. For each review the following questions were answered:

1. How many bibliographic databases were searched?
2. Which databases are mentioned in the review?
3. Did the authors attempt to identify unpublished trials and include them in the review?
4. What language restrictions were placed on the search?
5. Do the authors give a starting date and an end date for the search?
6. Do the authors quote any of the terms used in the search?
7. Do the authors provide the full strategy for at least one database - i.e. in sufficient detail for the search to be replicated?
8. Is there an explicit or implicit reference to publication bias, or any other comment on the search strategy?

Results

One hundred and sixty-five papers satisfied the inclusion criteria. The earliest was published in 1985, and the frequency increased to 36 in 1997. Most (135) were entitled 'meta-analysis', 29 were 'systematic reviews', and one included both terms in its title. The phrase 'systematic review' first appeared in a title in 1993.

Ten of the reviews (6%) gave no information on the databases searched, and 84 (51%) were based on a search of one database only. In almost every case this was MEDLINE, which was referred to by name in 153 reviews (93%). In all, 52 bibliographic and research databases were named. After MEDLINE, the most frequently named were EMBASE (mentioned in 28 reviews, 17%), Current Contents (19, 12%), SCI-search (12, 7%), CINAHL (10, 6%) and the Cochrane databases and trial registers (8, 5%).

Only 68 (41%) of the reviews stated explicitly that unpublished material had been included; 54 (33%) excluded unpublished material, and 43 (26%) gave no information. Fifty of the reviews (30%) were based solely on English-language material, and only 18 (11%) made it clear that there had been no language restrictions. Over half (86, 52%) made no reference to languages included or excluded. One hundred and thirty-one reviews gave some information on the dates covered by the search, with 109 (66% of the total) giving both a start and an end date.

Ninety-two reviews (56%) included at least some of the search terms used, but in only 56 (34%) did this appear to be a full list of terms, and in only 13 (8%) was there enough information to allow the search to be replicated. In most cases, even where an apparently complete list of terms was supplied, it was not possible to replicate the search because of lack of information. Typically, there was no indication of whether terms were entered as text words or as MeSH, or whether subheadings had been used, or whether MeSH terms had been exploded, or whether text words had been truncated, and there was generally insufficient information on how the terms had been combined.

Publication bias was referred to in 78 reviews (47%), but only 23 (14%) made any other comment on the comprehensiveness of the search or on the search strategy employed. This generally took the form either of an assertion of confidence that the search had been comprehensive, or a general admission that material might have been missed. In a few cases there was a specific reference to how the search could have been improved, for example by the inclusion of additional named databases or of non-English-language reports.

There was some evidence of a change over the thirteen years. The mean number of databases searched per review increased from 1.5 in 1985-94 to 2.5 in 1996-97. For the same spans of years, the percentage of reviews including unpublished material rose significantly from 32% to 51% ($\chi^2 = 4.324$, df = 1, $P<0.05$), and the percentage of reviews quoting search terms rose from 46% to 69% ($\chi^2 = 6.468$, df = 1, $P<0.05$).

Discussion

This study raises concerns both about the quality of the literature searches on which systematic reviews are based, and about the way in which the searches are documented.

The sample was restricted to reviews which included the terms 'systematic review' or 'meta-analysis' in their titles. Including reviews with other wording would be unlikely, however, to change the results. If anything, the use of these phrases by an author suggests an above-average awareness of the importance of a scientific approach to the review process, and including other reviews would probably result in a sample of reviews with less systematic literature search methods. On the other hand, the study did not include sources such as the Cochrane Library, where reviewers' search methods are generally more systematic and comprehensive, and are recorded in far greater detail, than in the journals examined here.

In spite of the evidence of recent improvements, many systematic reviews and meta-analyses published in the mainstream medical journals still appear to be based on poorly executed and inadequately documented searches. Especially surprising are the heavy reliance on MEDLINE as the sole bibliographic database, and the small number of reviews which include an adequate record of the search strategy.

As medical librarians, we should be working to improve the quality of systematic reviews. We should be involved in producing systematic reviews. We should draw up clear standards for the recording of literature searches, and we should help reviewers to adhere to them. Most of the published instructions on writing reviews are rather vague when it comes to the literature search, saying little other than that it should be comprehensive and unbiased, and that the sources, the search strategy and any time and language constraints should be recorded. What exactly is meant by 'recording the search strategy' is not spelt out, and reviewers are perhaps left following a formula without fully understanding the principles behind what they are doing.

We should make sure that the writers of systematic reviews are able to go beyond the formula, to produce reviews based on well executed and well documented systematic searches of the literature.

References

[1] Mulrow CD. The medical review article: state of the science. Ann Intern Med 1987;106:485-8
[2] Huth EJ. Needed: review articles with more scientific rigor. Ann Intern Med 1987;106:470-1
[3] Oxman AD, Cook DJ, Guyatt GH. Users' guides to the medical literature VI. How to use an overview. JAMA 1994;272:1367-71
[4] Undertaking systematic reviews of research on effectiveness; CRD guidelines for those carrying out or commissioning reviews. CRD Report no. 4. York: NHS Centre for Reviews and Dissemination, 1996

EUROPEAN UNION CONTRIBUTION TO AN INTERNATIONAL REGISTER OF CONTROLLED TRIALS

Carol Lefebvre
UK Cochrane Centre, Oxford, UK

Summary

Randomized controlled trials (RCTs) involving sufficient numbers of patients are essential to distinguish reliably between important effects of many forms of health care and the effects of biases or the play of chance. It has been shown repeatedly that if systematic reviews of RCTs, updated periodically, had been made from the beginning of series of related trials, reliable treatment recommendations could have been made available earlier, and resources for research could have been used more efficiently. Reliable systematic reviews are based on as high a proportion of the relevant evidence as possible. Searches of major bibliographic databases such as MEDLINE and EMBASE have shown to miss on average 50% of the studies in a number of clinical areas, and many important European journals, especially those not published in English, are not indexed in the major databases.

In 1994 the European Union funded a contract under the BIOMED Programme, to identify reports of trials from general healthcare journals published in Europe. By now 13,000 reports of trials are now identifiable in the Cochrane Controlled Trials Register (CCTR), which were not identifiable as trials in MEDLINE before. Extension of this contract for a further three-year period, in order to be able to search specialized general healthcare journals published throughout the European Union is expected in 1998.

An important discovery was made by colleagues who searched five leading general healthcare journals in German, when comparing studies reported in German with reports by the same authors in English-language journals. They found that only 35% of the German-language articles reported significant differences between the study and controlled groups. Conversely, 62% of the English-language articles reported significant differences between the study and control groups. These colleagues concluded that authors are more likely to publish RCTs in an English-language journal if the results are statistically significant. English-language bias may therefore be introduced in reviews and meta-analysis if they include only trials reported in English. It is therefore crucial that reports of trials published throughout Europe are identified and made available to those who are preparing systematic reviews and meta-analyses.

DES PRINCIPES DE LA MÉTA-ANALYSE NON STATISTIQUE POUR UNE REVUE CRITIQUE DE LA RECHERCHE BIOMÉDICALE

Françoise Pasleau, Catherine Delvenne, Nadine Cielniaszek
MEDICAL LIBRARY, UNIVERSITY OF LIÈGE, LIÈGE, BELGIUM

Abstract

In most circumstances, considerable time lags before results from biomedical research are integrated in general medical practice are inevitable. Several economic, technical factors and educational orientation are responsible for this gap. Effective information management at the institutional level could provide clinicians the means to adopt new perspectives. At present, the link between basic research and clinical application relies upon the motivation of individuals to develop new skills in literature retrieval and analysis and yet their occupational responsabilities inhibit this endeavour. Academic librarians, educated and trained in information and biomedical sciences, have a role in providing physicians with current and readily applicable knowledge from the critical analysis of the literature.

The Faculty of Medicine Library is developing a research programme to design an updated and comprehensive picture of the diagnostic and prognostic biological markers in the field of human prostate cancer. The final product is envisioned as a database accessible on the web. As this product is designed to have a direct impact on clinical decision making and patient care, it should guarantee thoroughness, relevancy and objectivity and not become yet another narrative review of the literature. Over the last decade, there is a move towards using statistical meta-analyses to synthesize literature. This has proven to be useful when similar strategies are used to produce similar quantitative outcomes that can be merged for statistical analysis.[1] Even though studies in cancer research assess the same model, they are often too fragmented or heterogeneous in their design, methods and instrumentation. Approaches have been developed to conduct non-statistical meta-analysis of such publications.[2] Quantitative and qualitative meta-analyses are based on common principles largely discussed in the literature, and are related to model development, literature searching, rating references for quality and annotating and synthesizing high quality references. In practice, these basic principles require translation into actual instructions adapted to every domain of biomedical research. Model definition is a very critical step that governs the quality of subsequent analyses. Specific examples illustrate the guidelines acquired from our experience.

Introduction

Le concept de la "Médecine Basée sur des Preuves" (EBM, Evidence Based Medicine), implique de systématiquement rechercher et évaluer les découvertes de la recherche biomédicale et d'en extraire des "preuves", à savoir des connaissances qui seront utilisées comme bases de décision clinique. En cancérologie, la prédiction à long terme de l'évolution d'une tumeur reste un problème difficile. Les études prospectives et rétrospectives des marqueurs tumoraux ouvrent sans cesse de nouvelles pistes, dont certaines se concrétisent par la mise au point de nouveaux tests de biologie clinique ou d'histopathologie. Nous proposons de centraliser à l'intention des cliniciens les informations utiles pour exploiter les résultats de ces analyses en vue d'évaluer le risque de rechute et de survie à long terme des patients et d'orienter les choix thérapeutiques. Notre projet est de créer un prototype de site web, consacré aux marqueurs du cancer de la prostate, qui se présentera comme une base de données bibliographique, avec notamment des liens vers des résumés structurés et des articles intégraux objectivant les preuves. Notre démarche devra répondre aux exigences de la méta-analyse.

Etapes de la démarche méta-analytique

En théorie, les démarches de la méta-analyse statistique,[1] de la méta-analyse qualitative[2] et de l'EBM[3] se composent de quatre étapes communes comprenant la définition d'un modèle, la sélection des informations en fonction de critères de qualité, l'extraction et la synthèse des données. La difficulté consiste à traduire ces principes en procédures précises et concrètes.

Un modèle est la description des relations existant entre des variables définies intervenant dans un contexte limité. Le contexte de notre recherche est celui de la transformation progressive d'une tumeur bénigne de la prostate en une tumeur résistante à l'hormonothérapie en passant par les stades de lésion prénéoplasique, de tumeur maligne et de tumeur avec métastases. Ces étapes correspondent à l'accumulation dans les cellules tumorales de mutations touchant des éléments de contrôle de la croissance et de la différenciation cellulaire, qui sont les variables de notre modèle. Le modèle doit être défini à priori car il servira ensuite à rechercher les informations pertinentes (étape 2) et à les associer pour produire une synthèse (étape 4). Il est donc le fondement de la démarche méta-analytique. Souvent, plusieurs cycles de recherche, lecture, analyse et synthèse sont nécessaires avant d'arriver à une description suffisamment subtile des relations entre les variables du modèle.

Sur base du modèle de la cancérisation de la prostate, nous avons établi une stratégie de recherche avec explosion sur 77 descripteurs MESH. Les citations extraites de MEDLINE et de PreMEDLINE (PubMed) ont été importées dans une base de données afin d'éliminer les doubles. Les citations ont ensuite été analysées pour leur adéquation au modèle. Les références non pertinentes ont été éliminées; les autres ont été classées par thème. La base de données est mise à jour mensuellement. Afin de garantir l'exhaustivité de l'étude, la recherche sera étendue à d'autres bases de données (EMBASE, EMBASE Alert, BIOSIS, Cancerlit, Physician Data Query).

CRITÈRES DE QUALITÉ

Les publications qui serviront de base à l'établissement de preuves doivent être sélectionnées en fonction de critères de qualité. Les protocoles de méta-analyse restent souvent imprécis sur la manière pratique de procéder à cette évaluation. Nous avons développé une grille à 24 entrées portant sur différentes caractéristiques des publications, à savoir: les références externes (facteur d'impact, "AIM" Journal), les objectifs, l'adéquation au modèle et la cohérence interne, le type d'étude (pilote, définitive, de validation, prospective, rétrospective, multicentrique), le type de publication (article, revue, essai clinique, méta-analyse, autre), l'échantillon (type, taille, sélection, groupe contrôle), la durée de l'étude, les méthodes, l'analyse statistique et enfin, la pertinence des conclusions par rapport aux objectifs annoncés et aux résultats rapportés. L'attribution de valeurs chiffrées en regard de ces différents critères permettra de calculer une cote globale pour chacune des publications et de définir un seuil d'exclusion. Il nous restera alors à définir une procédure de saisie et de synthèse des informations contenues dans les publications sélectionnées.

L'approche méta-analytique doit elle-même répondre aux critères de qualité suivants:
(1) le modèle et les critères de qualité doivent être définis à priori et ne peuvent être modifiés au vu des résultats; (2) tout amendement doit être solidement justifié; (3) chaque étape doit être documentée et décrite en détail; (4) l'évaluation des publications, l'extraction et la synthèse des données doivent être réalisées par des examinateurs indépendants.

Conclusions et perspectives

Notre projet tente d'apporter aux cliniciens une ébauche de solution au problème de recherche, d'analyse et de gestion d'informations adaptées à leurs activités, en vue d'améliorer la qualité des services rendus et de développer, à long terme, un véritable partenariat entre la bibliothèque et les services de la Faculté de Médecine. La création d'une équipe multidisciplinaire, associant des bibliothécaires et des biochimistes formés aux techniques des sciences de l'information, a sans doute favorisé le développement de programmes de recherche au sein même de la bibliothèque. Outre qu'elle participe à l'amélioration de l'image de marque de la bibliothèque, cette activité nous permet d'acquérir de nouvelles compétences qui se traduiront par une extension de la gamme des services offerts à la communauté scientifique. Nous nous efforcerons également de transmettre l'expérience acquise de l'analyse critique de la littérature, au travers des formations que nous organisons à l'intention des étudiants et des utilisateurs désireux de parvenir à une véritable maîtrise de l'information scientifique.

Références

[1] D'Agostino RB, Weintraub M. Meta-analysis: a method for synthesizing research. Clin Pharmacol Ther 1995;58:605-16
[2] Bland CJ, Meurer LN, Maldonado G. A systematic approach to conducting a non-statistical meta-analysis of research literature. Acad Med 1995;70:642-53
[3] Sackett DL, Rosenberg WM, Gray, JA, Haynes RB, Richardson WS. Evidence based medicine: what it is and what it is n't [editorial][see comments]. BMJ 1996;12:71-2

Chapter 5: FUTURE ROLES OF (MEDICAL) LIBRARIES

Introduction by the editor

The future roles of libraries and especially medical libraries will depend on many circumstances, not the least the expectations of our customers and the information technology available.

For the medical libraries worldwide the services and databases provided by the National Library of Medicine (NLM) in Bethesda, Maryland (USA) are of eminent importance. Supported by Federal Government Funding this library is able to provide and distribute services to all people working in healthcare worldwide. By providing access free of charge via the Internet to their databases and information sources the NLM will play a leading role in future developments in medical librarianship. The paper of Lois Ann Colaianni was well received: not only because the continuation of the NLM services on the web was annnounced, but also it was a stimulating and thought provoking presentation, of which only the more factual and tangible contents are herewith published. Arnoud de Kemp of Springer Verlag (Heidelberg, Germany) could, unfortunately, not provide the editor with the material of his presentation, but be convinced that his wittiful presentation gave us a different view on the scientific communication and publishing system.

For Bas Savenije, the library director of the University Library of Utrecht University, the most important issue to look at is not so much the organization **of** the library but the organizing done **by** the library. The added value of the gathering, combining, extracting, annotating and describing of information sources is the very important and creative aspect of library work. This creative work can only be supported by technology, but not replaced by it. Savenije foresees a reenchantment of the library: *Dreams take flight at the library....*

In his presentation Derek Law analyzes the elements that constitute the library paradigm and refers to the important elements of sustainability (permanence, availability and accesibility) which are necessary for scholarship. Without neglecting the important role local, national and international computer networks play in scientific communication, his analysis shows that the added value that has to be brought in by librarians that the overwhealming, rich and complex information sources offered by the World Wide Web will never replace library services. Internet and the library network will become complementarily knitted together.

THE NATIONAL LIBRARY OF MEDICINE: PLANS FOR INTERNATIONAL ACCESS TO ITS INFORMATION RESOURCES

Lois Ann Colaianni
NATIONAL LIBRARY OF MEDICINE, BETHESDA, MARYLAND, USA

Introduction

NLM is rapidly expanding Web access to its information resources. This means that I don't have to describe these resources in detail. I need to bring them to your attention. You can access these resources at your leisure and see how they work and how they can be useful. Web access is essential for you to serve your users adequately. Web access reduces, and in many cases eliminates, the barriers of distance and time. It also can reduce costs. Web access in a small village in Poland or Lithuania provides a health sciences librarian access to the same resources as the colleague in Paris or London.

PubMed and IGM

Both the, PubMed and the new Internet Grateful Med (IGM) search interfaces provide free access to MEDLINE. NLM expects to continue to provide free access to MEDLINE and citations from other MEDLARS databases via the Web. We have no plans to charge for Web access to our databases. What is the difference between PubMed and the new IGM? Users may like one better than the other because of personal preferences. The new IGM, which no longer accesses MEDLINE via ELHILL, should be available this summer, perhaps as early as July. PubMed and the new IGM will both have the links from the citation to the full text of the article on the publisher's Web site and the capability to "see related articles". I will talk more about the links to the full text when I talk about document delivery. The "see related articles" feature allows you to find the citation to "the perfect article" and ask the system to find more like it. The complicated mathematical algorithm for this feature considers the text words and MeSH terms. PubMed now has the capability for advanced boolean searching. The advanced searching features are being enhanced because former ELHILL users want the control they had to do precision searching.

The new IGM allows you to use the Unified Medical Language System with the French, German, Russian, Spanish and Portuguese translations of MeSH. This is helpful in case you forget the exact MeSH term in English but can remember the French word, or the word from one of the other languages. You can enter that term and retrieve using it. The new IGM also searches more MEDLARS databases, including OLDMEDLINE (1962-65), AIDSLINE, AIDSTRIALS, AIDSDRUGS, HISTLINE, HealthSTAR (health services research data) and others.

Access testing

Having an excellent database and a user-friendly search interface does little good if users cannot access the system easily and rapidly. Therefore, the National Library of Medicine is spending considerable effort to improve access. In the U.S. we are working with health libraries to assist them in getting connected to the Web. This involves convincing administrators of the value of the Web, ensuring libraries have the necessary equipment and connections, and testing the Internet/Web connections when there are access problems.

The Internet testing is grouped in two broad categories: user testing and technical (computer to computer) tests. In user tests, individuals log onto the Internet and conduct prescribed activities, timing each step. We also use some companies which automate the actions of a user, repeating these many times a day, seven days a week.

The technical tests NLM is conducting are bulk transfer capacity (a measure of the maximum size of the Internet pathway between two sites); reliability (sending a signal from one site to another to determine what percentage of time the pathway is working); latency (timing how long it takes for a signal to traverse a network path); efficiency (the percentage of packets successfully transmitted); and route stability (determining the number and identification of steps or hops in the transmission path). Generally these technical tests are done at set times every day, for weeks. Tests are being conducted not only in the U.S. but also with various International MEDLARS Centers and other locations around the globe.

We hear from some users that the Internet is slow. For example we in the United States have heard that the Americans slow down UK Internet service. The UK service begins to slow long before the U.S. workforce on the Eastern seaboard eats breakfast. Capacity starts to drop at 2 AM East Coast time, about the start of the UK business day, and starts to recover at 2 PM East Coast time, the end of the British work day. We need more access testing to determine where and when there are Internet access problems as well as attention to solving the problems, if the Web is truly to be a mass communication vehicle.

Document delivery

MEDLINE contains citations and author generated abstracts. As the publishers and aggregators increase the number of articles accessible via the Web and agree to link these to the citations in NLM's databases like MEDLINE, users can quickly link to the full text of the article. Publishers for 150 journals do provide such links for current materials. That means that about 3,700 to 3,800 do not. More are beginning to do so but until they do, and for the older literature, a document delivery system is needed.

U.S. and Canadian searchers use the Loansome Doc system through which they can request the copy of an article through their library. Loansome Doc is a play on the English phrase Loan (as in interlibrary loan) and lonesome (for the health professional away from an academic center) and Doc (documents or doctor). The system provides a user the way to find a medical library willing to serve him or her.

Approximately 48% of the PubMed and IGM use is from outside the U.S. and the usage is not centered in any particular country. Many of these users have been trying to use Loansome Doc. In response NLM is establishing the following process. An international user who searches PubMed or IGM and requests a document through Loansome Doc is sent to a Web page which asks if they are from outside the U.S. If so, they are sent to a screen, the text on which urges them to contact their local medical library. If their local library does not provide Loansome Doc or a document delivery service, they can obtain a list of International MEDLARS Center libraries and Canadian and American libraries which will serve overseas users by clicking on the appropriate link. Users are warned that there usually is a fee. The user must contact one of these libraries and establish a relationship for using their document delivery services. Eventually this list will also include libraries willing to serve only one country, like Poland or Armenia, where the librarians already have established some arrangements with libraries.

Why am I mentioning this at this meeting? First, I want you to know that NLM is receiving a number of requests for document delivery service from Europe. Second, NLM would prefer that users go to their local health libraries, the libraries you represent. Third, NLM is willing to work with some major health libraries in Europe as Loansome Doc sites to receive requests electronically from users searching the databases and fill them. Currently the Swedish and Italian MEDLARS Centers are Loansome Doc libraries for the Nordic Countries and Italy respectively. If your library has a major collection and has a large number of users who search MEDLINE using PubMed or IGM, and you would like users in your country or region to be able to use Loansome Doc to send requests to your library, please let me know.

Training

Because of the need to train librarians to search PubMed and IGM, NLM developed two new classes for 1998. The first is a one day "Making the Transition" course for experienced ELHILL searchers. The second is a two-day "Introduction to Web-based Searching." Between January and April almost 1,000 librarians were trained. The two workbooks can be downloaded from the NLM home page. We will be putting an HTML version of both workbooks on the Web soon along with some PowerPoint presentations. The PowerPoint presentations will be particularly helpful to train librarians in the use of enhancements which are being made to both systems. You are encouraged to use these to train yourselves and your staffs and neighboring colleagues. Using this information you will be as up-to-date as your American colleagues and ready to answer any questions your users may have. The workbooks can be located at http://www.nlm.nih.gov/pubs/web_based.html.

The Associate program. Each year NLM has a one year post-Master's in Library Science position for someone from outside the U.S. The successful applicants must pay their own round trip transportation, but receive a salary of approximately $31,000 for the year to cover living expenses. The associate must return to a job in their home country after the year. Their employer must agree to place them in a position which will allow them to use at least some of the knowledge and skills they have acquired. This is a good opportunity for an institution wanting to improve the information skills of its staff or develop a regional or country wide program to identify a staff member to apply for this program. The first half of the one year program consists of lectures and training in all aspects of medical librarianship and during the second half the associate selects a couple of projects to complete. In addition there are seminars, attendance at national library meetings and an opportunity to be in a class of seven or eight bright and talented U.S. medical librarians who also have competed successfully for the program.

Consumer health

Approximately 30% of the users of PubMed are members of the public searching for health information. The U.S. Government is interested in encouraging its citizens to be more knowledgeable about health matters so they will eat right, exercise, not smoke and generally behave in a way to preserve wellness and prevent disease. In order to assist members of the public to find helpful information NLM is doing three things of possible interest to you.

1. We have added to MEDLINE about 12 newsletters and journals on health written specifically for consumers. You will be able to retrieve just the special consumer health literature sometime this summer when a new feature is added to PubMed. This will also be accessible through IGM.

2. Web page. NLM has a consumer Web page under construction. We hope to link to other authoritative consumer health resources and would like to know about Web resources specifically for consumers which you think are particularly excellent.

3. NLM has a pilot project with over 30 public libraries to determine what assistance they need to improve the health information services they offer. The purpose of the pilot is to determine what would be needed to expand this to public libraries throughout the U.S. One obvious need is for training so that the public librarians can assist the public in searching MEDLINE and other NLM databases. We are developing brochures and posters to be used in public libraries to increase public awareness of free MEDLINE on the Web as a resource for answering medical questions. In our pilot project NLM is pairing each public library with a medical library to help with training and document delivery.

Integrated library system

NLM is acquiring an integrated library system from a commercial vendor this fall. This means that there will be some changes in our Online Public Access Catalog (OPAC). LOCATOR will cease some time this fall and the new OPAC will replace it.

Digital manuscripts project

The History of Medicine Division and the Lister Hill National Center for Biomedical Communications, the research and development division of NLM, are collaborating on a project to digitize major portions of the manuscript collections at NLM, including those of the Nobel Prize recipients who worked at the National Institutes of Health. These will be made available on the Web. This is an exciting project because for the first time, scholars and students anywhere will be able to search these collections by text words to locate the letters or memos in which they are interested. Links can be made to other Web sites with pictures or audio clips. I invite you to see the results of the pilot project for Dr. Donald Fredrickson's papers. Dr. Fredrickson is a former Director of the National Institutes of Health. The URLs for the overview of this project and the pilot are http://www.lhncbc.nlm.nih.gov/dlb/ and http://mhm.nlm.nih.gov/AA. The last item before turning to the future of medical librarianship, is exhibits.

Exhibits

NLM is spending considerable energy developing some very exciting exhibits. You can visit them on the Internet. The current one is Frankenstein which is available at: http://www.nlm.nih.gov/news/franken.html. We hope to do one major exhibit a year with information on the Web. It may give you ideas about something you could do in your library to connect the history of medicine, and art, with the current dilemmas of science so that users and others will begin to think about science and discuss it. We need to encourage the general public to learn more about science. In order to do this we need ways to explain scientific discoveries and dilemmas in terms that will interest and inform the public. Exhibits are a very visual way to do this.

Future of health sciences librarianship

I would like to raise three points about the future of health sciences librarianship. First: Health sciences librarians must continually be flexible about how we perform our fundamental mission - ensuring that health professionals, and increasingly the public, have easy access to authoritative health information while being true to the value system accepted by our profession. Many have already moved from doing searches to training others to do searches. Some are moving from training others to designing search interfaces, working with users to determine how and where they seek information. Notice the flexibility. Health sciences librarianship is not searching. It is not cataloging. Health sciences librarianship is ensuring that people get the health information they seek. There are many ways to do this. Our profession must include people who use different ways and we must be ever vigilant for new, improved ways to accomplish our mission.

The world of the Web ushered in the era of links. It is changing how we construct the bibliographic record for users now and in the future to identify the source of information so others can verify its existence. Think of the electronic journal which changes the layout of its home page. A paper journal which changes its cover may end up with a new title. Before the change the printed issues are cited one way and those after, another. But with the electronic journal, the earlier version no longer exists unless someone printed it or preserved the electronic bits and bytes. How will an article be cited? What about the links? Are they included in the citation as an expansion of pagination? Are they ignored? Look at the links in the BMJ to supplementary data. We must have more dialogs with users and publishers to reach common understandings about what is needed for current attractiveness and future finding aids.

This brings me to my third point, the need for collaboration. There is an enormous need for more interchange between us and publishers and editors, between us and our users, between us and decision makers, and so on. American librarians learned an interesting lesson in the 1980's. When CD-ROMs first came out, NLM set up an evaluation of the early MEDLINE products. A product was placed in a library and the librarian actively sought user feedback which was given to the producer of the product. Imagine! The librarian told the producer what worked and what didn't. The librarians didn't just vote with their wallet, they talked to the vendor. Surprise! The vendors responded by making changes so the system was more user friendly. This is the decade of customer service. Take advantage of it and communicate with the vendors.

We also need to collaborate with colleagues all around the world. The Internet makes this technically possible. The plethora of health information resources makes this necessary. Librarians must develop the relationships in order to work together to accomplish our mission. An outbreak of a disease in any part of the world which is not controlled because the health professional didn't know what to do, can spread easily throughout the globe, reaching each and everyone of us.

You may be disappointed that I have not ventured some technical predictions. We can manage these. We must remember our mission and use whatever useful new technologies are appropriate to accomplish our mission. We must build bridges, partnerships, in order to accomplish our mission. We must rethink what we do and how we do it. Those are the issues which will govern our future.

THE REENCHANTMENT OF THE LIBRARY

Bas Savenije
UNIVERSITY LIBRARY UTRECHT, UTRECHT UNIVERSITY, UTRECHT, NL

Introduction

Libraries have introduced a great many rules and procedures you need to familiarise yourself with, if you want to make use of the services. These rules are needed because of the manner in which libraries have solved the problems related to the explosion of information: the access to information has been rationalised in a one-sided way.

The future's library's challenge is to bring its content to live. What matters is not what you search, but rather what you want to create, i.e. the extra value that comes into being as soon as various information sources come together. With the help of information technology it will become possible to browse through information as though you were strolling among bookshelves in a multidimensional fashion. Thus, the connection with man's creativity can be restored: the reenchantment of the library.

Technological developments have a fundamental influence on many aspects of today's society. This influence is most apparent for those processes in which information plays a crucial role and, consequently, this also applies to libraries. Technological developments will change the traditional 'paper' libraries to libraries that are to a large extent digital libraries, and at least some of them will become completely digital. Of course we have to differentiate between different types of libraries and, within university libraries, between the different disciplines they provide their services for. But to a large extent these differences are only differences in the phase of transition. All libraries must and actually will use modern technology to change the way they are carrying out their traditional activities.

The nature of these developments imply that they represent not just 'a change' but a fundamental innovation. It will become apparent that they involve fundamental changes in the services and the library's attitude to the organisation and the people it is serving, and, consequently, also to the library's own strategy and goals. These consequences for the library are quite radical.

Obstacles for innovation

The radicality of these changes becomes even more obvious, as soon as we realise that a number of factors traditionally related to libraries and their organisation actually constitute an obstacle for innovating the library.

The first factor is the lack of flexibility in the library organisation as such. Customarily, the libraries have grouped their tasks according to rigidly defined function categories. The demands corresponding with these function categories have been strictly defined as well. Descriptions concerning the functions of subject librarian or catalogue librarian are examples of these categories. In practice, the rigid division and inflexible job descriptions do not contribute to a dynamic personnel flow.

Secondly, as soon as the average library staff member becomes confronted with the prospect of change, he tends to be somewhat conservative and cautious. Of course his cautiousness is related to the nature of his profession. In his job, the librarian is concentrated on the task of preserving. Therefore, he is always alert when it comes to protecting the cultural heritage.

In the third place, innovations as such do not easily find a firm holding within the entire library organisation. This circumstance is related to the position occupied within the organisation by the activities that are connected with information technology. Many libraries have had a department for information technology since the first computerisation wave, its responsibility being the supervision of computerised library systems and its proper functioning.

In many cases, one of the activities this department is requested to instigate (or has chosen to create for itself) is the testing of new technology examining its usefulness for library purposes. Thus, the department in question becomes a centre of innovation within the existing organisation. This turn of events may bring along the risk that it eventually results in the creation of an electronic library within, or rather in addition to the traditional library, where the library's strategy should be aiming at an integration of traditional and new tasks.

Clearly, these circumstances are in obvious contrast with the requirements innovation and change demand from library personnel. But nevertheless they will be confronted with a situation in which their position in the process of information provision is no longer certain. Traditional distinctions and boundaries will fade. This goes for boundaries between the library and other organisations in the information business, as they are traditionally described in the information chain. But also the boundaries between the library and the functions it is serving with information are disappearing.

The information chain

The role of the library is often described in terms of a link in the so-called information chain. For readers who are not familiar with the jargon, the accepted definition of the information chain is as follows: "An infrastructure consisting of a chain of groups who each fulfil one or more functions in the process of supplying information by using the available means." This process stretches from the production of information to its consumption. Traditionally, the various stages have been strictly distinguished in terms of the chain's main functions, i.e. subsequently in the production, distribution, acquisition, and consumption of information.

At the moment, we can notice several problems connected with the information chain. Usually, the chain is represented graphically. This traditional representation used to be comparatively simple. Lately however, it has grown more complex due to the pressure of an ever expanding information stream and as a result of various technological developments. It is as if the chain is about to explode. Even so, this metaphor of an exploding chain or cycle is not appropriate. The chain is not bursting at all. What is erupting, though, is the amount of information as a result of the way it has been transferred.

Yet, the functions within the traditional information chain, i.e. production, distribution, acquisition and knowledge consumption, could all be carried out at a so-called integrated work site. In this context, therefore, the use of a metaphor describing an imploding chain would be more suitable, since due to the pressure exerted by the environment, the system has started to shrink.

The configuration of functions within the information chain has become subjected to change, whilst within this changing constellation, all the parties involved are struggling to determine their own position. At the moment, for instance, both universities and publishers are instigating all sorts of arrangements between themselves on how they are to explore their new roles in unison. There is considerable danger, however, that they will remain stuck within the traditional chain.

In my opinion it would on the long run more effective to experiment in an innovative and creative way with new roles instead of the adherence to traditional patterns. All forced attempts to preserve the old structure will not only impede development as such, but will also expose it to the increasing danger of its arbitrary disintegration.

A conclusion from this analysis, in my opinion, would be that the libraries should aim at becoming electronic document publishers, instead of merely relying on agreements with commercial publishers.

Library activities as a directly productive force

The second important development is related to the traditional way in which the library tasks have been considered to be some kind of overhead. This idea is due to become obsolete rapidly. In time, library tasks will be regarded as directly productive forces. We must realise that it has become increasingly difficult to distinguish between the actual provision of information and the various processes in which this information is used. In the case of the university library, the primary university tasks are training and research. The fundamental aspect of training is the transfer of knowledge from teacher to student. The once clear distinction between knowledge transfer through teaching on the one hand, and the provision of information by the library on the other is fading as a result of the deployment of information technology in education. More and more, library services are blending with the teaching process.

A similar trend can be observed within the process of research. Here, the fundamental stages are the identification of sources, the exchange of information between colleagues, the interpretation and analysis of data, the dissemination of findings. In this case, the boundaries between information provision and the various stages in the research process are becoming faint as well. Similar tendencies have become apparent in other primary processes supported by library tasks, for example in policy-making and legal consultancy.

In general, we may establish that library functions are progressively integrating with the primary processes they are serving. This implies that the library tasks can no longer be considered some sort of overhead services. On the contrary, they are developing into a directly productive force. And I would like to emphasise that, in order to properly determine the relevance of certain information amidst this vast available reservoir of data, it is imperative to acquire a thorough knowledge of the discipline in question.

About procedures and regulations

At the university, the library has the task of providing scientific information for the benefit of education and research. The library selects, collects, preserves and provides access to information sources. Since this information functions as knowledge in the educational and scientific research process, it has to have a key role. To reach this objective, it is necessary that the information provision is adapted to the manner and situation in which it is used. This, of course, implies that involved library staff needs to be familiar with the user's requirements. Only then the library will be able to provide the information with extra value which is needed for applying it in both primary processes.

In the past university libraries have taken great pains to improve the application of its services in education and research. However, the instruments the library has created for this purpose comprise a large number of procedures and regulations. That is, rules the user needs to grow accustomed to if he wishes to find his way within the library. The following examples are intended to illustrate this fact.

The library's contents are described in the catalogue that is organised alphabetically and according to subject. Presently, it has become possible to consult other library catalogues, either at your own library or at your own desk or working place. You can even order documents from other libraries. This is a step in the right direction, since it is a step towards the virtual library of the future, assuring us the availability of relevant information, irrespective of the place where this information is stored. Nevertheless, when considered from these new developments' perspective, the current character of the catalogue seems to be somewhat awkward.

Let us, for instance, have a look at the unified Dutch Library catalogue. Oddly enough, this register does not contain a complete overview of all the information published. When consulting this catalogue, the user can only access the combined inventories of a limited number of libraries, who have agreed to integrate their respective indexes. Thus, when living near the Belgian or German border, you can never be certain whether this catalogue gives you information considering the contents of the nearest scientific library. Also, it does not even provide information on the inventories of various scientific institutes not belonging to a university.

Even more deplorable is the fact that this catalogue does not refer to available documents which have not (yet) been collected by the participating libraries. Fortunately, there is another way of finding out whether any material has been published about a certain topic. This is by referring to a bibliography, that is, if there exists one on the subject in question. However, bibliographies also have a reputation for not being very useful when it comes to indicating the exact location where the particular information or documents can be actually found. To this end, you need to turn to the catalogues once again. There are sufficient examples demonstrating that it is virtually impossible to achieve the required result.

The library also uses a system of subject headings, which originally were designed to provide some help when searching for information. Like categorising, subject heading amounts to arranging information according to certain categories, presupposing a more or less rigid system of categories. But in effect, there are no categories at all. There is only a continuous flow. Moreover, the conceptual scientific landscape is in constant motion as well.

Of course, we must take into account certain differences between various disciplines. But we should also realise that the boundaries between them do not have a permanent character. Specialised subject librarians, having finished their curriculum several years ago and not actively participating in the research process, are no longer able to cope with the system itself, nor with its application.

There is another point of view from which the library's classification methods may seem to have a rational appearance, though in practice, they prove to be not quite as effective. The classification system can be useful if you have a specific question and you are looking for a specific answer. However, scientists do not just have simple questions. They usually deal with problems that only with the greatest of effort, can be translated into questions. The action nowadays referred to as browsing may be useful in that it helps them formulate new and fruitful ideas.

Naturally, I am not suggesting that all library activities involved should be cancelled, nor do I intend to say that they are useless. They are important activities which are valuable for our users. On the other hand, they are time-consuming too, both for the library and its users. Furthermore, they tend to be of a bureaucratic and procedural nature, qualities that even further limit their effectiveness.

From these trends we may conclude that it is the library itself that has introduced and self-imposed a number of rules and procedures which are far from being self-evident. As a matter of fact, the use of library facilities has become rather complicated to such an extent, that users need instructions in order to properly make use of its services. Worse even, these instructions necessitate the training of special instructors who are to coach the users. Basically, that is the reason why we have set up library instructions, since the use of the library cannot do without it. It is a situation — if I am allowed to say so — the library needs not be very proud of.

Reenchantment

As we have seen, the library has introduced a great many rules and procedures you need to familiarise yourself with if you want to make use of library services. If a scientist has a specific problem, these rules prove to be rather inconvenient for solving it. It seems, therefore, that generally the access to information has been rationalised in a one-sided, one-dimensional way only. I am convinced that this situation can be improved by means of information technology.

Surely, one could consider the application of this new technology as a mere continuation of the rationalisation process. Yet, this would be a one-sided observation. Soon it will become possible to link scientific intuition to technological achievements. Scientists and students will be able to browse through information as though they were strolling along bookshelves in a multidimensional fashion.

The future library's challenge is to bring its contents to live. We must create a library that is not merely a guide for receiving insight into the current way of organising information. The future library should also be helpful in establishing new methods of organisation. Search engines must not be designed to exclusively retrieve answers to specific questions. What matters is not what you search, rather what you want to create, i.e. the extra value that comes into being as soon as various information sources come together.

Such a library can be represented in terms of a philosophical parallel. For instance, as the realisation of the ideal presented by Leibniz. The philosopher Leibniz commenced his career as a librarian and he strove towards creating an encyclopaedia in which all knowledge was to be rationally gathered and interlinked. Referring to Leibniz's ideal, we could regard the library as an encyclopaedia of the sciences, as an encyclopaedia being endowed with a richly layered multidimensional order.

Modern information technology can and must be deployed to bring the library closer to scientists, teachers and students, in terms of both space and content. Thus, the number of rules and procedures, however rational they may seem to be, will be automatically reduced. Logistic automation has in effect created the large gap that exists between service and creativity. We may see in this a parallel with Weber's 'Entzauberung' or disenchantment in English. This disenchantment of the library is caused by the manner in which we have decided to resolve the problems related to the violent explosion of information. A solution that in practice amounts to stacking information in such a way that it can be accessed by means of complicated logistic procedures only. This has inevitably led to a widening crevice between information and the individual's creativity and his values.

The original connection with man's creativity can be restored by introducing sophisticated search engines that carry information to the user's working place at dazzling speed. This development suggests that using library services will become easier in the future, since these services are to be directly linked to the user's actual requirements.

In South Africa a saw a large picture in the children's department of a public library. When we transform the meaning of this picture to the scientific library, it very well illustrates what I mean to say about the library's future: "Dreams take flight at the library". This will be possible with the help of new technologies. And this will eventually result in the reenchantment of the library.

NET-KNITTING: THE LIBRARY PARADIGM AND THE NEW ENVIRONMENT

Derek Law, Tony McSean
[1]KING'S COLLEGE; [2]BRITISH MEDICAL ASSOCIATION, LONDON, UK

Introduction

It is the purpose of this paper to argue that librarians have been blinded to its basic flaws by the gaudiness of the Internet and that we are confusing sources and resources. The Internet shows none of the features required for scholarly communication and whether or not we believe this will change, we should be developing models which offer electronic services as a viable and reliable resource.

Although the Internet is of some age in the dog years which pass for computing time, the World Wide Web is relatively new, with the first web browser dating only from 1994. In the four years after that it achieved a phenomenal acceptance, in what Paul Evan Peters called the largest mass migration in human history. It was adopted by fifty million users in fifty months. Radio took 38 years to gain such an audience and television some thirteen years. Currently it has some seventy million users. And yet it lacks the important elements of sustainability necessary for scholarship:

- Permanence
- Availability
- Accessibility

The Web is in fact a four year old experiment, not a robust service. Not for nothing is it called the World Wide Wait. Not for nothing has a Dilbert cartoon appeared noting that all the time saved through automation and computers in the last fifty years has been entirely outweighed by people sitting in front of pc's waiting for web pages to load. A variety of issues reflect the very real difficulties of the Web for scholarship.

Identifiers and naming

The continuity of citation is central scholarship. In a print on paper world we take it for granted that a scholarly paper can cite Vesalius, Lister or Suzanne Bakker and that other scholars or libraries can trace and find these publications or data. That stability does not exist on the Internet where there is a basic need to reference objects as they move and change over time and place. Rather resignedly we simply note the impermanence of URLs. Nor is their any consistency over who may name objects since it appears that anyone can. This in turn removes one of our marks of quality. Authorship, ownership and impartiality are easily disguised. Worse, there is no expectation of who will maintain naming over time. It is our experience that libraries, even national libraries are as guilty as anyone else in having created a fluidity that sits uneasily with scholarship. Commercial publishers have created Digital Object Identifiers, but it is not at all clear that they are usable in the very substantial area of primary sources and grey literature.

Metadata

This appears to be under better control by our profession as the Dublin Core now involves Europe, USA and the Pacific Rim. But there is still basic work to be done on how to describe new genres of multimedia and how to describe new services. What kind of record are we to create for a changing and dynamic resource. We also need to describe the terms and conditions of use and at present these vary between locations, between user groups and over time. For example, an electronic textbook may be licensed to be available only to first year anatomy students in the summer semester.

Authentication

This is important for electronic commerce, but there are no good ways of proving membership of the data club when away from home. This is perhaps no more than irritating. More importantly once membership is established through some form of individual log-on, are we willing to give up the anonymity of the user? Most libraries consider it a matter of professional ethics not to reveal who has used what library material, unless a criminal offence has been committed. Some users, particularly those working with pharmaceutical companies, regard their library use as commercially sensitive. Are we really willing to cede this anonymity to gain access to electronic data?

Distributed search and indexing

This remains a very big issue with a great deal still to be done technically. Web indexing systems are breaking down as their architecture collapses under the weight of data. A simple quite specific search will frequently produce over a million hits, listed in no discernible order. There were 320 million web pages on the Internet in May 1998, of which no more than 34% are searched by the best search engine - and there is no readily available way of discovering which 34%!

Rights management systems

These are being designed largely at the behest of commercial organisations in ways which mirror the power and needs of the entertainment industry. And yet from the scholarly perspective there are at least three major areas of philosophic contention.

PRIVACY

As mentioned above, the right to anonymity is both an academic requirement and has been an obligation from the library to its users. Not only is such privacy under threat, there is the further possibility that usage information could be sold on to third parties as marketing information.

PRESERVATION

Publishers have never had a responsibility to preserve their publications, yet we have no general legal deposit for electronic publications, even if we had a definition of what constitutes an electronic publication. As publishers typically lease rather than sell electronic data, such material must be considered at risk. In any case the technology for preserving electronic material is far from robust. Who is to preserve what remains a major, undecided issue.

FAIR USE

The concept of fair use for private study and research is an important one. Yet rights management systems which prevent general browsing take away that right. Commercial publishers feel it inappropriate to an electronic environment; scholars might beg to differ.

Network topology

In Europe, at least since the time of the first Bangemann Report this has been assumed to be a matter for the commercial marketplace. Yet scholarship, unlike commercial markets, is both global and goes into uneconomic areas. Problems arise at both extremes of need. On the one hand high technology scholarship demands very high bandwidth computing at the leading edge of technology. Yet the report on the (in academic terms) quite modest Ten-34 Project to link European Research Networks found that such links were not available commercially. At the other end of the spectrum, the commercial marketplace will not put adequate technology into non-commercial markets. That is to say that there are large parts of the world where networks and network services will lag impossibly if left to purely commercial motives.

Preservation and archiving of electronic information

This is commonly acknowledged to be one of the hardest of areas to resolve for all stakeholders, one fraught with technical, legal and operational problems. Some technical preservation centres have been running for over twenty-five years. They have produced no magic solutions and little comfort in proving that the technical problems are very difficult and very expensive to resolve. Some progress is being made on electronic legal deposit where useful dialogue has opened up with the publishers. But it must constantly be re-emphasised that much of the material we will wish to preserve is non-commercial. Nor is it self-evident who should conduct the preservation. The national libraries might manage the process but it seems safe to assume that issues of institutional continuity will be even more important than in the paper environment, where company take-overs and bankruptcies, incompetence, indifference and even malice have put many historic collections at risk over the years.

Instructional media, courseware and new media

Libraries need to rethink their roles and mission in relation to electronic material. This applies both to external material and to internally produced material. In the case of external material librarians must consider not just purchasing licences to make titles available (or ignoring them while departments make the purchases). We would argue that they must consider the relative costs and merits of remote access, local mirroring, consortial purchasing and so on. And this must sensibly involve the total cost including network charges. Even for "free" sites such as pre-print archives it is important to establish whether the archive has a more appropriate European mirror site which turns it from a variably available source into a reliable resource, saving the organisation many hours of waiting for screens to load. In terms of access how far should library staff surf the web to catalogue and record useful sites or e-journals and start to provide information on what is available rather than what is possessed.

Internally the Library has to clarify its role in relation to electronic information. Is it the institutional provider and/or archive for all instructional material created locally? If so, how far does the remit extend? Does it include, for example, collaborative data analysis and its records or knowledge representation and its re-use? Even if the library is not meant to cover this type of activity does it or should it have a role in ensuring that standards are met by the organisation as a whole for issues ranging from standards used to intellectual property rights.

The new media require a major redefinition of the library's role. Even if the outcome is to leave the libraries role as it was, at least the organisation will have ensured that it has a series of policies and responsibilities in place for dealing with electronic material.

Scholarly communication

There is a real threat of what has been called cybercolonialism, the overt or covert preference for one set of resources over another. This is compounded by our own willingness to confuse sources and resources. As an example of this it is worth examining a language neutral discipline such as mathematics and comparing the treatment of major and very longstanding east European journals from universities such as Cracow or Warsaw. This will appear in European gateway sites but not North American ones. This problem is worsened by an increasingly common practice - often fostered by search engines - of preferring to use American websites. These may provide better or richer sources but if slow to the point of unavailability for much of the European day are in truth inadequate resources or services.

Two key issues are standards for version control and mirror sites. Originators of data, jealous of its quality are often unwilling to entrust it to third parties without prolonged negotiation. And yet mirror sites are a very economic method of improving network performance. An obvious solution is a set of standards or kite-marking to indicate the quality of potential mirror hosts. This would reassure not only the data supplier but also the data - user, who must at present also rest uncertain of the version of the document which is available.

It is also regrettable that the debate on electronic publishing has been so dominated by the STM commercial model. STM publishing while undeniably important represents only a fraction of the annual acquisitions of most universities. Even in scientific libraries significant quantities of non-commercial material or small learned society material are acquired and this may be expected to grow in an electronic arena. And yet it is not self-evident that systems and practices designed for electronic commerce sit comfortably with the needs of scholarly discourse. Yet at present very little thought is being given as to how we support the scholarly infrastructure of the small learned society or the science and medicine of developing countries.

There is a further category of material at risk, what Clifford Lynch of CNI has called endangered content. Computer Science, a discipline founded and maintained on a non-printed tradition has reached a point where its pioneers are retiring and dying. As a discipline it has only just begun to realise how much of its common heritage it may need and may already have lost. Great efforts are now being made to salvage this position. It illustrates perfectly that in an electronic environment new thought must be given to how we record and locate a discipline. We cannot wait for paper archives to arrive on the death of great men, nor are laboratory books now the only source of laboratory data. A complete reappraisal is needed of how primary research data and even the e-mail of scientists, of bulletin boards and discussion groups is to be maintained to show the traceable path on which science depends.

Network management

As already remarked, the United States becomes a virtual country for most of Europe in the afternoon, as the bandwidth clogs and slows with traffic. It is claimed that costs are dropping and so we can simply buy more bandwidth. It is more likely that the UK experience is typical. For the UK academic community, the cost per bit of international traffic halves each year - but the traffic trebles, inexorably increasing the bill to a point where restraint has to be applied. It has been interesting to see the reaction to this in Australia where costs are passed on directly to universities. In 1998/9 Australian Vice-Chancellors have introduced schemes in which hits on non-Australian web-sites will be charged at twice the rate of local web-sites. This clearly recognises the distinction between sources and resources and aims to manage traffic in sensible ways. We may expect others to follow this model.

The library paradigm

Although Australian universities have adopted a model for managing network topology it is not clear whether that model has any theoretical underpinning. We would then wish to suggest that the current model of unbridled access to the anarchy of the Internet is not the only or the best model for managing electronic resources. Intranets and/or regional networks are being created which form more appropriate boundaries for electronic resources. As the cost of filestore drops very quickly it can often be shown to be economic – not least of time – to mirror resources on the local network. Further, the ease of access to electronic resources allows us to revisit the issue of access versus holdings strategies – where access has held sway for some time as a professional dogma – and argue that holdings strategies may again be appropriate in an electronic environment. When managing information, what organisations have never done is line all employees or students up (at least metaphorically) at the start of the financial year, give them one thousand guilders and told them to acquire anything they liked that might help with their work. Instead they have identified the material relevant to the work of the organisation, collected as much of it as they could in one place, employed professional information specialists to manage it and make it available, and arranged controlled access to the information which cannot be held locally for those who can show they require it. This does not prevent individuals using other channels from public libraries to bookshops for any other information they choose. We would then argue that this model of the library provides a perfect paradigm for the management of networked resources.

Table 1: The library paradigm for network management

LIBRARY CORE ACTIVITY	INTRANET CORE ACTIVITY
Acquisition	Resource Discovery
Collection Building	Local Fileservers and Mirrors
Classification	Knowledge Management
Preservation	Long-term Data Sinks
Inter-Lending and Document Supply	Controlled Internet Access
User Instruction	User Instruction

We would contend that there has been an all too ready acceptance of the Internet. Its undoubtedly huge impact on the availability of current information has dazzled us to its flaws as a medium for scholarly communication. It is important to revisit the information needs of our organisations and of scholarship and to re-interpret them in the light of the possibilities and limitations of networks. The model proposed above then describes how in a local context we can take control of the environment and use it positively, acting collectively to meet institutional need.

Chapter 6: NEW SERVICES

Introduction

In the former chapters the changes taking place around the medical libraries was investigated and discussed: the legal aspects of copyright and licences (Chpt. 1 p. 5); the changes in scientific communication by the introduction of information technology (Chpt. 2 p. 19); the political changes that create a higher need and the right for the public to get informed about health, health care and medical information (Chpt. 3 p. 35); the changes in the practice of medicine stressing the importance of making use of available evidence, with the Cochrane Collaboration as the most visible exponent (Chpt. 4 p. 59).

In chapter 5 (p. 85) the broader view on the changes in medical librarianship and the roles of the medical library were given. In the following chapters more specific examples of changing roles will be presented. After this chapter of new services, there will be examples from the veterinary (Chpt. 7 p. 129), medical school (Chpt. 8 p. 153) and nursing libraries (Chpt. 9 p. 171), followed by examples from academic libraries that have a strong user education commitment (Chpt. 10 p. 183).

The new options and therefore new services for medical libraries are the subject of the presentations of Ulrich Korwitz, Grete Bjørkenes, Ronald van Dieën, Nico van Putte, Maria da Luz Antunes, Veronica Fraser, Giovanna Miranda, Glenda Myers and Marc van Kuik in this chapter.

What kind of options do medical librarians have to change library services and to add value to their work? The first paper explains why citation analysis is an important tool in evaluations of scientific performance and how the librarian could support this process in his/her institution by knowing the details and limits and by adding and creating information by using bibliometric methods themeselves. Of interest is also the paper of Tom Roper (p. 135) showing the relevance of citation analysis to map communication and information flow within a specific subject field; the so retrieved information can be of practical use in collection development strategies. In order to improve the quality of library work it is essential to investigate the information needs and behaviour of the users.[1] According to Leo Egghe this kind of library research also part of and must be included in bibliometrics.[2]

In the second paper of this chapter Grete Günther Bjørkenes reports on how the quality handbook was set up and used in the library of the County Hospital in Østfold (Norway). Gerhardus van Dieën explains how the work on quality management fits into the activities of the professional association of the Dutch biomedical librarians. Nico van Putte reports on the outcome of a project of changes in a pharmaceutical industry library. The papers of Maria da Luz Antunes, Veronica Fraser and Giovanna Miranda underline the importance of medical librarians working in close cooperation with the medical doctors and users of the library. And the last papers of Glenda Myers and Marc van Kuik explain how social and political changes influence expectations about the services of the library and the changes in library policy that must necessaryly follow.

To summerize: in this chapter several examples are given on how colleagues made the change in their library. Sometimes new services are additional to existing services, often they replace existing services, but in most of the cases they are the same (traditional) services but offered in a slightly different way. So do not hesitate: read the following papers and start your own local or regional project to make a change.

References

[1] Urquhart CJ, Hepworth JB. Ebhancing the value of a health library and information service to clinicians. In: Bakker S (ed) Health Information Management: What Strategies?. Dordrecht: Kluwer, 1997. p. 61-63

[2] Egghe L. Quantitative aspects of the management of health information. In: Bakker S (ed) Health Information Management: What Strategies?. Dordrecht: Kluwer, 1997. p. 282-289

CITATION ANALYSIS OF BIOMEDICAL PUBLICATIONS: A CUSTOMER ORIENTED SERVICE IN MEDICAL LIBRARIES

Ulrich Korwitz
GERMAN NATIONAL LIBRARY OF MEDICINE, COLOGNE, GERMANY

Introduction

About ten years ago, being a librarian of a medical school in Germany, I was asked for the first time by the dean of the medical faculty to help evaluating the scientific work of applicants for professor's chairs. I reacted very reservedly at that time. Until then, I had understood my professional role as an administrator of the mass of incoming literature not regarding the individual paper and even less helping to assess the quality of individual authors.

But times have changed: formerly we were curators of the medical book and journal heritage, today we regard ourselves as service agents for the supply of information and literature for all kinds of customers. Formerly the customers needed us to get the information and literature, today they increasingly find their ways to the information and full-texts by themselves and we have to justify our role and our institute. We can do this by understanding the current needs of our customers and offering value-added services or even expert opinion to them.

What is such a current need and how can we as medical librarians help? It is a trend in Germany and other European countries that scientists and scientific institutes even at universities have to proof the impact of their work. Money for research is not abundant any more and the times of working quietly in an ivory tower are gone. Criteria for the internal distribution of funds are set up by university committees and by councils in research institutes. What counts are national or international prices won, doctoral or habilitation theses completed successfully, the number of guest scientists attracted and money received from the industry.

Research performance

The most important criterion however is the performance of members of the institute in the field of scientific publication. "Publish or perish" is still a dictate for every scientist in the biomedical field. But the number of publications placed in scientific journals alone is not relevant any more. It becomes more and more important to know where to publish. Which journals are read by the scientific community? What are the journals with the highest impact in the different fields? Where should manuscripts be submitted? How can the relevance of individual publications be recognized? These are the questions raised daily by customers in our libraries. And medical librarians can help to answer these questions using simple bibliometrical analyses. This is a value-added service for scientists, for administrative institutes in universities and for publishers.

BIBLIOMETRIC ANALYSIS

To do bibliometrical analysis is not very difficult. Publication lists of authors or institutes can be compiled by using biomedical databases. The tools for citation analyses are prepared by the Institute for Scientific Information (ISI) in Philadelphia, USA. They allow to identify high impact journals on one hand and determine the relevance of individual publications on the other.

The most important tool for evaluating the relevance of journals are the "Journal Citation Reports" (JCR).[1] They were published as a paper supplement to the "Science Citation Index" (SCI) from 1975 to 1989 and as a microfiche supplement since 1990. Beginning 1995, a CD-ROM with the same data but better search capabilities can be purchased. The JCR data are not available via the Internet.

The JCR (the most recent edition with data for 1996) provide ranking lists of 4.779 source publications (journals) with information about the number of citations on papers in these journals. The idea of Eugene Garfield, the founder of ISI and the SCI, was to determine the relevance of a journal by counting how many citations papers published in this journal get.[2] This seems to be a striking idea: the more important a journal is the more frequent articles in this journal are read and cited. So if an author is successful in getting his paper placed into a journal he profits from the relevance and reputation of this periodical.

- # Self citations
- # Citation rings ("If you cite me, I cite you")
- # Publications in monographs, congress reports, etc. do not count
- # Compilation of the source journal list
- # Journals not indexed in major databases
- # Under-representation of non-American journals
- # Language bias
- # Overstressing of review journals
- # Underrating of clinical journals
- # Different citation practice: no comparison allowed between different disciplines
- # Different half-time of knowledge in different disciplines
- # Journal title changes/splitting up in sections
- # Newly founded journals not included with all issues
- # Circulation of a journal
- # Costs of a journal
- # Mistakes made by ISI (e.g. letters/editorials not always excluded; arithmetical errors)
- # *"To be cited does not mean that a publication was significant"* and *"To be an uncited scientist is no cause for shame"* (Garfield 1991)

Arguments against the simplified use of the "Impact Factor"

Besides the list of numbers of citation for articles in the 4.779 source journals, Garfield developed other bibliometrical factors: the "Impact Factor", the "Immediacy Index" and the "Cited Half-life Index". The most famous of these factors and indices is the "Impact Factor" (IF). The IF considers not only the number of citations for papers in a journal (a) but also the number of original papers which were published in the journal itself (b). It is built by dividing (a) by (b). The list of journals sorted by the IF is often taken as a direct relevance scale for scientific institutes or researchers. The IF for publications of all the authors of all departments of an institute are added up separately and the money for research is distributed to the departments proportionately.

FINANCIAL CONSEQUENCES

Money distribution by using citations? One might say: "Is it really so simple and evident?" As this method is gaining more and more importance warning voices are being raised.[3,4] Table 1 shows the main arguments put forward against the unreflected usage of the IF.

In Germany, several scientific medical societies decided not to consider the "Impact Factor" as main criterion for the quality of research any more. Other societies are setting up their own ranking scales of journals including nationally important journal titles in their fields of research which are not to be found in the JCR lists. Others finally remind us that there is more than the pure "science impact". No doubt, it is important to proceed in scientific research but isn't it equally important when research results in practical application or in health policy decisions? The "practice impact" and the "policy impact" of research work should not be overseen.

Librarian added value

Nevertheless, our customers will ask for the journal ranking lists, mainly the alphabetical list, the list of journals sorted by impact factor and the subject category list. The subject category list allows one to find out which journal is highly respected in a specific field. Presumptive authors need it to find out where a paper should be submitted and editors and publishers need it to see where their journal stands within the international journal community. However, as it is not quite clear how the categories in the "Subject Category List" are built this list has to be interpreted with special caution.

In general, I would strongly recommend not just to pass the lists to our customers without any comment (like a copy of a journal article) but to ask for what purpose they need it. So we can better help them to find the best listing, help interpret the lists and identify the pitfalls. In Cologne, we generally add some information about the interpretation of the IF including a short bibliography of articles with critical voices about the IF and, if possible, personally explain how to deal with the lists.

CONSTRUCTED IMPACT FACTOR

But we can do more for our customers. One major point of criticism is that nationally important journals are not indexed in the SCI and by that are not included in the IF list. We can construct impact factors for such journals not included in the JCR. The source listing of the JCR includes only 4.779 journals whereas more than 7.000 unique journals are continuously indexed in MEDLINE, EMBASE and BIOSIS. Our colleague Johannes Stegmann from the Library of the University Clinic Benjamin Franklin in Berlin shows in a letter in Nature how to proceed in a simple way using several biomedical online databases and SCISEARCH, the online version of the SCI.[5]

PERSONAL CITATION INDEX

Realizing the pitfalls in utilizing the IF listings several universities and research institutes turned to another evaluation method. They ask their scientific staff or applicants for their "personal citation index". The index can be determined by adding the citations the person in question received using the SCI. ISI offers such a "Personal Citation Report" for 295 $ per name. We can help our customers to avoid this expenditure by setting up such a report by ourselves. We will need the name of the person and all surnames and initials (and the institutes he was affiliated with in the last years). Special attention has to be paid when the person's name has any peculiarities (like the German "Umlaut" in "Müller"). We will have to find out how these were "transliterated" in the journals he published and in the SCI ("Müller" -> "Mueller" and "Muller"). Using the SCI we can now hand-search the citations and adding them finally. Alternatively, we can turn to the CD-ROM-product or the SCISEARCH database. Attention has to be paid when the author in question is not the first mentioned author of a paper: not every database allows one to find his citations in that case.

When preparing the personal citation report self citations should be marked. Authors have to include self citations in their papers because they have to refer to their own previously published papers. But self citations will not be considered for official purposes, generally. Within the "Personal Citation Report" we should (on demand) also mark repeated citations of colleagues of the person in question. By that citation rings may be identified and such citations can be eliminated.

INSTITUTIONAL CITATION REPORT

Also we can offer an "Institutional Citation Report". ISI's price for such a report depends on the number of papers indexed at an institute (9.000 $ for 35.000 papers). We can do this free of charge or charging only the online costs for the institutes we care for. What we need are the variants of institutional names used by the authors in their papers. Then we can hand-search for the institute or turn to the CD-ROM product or SCISEARCH to get a list of the original papers and finally search for citations to these papers.

To publish in the top journals is indispensable, to be cited is important, too. But it becomes more and more important in what journal a scientist was cited: so "Personal and Institutional Citation Reports" are incomplete without lists of the citing journals and indicators of the impact of these citing journals. Here again the IF gets involved.

Conclusions

Giving advice how to use the JCR lists wisely, determining impact factors for journals not included, preparing personal and institutional citation reports: these are value-added service products for our customers. Who else than a biomedical library could provide such professional information and explain the facts and identify the pitfalls? We can help our customers and ourselves: offering value-added and individual service will help in answering the question "what is a biomedical library useful for": in these hard times of justification we must offer better and extended service - so we will achieve in making the library and ourselves irreplaceable.

References

[1] Science Citation Index: Journal Citation Reports (JCR): a bibliometric analysis of science journals in the ISI database. Philadelphia: Institute for Scientific Information (published annually)
[2] Garfield E. The impact factor. In: Current Contents. Life Sciences 1994;37(25):3-7 (Also: <http://www.isinet.com/essays/essay7.html> (Last chequed: 6/7/1998))
[3] Seglen PO. Why the impact factor of journals should not be used for evaluating research. BMJ 1997;314:498-502
[4] Op 't Hof T. Sense and nonsense about the impact factor. Cardiovasc Res 1997;33:1-7
[5] Stegmann J. How to evaluate journal impact factors. Nature 1997;390:550

QUALITY HANDBOOK: A TOOL FOR RAISING THE EFFICIENCY OF LIBRARY WORK

Grete Günther Bjørkenes
ØSTFOLD FYLKESKOMMUNE, SENTRALADMINISTRASJONEN, SARPSBORG, NORWAY

Introduction

Are our workplaces for the staff or for the users? This question was asked last June in "Synopsis" the journal of the National Office of Research Documentation, Academic and Special Libraries, by its Acting Director General; Kirsten Engelstad. There is no simple answer to that question. As she continued; a good, secure and stimulating workplace is important to the staff, but most workplaces are dependent on customers or a market. The staff of special libraries have become increasingly engaged in orientating their activities towards good customer service.

For a long time librarians were occupied with internal library systems and co-operation between libraries. The users benefited, of course by those efforts. One could hardly meet a more enthusiastic and idealistic occupational group. But it was not until the libraries turned their attention to leadership, organization, customer handling, benchmarking and marketing that this became important.

The quality of the service has been more and more the question when librarians meet. In Norway this issue is also one of the main tasks for other organizations, for example, the hospital of which our library is a part. Securing quality and improving the service is what we have aimed at, all the time, but the new way to work, is to document what you do, do what you document and let the user know what they can expect of their libraries. As a service organization our library should develop, establish, document, implement and maintain a quality system as a means by which stated policies and objectives for service quality may be accomplished.

Increasing efficiency

The main goal for the librarians at the County Hospital of Østfold in order to start the work on a quality handbook ,was to increase the efficiency of the library. We very soon discovered that measuring quality became important and led to better service for the users, a better work environment for the staff, greater enthusiasm for the work, and a more efficient library as a whole. It was a great task to start and took us about 1½ years. We celebrated when the book was finished. But we knew already then, that this work will never be finished, if you want a handbook like this to be a help, both in daily work, and in the planning for the future of the library.

It has to be revised every year, and one may ask if the work is worthwhile. Especially the way we have done it, with great stress on the practical work involved in the procedures, and also with separate manuals for special equipment. I would immediately say YES. Especially when one has a small staff. The staff in our medical library consists of two librarians in full time positions and one part-time, and one part-time clerk.

It is of great value when we get a new employee, a student doing a practical period, or during vacation time, when we all have to fill in for one another. We have experienced this during a year or so, and so far we can't imagine to be without it.

The practical work with the quality handbook

We started to list all the functions in our library, and to which staff category they were connected. Then each of us described in detail the way we did the various tasks. We then had weekly meetings, presenting the descriptions, discussing them and confirming the result. This is a critical point. All members of the staff must agree on, or give their assent to, the procedures, if the work is to reach utmost efficiency. Step by step we wrote down the final guidelines for each function and made special procedures for each.

PROCEDURES

These are written statements which specify the purpose and scope of activities in the library. They define how the activities are to be conducted, controlled and recorded. All documentation should be legible, dated (including revision dates), clear, readily identifiable and carry authorization status. When we described the purpose for each procedure in this way, we used the opportunity to think if we really did the tasks in the most efficient way. We asked each other all the time: why do we do this the way we do? Are there any other solutions? The question of quality and efficiency was the guideline all the time. In many senses we really came up with new and better solutions. We also had to think through and describe the primary goals for all library functions and find quality objectives to achieve them. At this point we were also in contact with other medical libraries to find out if they had good routines that we could benefit from. We participated in several seminars and workshops on quality management and quality assurance, not only for libraries, but also for other service organizations and businesses. It was of especial interest to learn more about service management in general, and how the service business thinks about their customers. In professional marketing, modern salespeople no longer only show the varieties of choices and give information on their products, but they now go out to the customers individually and learn what each of them especially need and want. We also read and learned about Total Quality Management. The way we see it, it is impossible to work with quality systems without implementing Total Quality Management. The philosophy behind this management theory is part of our foundation. Lesley and Malcolm Munroe-Faure are authors we can recommend in this area.[1]

STRUCTURE OF ORGANIZATION

After having written down all the functions and procedures with quality objectives, we also wrote a chapter on the structure of the organization of which the library is a part - the hospital - and defined who our users are, and in what manner we are going to give them service. We do not have the capacity to give service to all that call or visit us, so to define what we can do for the users, is a challenge for us.

PRIMARY GOALS AND STRATEGIES

A chapter on the primary goals and strategies to achieve them was also written. We defined goals for the media collections, for the use of the collections, for our own databases, for the reference service, information retrieval, for the information and training of the users, and for the development of the staff. Particularly at this point it is very important to have the needs of the users strictly in mind all the time. The quality of our service is to be defined by the user and it is of utmost importance to the efficiency of our work to find the right level. A great emphasis on systems and accuracy may be the dream of some librarians, but it is not always to the benefit of the user. The user's perception of service quality is acquired through communication with the library personnel and facilities, and it involves listening to them and keeping them informed. We must ensure that users are aware of the contribution they can make to service quality. In this respect their opinion is of great value.

PERSONNEL DEVELOPMENT

The most important resource in any organization is that of the individual members of personnel involved. This is especially important in a service organization where the behaviour and performance of individuals has a direct impact on the quality of the service. We have therefore established planned actions for updating the skills of the personnel and have implemented career planning and development. We have also stated ethical rules for behaviour and communication with the users.

Service quality improvement

The whole idea of a quality handbook is a continual evaluation of the service processes in order to identify and actively pursue service quality improvement. Identification and reporting of nonconforming services, is the duty and responsibility of each individual in the library. Action should be taken to record, analyze and correct it when nonconformity is detected.

When our quality handbook was revised this winter for the first time, we went through all the procedures, analysed them thoroughly, and made corrections where we had come up with better solutions or where the procedures or part of them had failed, according to their purpose. We then made an evaluation report, and also revised our goals for the next year. At this stage, we knew quite a lot about our work down to minute details, and through good communication with our users over years, we also knew a great deal about their needs. But this was of course based on assumptions. The user's assessment is the ultimate measure of the quality of a service, and their satisfaction should be consistent with the professional standards and ethics of the library. We then carried out a survey amongst our users to find out about our service quality. But to describe and analyze this survey would be the theme for another presentation.

Reference

[1] Munro-Faure L. Implementing Total Quality Management. London: Longman group, 1992

STRIVING TOWARDS TOTAL QUALITY MANAGEMENT IN DUTCH MEDICAL LIBRARIES: 1987-1998

Gerhardus J. van Dieën
MEDICAL LIBRARY, SOPHIA HOSPITAL, ZWOLLE, NL

Medical library standards

Since 1987, Dutch medical librarians have been working to improve quality and professionalism in their field. In the light of a number of milestones in the past years, I should like to show you how we are striving towards total quality management.

In order to strengthen the position of the medical library in general hospitals, the Royal Dutch Medical Association (KNMG) and the Dutch Hospital Institute (NZi) created a committee in 1985, which was asked to develop standards for the functioning of these libraries. The committee's report contains standards which should be considered as basic requirements.[1]

The guidelines were written by doctors. Only two medical librarians were involved as advisors, namely mrs. E. Biekart-Hanhart and mr. J. Sennekool, from the Sophia Hospital in Zwolle and the Medical Centre in Leeuwarden, respectively. Although the librarians were not fully content with the report published in 1987, it was nevertheless gradually accepted by the boards of hospital directors and the medical librarians. The librarians themselves, employed in psychiatric clinics, rewrote these guidelines in 1991. They updated the guidelines, made them more functional and more oriented towards their own working environment, the psychiatric clinics.[2]

The librarians of the general hospitals also wanted a thorough revision of their guidelines, but since the KNMG and the NZi no longer wished to cooperate, they had to rely on themselves. The idea was that if we, as librarians of the general hospitals organised in the Dutch Association of Librarians (NVB), Section Biomedical Information (BMI), would present guidelines of high quality, the working environment (at management level, e.g. boards of hospital management and personnel management) would accept these guidelines automatically as being a form of professionalization.

Refresher courses and continuing education

The Commission Training Requirements, later renamed the Commission for Refresher Courses and Continuing Education, was found in 1991. In its report[3-6] this commission described the various requirements that medical librarians would be expected to satisfy. Subsequently, each group of requirements was looked at to see if the relevant courses were available. As a result of the work of the commission, a number of separate modules have been developed in cooperation with the *Haagse Hogeschool* and the *Hanze-Hogeschool Groningen* (departments of librarianship). Together these modules make up the *Post-HBO Cursus Biomedische Informatie*.

1. CD-ROM and biomedical information;
2. Dutch information sources;
3. structure and organisation of the Dutch Health System;
4. management of biomedical information supply;
5. international sources and information accessing methods.

These courses are regularly repeated and new modules, for example about performance measurement, are being developed.

Recognition and registration

Partly due to these developments regarding education, the working party 'Recognition and Registration' (1993-1994) has discussed whether recognition and/or registration of the developed course would be possible. It appeared that recognition and/or registration was neither possible within the *Wet Beroepen in de Individuele Gezondheidszorg* (BIG) nor within the *Kwaliteitswet* (Quality Act). Possible recognition can only be given by the working environment (at management level).

Quality assurance

After the fourth European Conference of Medical and Health Libraries in Oslo in 1995, the Commission on Quality Assurance was founded on the initiative of the Commission Refresher Courses and Continuing Education. In the Netherlands the Accreditation List presented by Anne FitzGerald was soon called the Oslo List.[7,8] On the basis of the American[9] and Canadian[10] checklists the Dutch Commission on Quality Assurance compiled its own list.[11]

PACE (FOUNDATION FOR TRIAL PROJECT ACCREDITATION)

The *Stichting Proefproject Accreditatie* (PACE) was founded in 1989. Its aim was to meet the Quality Control Standards as well as an accreditation systematics on behalf of Health Care Institutions in the Netherlands.
After having pressed their case long and hard, the medical librarians were formally allowed to have a commission of the NVB/BMI formulate their own Quality Control Standards in cooperation with PACE.[12]

On 23 April 1997, the library of the Sophia Hospital in Zwolle was the first medical library in the Netherlands to participate in a (test) visit by PACE. The reward was a certificate.

INK: INSTITUTE OF DUTCH QUALITY

Nevertheless, most hospitals today prefer the so called INK-model of the Institute of Dutch Quality.[13] This model has been derived from the Self Evaluation Model of the European Foundation for Quality Management (EFQM).[14]

The INK-model has the same two main groups, Organisation and Results, which can also be classified in nine categories: Leadership; Personnel Management; Policy

& Strategy; Resources Management; Procedures; Employee-Satisfaction; Customer Satisfaction; Evaluation of impact on Society and Business Results.

All attention for PACE or ISO has not been in vain, because this attention may be a good start towards total quality assurance. Moreover, the ISO-9000 systematics will be changed within two years. Amongst other things, a path to excellence will be added, through which the system will bear more resemblance to the INK model.

Guidelines

Momentarily the Commission on Guidelines has almost finished the revised edition of the report Guidelines from 1987. It is to be expected that this report will be submitted before the end 1998.

Future

Given the fact that the medical librarians have so far only dealt with the main group Organisation, in which it is difficult to measure the quality results, I myself am working on the implementation of a Dutch version of the Rochester Study at present.[15] In addition, the Project Bureau for Information Management (NBBI) has plans to set up a bench-mark system for libraries.[16]

References

1 Richtlijnen medische bibliotheken in algemene ziekenhuizen: een rapport van de Commissie Richtlijnen Medische Bibliotheken. Koninklijke Nederlandse Maatschappij tot Bevordering der Geneeskunst; Nationaal Ziekenhuisinstituut, 1987

2 Normen & richtlijnen voor bibliotheken in psychiatrische ziekenhuizen: een rapport van de Werkgroep Normen & Richtlijnen Psychiatrische Bibliotheken, 1991

3 Bakker S, Blijdenstein L, Dieën R van, Geertshuis G, Mertens M, Sennekool J. Opleidingseisen medisch bibliothecarissen: rapportage en advies van de Werkgroep Opleidingseisen van de Afdeling Biomedische Informatie van de NVB aan het bestuur NVB/BMI, 1992

4 *idem, main parts translated in french:* Exigences de formation des bibliothecaires médicaux: rapport et recommendations du groupe de travail exigences de formation de la NVB/BMI, 1992

5 *idem, main parts translated in english:* Training qualifications for medical librarians: report and recommendations of the study group training qualifications of the NVB/BMI, 1992

6 Bakker S, Geertshuis G, Mertens M, Sennekool J, Dieën R van, Blijdenstein L. Medical librarians: education and professional quality. Strategy to improve professional image, social status, self-esteem and job salaries. In: Bakker S, Cleland MC (eds). Information transfer: New age - new ways: Proceedings 3ECML Montpellier, France, September 23-26, 1992. Dordrecht: Kluwer, 1993. p 91-94

7 FitzGerald A. Maintaining quality: the accreditation experience. In: McSéan T, Loo J van, Coutinho E (eds). Health information - new possibilities: Proceedings 4ECMHL, Oslo, Norway, June 29-July 2, 1994. Dordrecht: Kluwer, 1995. p 60-62

8 Accreditation of libraries in support of postgraduate medical and dental education. COPMED in consultation with NHS RLG, 1992

9 Standards for hospital libraries. Medical Library Association, 1994

10 Standards for library and information services. Canadian Health Libraries Association, 1995

11 Kwaliteitschecklist medische bibliotheken. Commissie Kwaliteitszorg NVB/BMI, 1996

12 Kwaliteitsborgingsnorm medische bibliotheken. In: Toets uw eigen instelling: een leidraad om de kwaliteit van dienstverlening bij de instelling te beoordelen, waar nodig te verbeteren, en te verankeren in de organisatie. Pace, TNO, 1996 [cd-rom]

13 Handleiding postitiebepaling & verbeteren: zorg-instellingen: bewust werken aan verbetering van resultaten. Instituut Nederlandse Kwaliteit, 1998

14 <http://www.efqm.org/>

15 Marshall JG. The impact of the hospital library on clinical decision making; the Rochester study. Bull Med Libr Assoc 1992;80:169-178

16 Frowein C. Benchmarking voor informatiedienstverleners. Informatie Professional 1998;2(3):21-27

THE DEVELOPMENT OF A STRATEGIC PLAN FOR THE SCIENTIFIC INFORMATION PROVISION OF A PHARMACEUTICAL COMPANY

Nico van Putte
DEPARTMENT OF SCIENTIFIC INFORMATION, N.V. ORGANON, OSS, NL

Introduction

Scientific information presented in journal articles, patents and other publications is of essential value for the innovative pharmaceutical industry. Such information plays a crucial role in the research for and development of new pharmaceutical products, in the registration of new products in the different countries and in the support of new and existing products on the market. Stronger competition between pharmaceutical companies and rapid developments in the area of scientific information have made a pro-active approach of the scientific information provision of a pharmaceutical company increasingly desirable. Therefore Organon has developed a vision on its scientific information provision for the forthcoming years and has laid down this vision in a strategic plan.

ORGANON

Organon is a medium-size, Dutch pharmaceutical company located in Oss and a business unit of the parent company Akzo Nobel. World-wide it has about 9,000 co-workers. About 2,000 of them are working in The Netherlands and about 1,500 in Research and Development. Subsidiaries can be found in more than 50 countries.

Scientific information is not only of value for people working in the R&D laboratories, but also for co-workers of the Clinical Development Department, the Registration Department, the Patent Department, the Medical Services Department and several other departments, both in The Netherlands and abroad.

THE INFORMATION DEPARTMENTS

Within Organon, scientific information services are mainly supplied by the InfoCentre in Oss. This is the central information department of the company with about 30 co-workers divided over four different groups: Library Services, Information Services, Database Services and Imaging Services.

Library Services is carrying out the traditional library tasks such as the collection, registration, distribution and storage of books, journals and other information sources.

Information Services consists of a group of information specialists, who take care of the patent and literature searches and alerting services in the various scientific disciplines such as chemistry, biotechnology and medicine.

Database Services is responsible for the databases supplied to the end-users through the local network as well as for the end-user support. Databases are not only available on CD-ROM such as MEDLINE and Current Contents, but have also been developed in-house, especially for the literature on the company products.

The fourth group, Imaging Services, supplies photography, desktop publishing and similar services.

However, information services are not only supplied by the InfoCentre but also by some other departments such as the Marketing Research Department, which is responsible for commercial information, and the Research Information Management Group, which is responsible for the internal research information. Moreover, the major local companies have their own small information units.

Changing environment

In general, co-workers of the pharmaceutical industry are living in a rapidly changing environment. Due to a stronger competition e.g. a shorter time to market is required for new products in R&D. New developments, e.g. in information and communication technology, have an influence on the work of many people. Many co-workers also have an increasing need for information and show an increasing tendency to self-support with regard to their information provision. However, due to an ongoing information explosion there is also a real danger of information overload for many of them.

The rapid developments which are taking place in the information world have made it a real challenge nowadays to find the right answer to these development in due time. Therefore a pro-active approach is required so that information departments can be involved in a timely implementation of these developments in the company and the company can have a maximum benefit of them.

Many developments concern the so-called electronic library with electronic journals and other electronic information sources, but other aspects of the information provision of the company such as competitive intelligence and knowledge management should also be followed closely.

Strategic plan

A few years ago we decided at Organon to lay down our vision on the scientific information provision of the company in a strategic plan, so that it would be clear to the whole company which policy we would like to follow in the next few years. Important strategic issues for such a plan were the role of information professionals and end-users, the relation between information services and IT services, the use of electronic and printed information sources, the use of internal and external information services, the use of scientific and non-scientific information services and the relation between costs and benefits. New developments would of course receive special attention.

Initially the plan was restricted to the scientific information provision of the R&D organization in Oss. However, in the mean time the plan has been expanded to the R&D organization abroad and a second, slightly different plan has been developed for the Marketing organization. Although the plans have been limited to the external scientific information provision, the relation with the internal scientific information provision (based on internal research data) and with the non-scientific (viz. commercial) information provision has also been described.

The following procedure has been used in the development of the plans. First, a draft has been written based on our own knowledge and experience. This has been discussed with a few key persons in the organization. Thereafter a more definitive plan has been prepared and this has been presented to the managing director for approval. Finally the plan has been distributed to all responsible managers in the organization.

CONTENTS

The whole plan has five chapters. The first chapter is an introduction, in which the significance and scope of the plan and some new developments are described and in which some definitions are given. In the second chapter the policy for the next few years is outlined and in the other three chapters the consequences of this policy for respectively the end-users, the InfoCentre and some other departments are mentioned.

The main elements of the policy are the electronic information provision via the Intranet, the central role of the end-users, the support given by the InfoCentre and other information departments, the integration of the information services of the different locations and the co-operation between all parties involved.

IMPLEMENTATION

It is important that a plan after its development and approval is implemented properly. However, a strategic plan does only mention the ideas for the next few years and no concrete action steps. Therefore it has been arranged in the strategic plan that the InfoCentre together with the other information units will develop an operational plan annualy in order to realize the ideas. Action steps should of course also be mentioned in the operational plans of other departments such as the automation department.

The strategic plan itself is maintained by annual updates, in which new developments are incorporated.

Conclusion

The development of a strategic plan is not a simple task because it requires a lot of study and a lot of discussion. However, when it is ready, it offers several advantages. Within the company there is one policy, which is supported by the management, so that there are no different opinions about the future direction of the information provision. New developments are easily picked up and decisions are made more easily than without a plan. There is a better co-operation between the parties involved and usually there is also more recognition of the value of information departments and a higher motivation of information professionals. This all, of course, is of benefit to the company as a whole.

LE DOCUMENTALISTE-CONSULTANT

Maria da Luz Antunes
INSTITUTO DE CLÍNICA GERAL DA ZONA SUL, LISBON, PORTUGAL

Summary

The health documentation centers should assure the users specific training as information consumers. The librarian is a true expert on the information sources that can turn a poor and badly request in references of keywords on a research based on databases and Internet. On the other hand, the librarian can assure medical training on a specific research methodology, and documental research on databases. The orientation in the structural and methodological plan, the scientific support, the bibliographic revision following the bibliographical rules suitable in each thematical study should demonstrate the constant presence of the librarian near the user - the medical doctor.

Résumé

Les centres de documentation médicales doivent assurer la formation des utilisateurs en tant que consommateurs de l'information. Le documentaliste est le vrai connaisseur des sources d'information et remplace une demande mal structurée et pauvre en références de mots-clé par une recherche sur les bases de données et sur l'Internet. Par ailleurs, le documentaliste peut assurer la formation des médecins dans la méthodologie de la recherche scientifique et dans la recherche documentaire axée sur les bases de données. L'orientation dans le plan méthodologique et structurel, l'appui scientifique, la révision bibliographique selon les normes bibliographiques adéquates à chaque thématique d'étude doivent manifester la présence constante du documentaliste auprès de l'utilisateur - le médecin.

CONFIANCE = TRUST

Aujourd'hui, on demande au documentaliste plusieurs qualités pourqu'il puisse assurer le pont de liaison entre l'utilisateur exigeant, toujours en recherche d'information actualisée, et l'information préférablement électronique, actuelle, rapide.

Qualités du documentaliste

Le documentaliste doit avoir:
- attitude flexible devant l'explosion de formats électroniques et les autoroutes d'information
- curiosité exploration constante sur l'Internet
- appétence par les technologies en disponibilisant son expérience pour l'utilisation et pour l'évaluation des technologies appropriées à la consultation, tennant compte la pérmanente évolution de l'information électronique
- créativité
- expérience en communication et connaissance de plusieurs protocols de recherche, coûts d'accès, d'abonnement...
- relations publiques à promotion des ressources d'information
- savoir faire la réponse aux innovations
- familiarité incitation à la consultation des sources d'information électroniques
- information actualisée et rapide
- crédibilité: connaissance du langage médical, interactions et processus
- compréhension des contenus médicaux

Identification et recueil d'information

- compréhension de l'information sélectionnée et filtrée
- élaboration de bref résumés = description de la découverte

Conclusion

Le documentaliste comprend l'importance de la nomenclature des systèmes d'autorité utilisés dans les systèmes d'information. Le documentaliste est, donc, le pont de liaison entre les technologies d'information et le consulteur-médecin, puisqu'il a les connaissances et la formation nécessaire, puisqu'il connaît les besoins d'information aux soins de santé.

Bibliographie

Low K (ed.). The Roles of Reference Librarians: today and tomorrow. New York: Haworth Press, 1996

Thompson ML. Characteristics of information resources preferred by primary care physicians. Bull Med Libr Assoc 1997;85:187-92

Giuse NB. Advancing the practice of clinical medical librarianship. Bull Med Libr Assoc 1997;85:437-8

Giuse NB, Huber JT, Kafantaris SR, Giuse DA, Miller MD, Gilles DE Jr, Miller RA. Preparing librarians to meet the challenges of today's health care environment. J Am Med Inform Assoc 1997;4:57-67

A NEW NHS: A NEW ROLE FOR LIBRARY SERVICES

Veronica Fraser
NHS Library Adviser, Skipton House, London, UK

Introduction

As the National Health Service (NHS) celebrates its 50th birthday and, incidentally, the appointment of the first professional librarian to the Ministry of Health, a series of Government Papers signal important developments in health care in the UK. Librarians are poised on the threshold of an expanding need for high quality, evidence based information with new roles and new skills required if they are to deliver the new NHS.

Primary Care Led

The New NHS announces the evolution of Primary Care Groups which will increasingly take over the role of commissioning health services for their local communities from Health Authorities. As their role develops, both Health Authorities and Primary Care Teams will have a greater need for a wider range of information than is currently available to them.

Primary Care staff often have poor access to the health care knowledge base and the new NHS Information Management and Technology Strategy (IM&T Strategy) offers the possibility of harnessing information and communication technologies to deliver services to this key group of health care staff. The NHS Information Zone is already in existence and NHSNet will link community and acute staff across the UK by 2002.

Working together to reduce health inequalities

The new NHS promotes multiprofessional working within the NHS and partnerships with higher education, local authorities and the private and voluntary sector outside. Librarians will need to develop existing and fresh networks in order to avoid duplication of, or gaps in, services.

Service excellence

Quality will be at the heart of the new NHS. Continuous improvement in service quality and safeguarding of standards will be reinforced by establishing a duty for quality assurance to be known as clinical governance. Librarians have a key role to play in the success of this at local level by demonstrating their role in the provision of up-to-date evidence on which decisions should be made.

New roles - developing skills

The new national library policy issued in November last year, *Library and Information Services Health Service Guideline (97) 47* emphasized the role of library staff and the skills needed for speedy access to information in support of research; education and training; management decision making; continuing professional development; for patients and carers; and for promoting healthier lifestyles.

Librarians increasingly need to develop their skills as expert searchers, in critical appraisal and as teachers of information skills to other NHS staff. Additionally they will need to be confident problem solvers and facilitators who are also competent business managers with a portfolio of interpersonal and managerial skills.

SCIENTIFIC INFORMATION STRATEGIES: "DISINTERMEDIATION" OR A NEW WAY OF INTERMEDIATION?

Giovanna F. Miranda, Jeannette Ginestet, J. Timmermans, I. Aragon, D. Nisato
[1]SANOFI WINTHROP, SCIENTIFIC INFORMATION DEPARTMENT, MILANO, ITALY; [2 3 4 5]SANOFI, MONTPELLIER, FRANCE

Summary

The library and scientific information department in pharmaceutical firms play an important role in relation to basic knowledge. New technologies and new facilities call into question the role of librarians and information professionals from their present role as intermediates to a situation in which there will be no need for intermediation (i.e., "disintermediation"). "Disintermediation" in information management looks like the future. Librarians and information professionals need not feel threatened by this new scenario, but they do need to rethink certain strategies, acquire new skills and reformulate their own identity. They must focus on understanding the customers's expressed and latent needs and offer new solutions. They must shift from the traditional role of capturing, sorting, organizing and disseminating literature to analysis of resources and educational initiatives. Training users in new technologies, helping them identify internal and external information resources, nurturing users information searching skills and boosting the effective use of literature (e.g. building personal digital reprint files) are only some of the new challenges. In the "Internet information era", librarians and information professionals have to acquire other management skills such as resources analysis, continuing information, communication, knowledge management and outsourcing. Our cooperation with Sanofi Research Cardiovascular Department was discussed as one example.

POLITICAL, ECONOMIC AND SOCIAL CHANGE: TAILOR-MAKING A LIMITLESS LIBRARY SERVICE

Glenda Myers
UNIVERSITY OF THE WITWATERSRAND HEALTH SCIENCES LIBRARY, JOHANNESBURG, SOUTH AFRICA

Changes

The political and social changes in South Africa since 1994 are well-documented. Demographic student patterns at universities are altering radically with the admission of educationally-disadvantaged students from secondary educational facilities which are still suffering from the legacies of apartheid. The education system as a whole is struggling to redistribute funding and facilities more equitably throughout the country's nine provinces, while universities are undergoing radical changes to funding patterns. In addition, both the private and public sectors of the country's health system are in the process of major restructuring towards a focus on primary health care, with a mandatory extra year of community service soon to commence at intern level.

The library

The University of the Witwatersrand Health Sciences Library (WHSL) in Johannesburg serves a user population of some 8000 people, drawn from academic, provincial and private practice. Management of the change process within the health and education sectors at WHSL now actively incorporates both free as well as fee-based activities, in addition to cross-subsidisation of services across public/private sector lines. This latter activity has been facilitated by the incorporation of Southern Africa's first wholly-owned, subsidiary, for-profit company, the Wits Health Consortium (Pty) Ltd. Although the Consortium was initially developed to establish a mechanism through which to conduct contract clinical research, it is constantly identifying value-adding partners and developing new ventures with these partners. WHSL has been identified as a significant value-added partner, and is developing continuing professional education programmes in the area of electronic information retrieval in conjunction with academic staff and private sector companies.

The strategy

In conjunction with these tailor-made services, WHSL is also working with the Faculty of Health Sciences to introduce a new, hybrid curriculum from 1999, incorporating elements of problem-based learning and evidence-based medicine, in addition to the more traditional curriculum activities. It is likely that the Faculty will concentrate on clinical training only in the near future, and will accept into the Faculty students with any undergraduate degree. WHSL is addressing the problems of a changing curriculum by using the opportunity to redefine the entire organisational structure and traditional functions of the library, in order to maximise the benefits of changing technologies at the same time. Once again, this process has been facilitated by the transfer of an extra post from the Faculty to WHSL, at the level of deputy librarian, in order to further encourage the use of multimedia products and to continue to incorporate training in electronic use and evaluation of information. Focus on high-tech systems does not preclude the needs of the primary health care sector, however, which have not been ignored, and an outreach programme has been introduced this year to postgraduate students of the Department of Community Health, who are based throughout Southern Africa. This outreach service will be extended to interns in their community service year as well from 1999, and incorporates design of web pages appropriate for district health nurses and community health education programmes.

Mutually beneficial schemes, such as the appointment at WHSL of library staff on the payroll of other institutions, in return for the use of the library, or library staff appointed from wholly self-generated funding are some of the other strategies which have long been in place to counter economic stringency. Taken altogether, these services, tailor-made by a library in transition from a traditional academic service to one which serves the needs of a wide variety of users in the health sector in the province of Gauteng, are dynamic in nature, and will ensure the strategic and economic survival of WHSL well into the 21st century.

BROADENING THE COLLECTION IN A VIRTUAL ENVIRONMENT: CHALLENGES FOR A SMALL LIBRARY IN THE 21ST CENTURY

Marc van Kuik
National Institute for the Victims of War (ICODO), Utrecht, NL

Summary

Broadening the collection is usually not the objective of a special library. In most cases literature on just one subject of interest has been collected. At present modern technologies are playing a big - although sometimes still uncertain - role in collecting literature. Internet has made the access to other databases (e.g. MEDLINE and DIMDI) and other collections (e.g. KNAW Library, now part of the NIWI) even for small libraries within their reach. This makes it easier to find and collect literature, but it has also risen the problem of selection, especially in the case of broadening a collection. In the library handbooks and literature the problem of broadening a collection is emphasized, making a difference between macro- and microselection. The practice of the library of ICODO (National Institute for the Victims of War) has been evaluated in this context.

In 1996 the statute of ICODO was changed to incorporate her present knowledge of war victims in the Netherlands into the field of other victims of violence like, for example, refugees from the former Yugoslavia. The library, which is specialized in the psychosocial consequences of the Second World War, started her services in the 80's. Nowadays it is internationally renowned for her collection on posttraumatic stress disorder (PTSD). The library first collected only books and articles, later on newsclippings and videos, and now uses modern media like Internet and CD-ROM. The collection is of peculiar interest because it covers different fields: medicine, antropology, sociology, psychiatry, psychology and history. This is highly appreciated by the users of the library. The broadening of the collection is an opportunity for an evaluation on how to select and collect literature into the 21st century, specially from electronic resources like Internet or CD-ROM.

A literature search in LISA (Library Information Science Abstracts) led to the following conclusions:

1) a collection development profile through the Conspectus method is a good base for broadening a collection, and
2) the same criteria for selecting "older" resources like books and periodicals are also effective in selecting new media materials.

Chapter 7: VETERINARY LIBRARIES

Introduction

The subjects to be discussed among the colleagues of veterinary libraries are not so much different from those of relevance to other biomedical and allied health librarians. Nevertheless a special interest group of veterinarians has a right to exist because of the mixture and interdependence of several factors influencing library services. Economical and juridical apects in animal health care are more prominent and of a different kind than in human health care; governmental regulations regarding animal husbandry, industrial interest of producing food of animal origin, those are mingled with the education and training of veterunary students and junior faculty. Most countries have only one or just a few veterinary institutions with libraries which causes that cooperation for our verterinarian colleagues is almost synonymous with international cooperation.

The contributions of Theodora Oker-Blom c.s. and of Gerdien de Jonge & Theo Elsinghorst deal with international cooperation and the benefits for participating libraries.

The paper of Tom Roper illustrates how scientific communication in a field such as veterinary sciences can be studied and how the results of citation analysis can be used to understand if and how relations exist between different areas such as biology, medicine, animal health and grey literature.

Doris Reinitzer and Hans Kuiper describe user needs and how the library can contribute to training and education in searching and finding relevant literatue. These examples do not differ much from the experience of colleagues in other school libraries: be it medical or nursing (see chapters 8, 9 and 10).

Guus Mathijsen, retired but still very active in the field of History of Animal and Veterinary Sciences, pleas for more and better awareness towards the history of librarianship, especially veterinary libraries and librarians. The same holds true for other fields of librarianship, e.g. nursing, pharmaceutical. A lot of information is gathered and many aspects of medical librarianship has been studied, not the least by activities of the National Library of Medicine and the Medical Library Association in the United States of America, but a strong bias towards medicine and the USA can be noted.

INTERNATIONAL COOPERATION AND STRUCTURED ACCESS TO QUALITY INFORMATION

Teodora Oker-Blom, Sinikka Suckcharoen, Kristiina Hormia-Poutanen
[1 2]VETERINARY MEDICINE LIBRARY; [3]AGRICULTURAL LIBRARY, UNIVERSITY OF HELSINKI, FINLAND

Introduction

A subject gateway, or subject-based information gateway (SBIG) as we describe it here, is a facility that allows easier access to network-based resources in a defined subject area. The more advanced gateways offer an enhanced service via a system consisting of a resource database with various indexes, which can be searched and/or browsed through a Web-based interface. Each entry in the database contains information about a network-based resource. This could be a Web page, Web site, document or database. The sources are selected, described and catalogued using a template and classified and indexed to a database. An example of a subject-based information gateway is OMNI, UK's independent gateway to high quality biomedical Internet resources, which has been presented at earlier EAHIL conferences. Another example is NOVAGate.

Nordic cooperation

NOVAGate is a Nordic Gateway to Information in Veterinary Medicine, Agricultural Sciences and Forestry. It is a quality-assessed database of Internet resources, aimed principally at higher education and research. The database is being developed and maintained by the libraries of the NOVA university. The NOVA university is a cooperative project between the veterinary and agricultural universities in the Nordic countries. The cooperating libraries are the Danish Veterinary and Agricultural library, the Veterinary Medicine Library, the Agricultural Library and the Library of Forestry, all at the University of Helsinki in Finland, the Norwegian College of Veterinary Medicine and the Agricultural University of Norway and the Swedish University of Agricultural Sciences. Our colleagues from Iceland will join the project later.

The project was initiated by the Agricultural library of the University of Helsinki in late 1996. Economic support has been applied for and received for 1997 and 1998 from the Nordic Council of Ministers. The participating libraries have also supported the project substantially by covering travels, equipment and staff time.

At an early stage a conference was arranged, where representatives of similar projects e.g. EEVL, SOSIG, EELS, the EU's DESIRE and the Nordic metadata project presented their views and experiences. On this basis the project structure and elements were envisaged and the project organisation was settled.

A steering committee and an operational committee with representatives for all participating libraries are carrying out the project. Two to four meetings per year have been arranged as well as some training sessions in cataloguing on Nordic and local level. The main means of communication is the network. The NOVAGate project has established an e-mail conference and a homepage. At the well-structured homepage one can easily find the project plan, the e-mail correspondence archive, the minutes of the meetings, the annual reports etc. The experiences of network communication are good. Every participant gets current information and has the possibility to give their opinion. However, it was noticed that it is very important that the project coordinator has the last word and clearly states the final decision. The network communication does not compensate meetings in a multicultural, multilingual setting.

The project elements that had to be dealt with were:

1) technical structure: software, hardware, platform, tools
2) content, coverage and quality criteria: i.e. authority and reputation of source, accuracy, currency etc
3) subject structure, cataloguing policy and language: classification, indexing, depth of cataloguing
4) form criteria: ease of navigation, provision of user support, use of standards, aesthetics (marketing, use, evaluation)

TECHNICAL STRUCTURE

The software chosen for NOVAGate is ROADS (Resource Organisation And Discovery in Subject-based services), created in the United Kingdom. About 20 subject gateways use ROADS today. The records in ROADS databases are stored in templates based on the IAFA template. It gives the creator the possibility to produce a flexible but also comprehensive entry. The software toolset includes a number of facilities to assist cataloguers in data entry, for instance a cataloguers interface with indexing facilities.

The search mechanism is based on the WHOIS++ protocol, which provides separation between the user front end and back end search engines and supports a variety of strategies for searching single and multiple services. The pilot system is mounted on a PC at the Swedish University of Agricultural Sciences, who have been responsible for technical management and support. That has been an economically rational solution for the project.

The experiences of ROADS are good. However it was not designed for multilingual purposes, a unique quality of NOVAGate. The second version of ROADS, which will be released in July 1998, will hopefully support the multilingual approach.

CONTENT, COVERAGE AND QUALITY

The subject coverage of NOVAGate corresponds to the subjects taught and researched at the NOVA universities. The resource types selected and catalogued so far are services like databases, organisations, library catalogues, electronic journals, training materials and documents. The system allows a broad range of resource types to be catalogued in the future. At present only sources of Nordic origin are added, but the scope of the project is to also include electronic resources from other countries. Could this possibly be taken care of by cross-searching national subject gateways?

The contents of each resource is judged against a set of quality criteria. The extensive list of quality selection criteria developed by the EU project DESIRE (Development of a European Service for Information on Research and Education), has formed the basis for judgement. They list the groups: (1) scope policy, (2) content criteria, (3) form criteria, (4) process criteria and (5) collection management policy. The content criteria to consider are: validity, authority and reputation of the source, substantiveness, accuracy, comprehensiveness, uniqueness, composition and organisation, currence and adequacy of maintenance.

There is of course no global standard or unified way of whether a resource is of sufficient relevance and quality to be catalogued by a subject gateway or desription of how resource descriptions should be written, but we have tried to discuss this thorougly, tried to put the information into the guidelines of NOVAGate cataloguing and thus hope to reach some kind of consistency. This has obviously been one of the more difficult matters. The description of each resource will, if necessary, include some comments on the quality, since all organisations, considered to be important to include, have not developed their web sites enough yet.

SUBJECT STRUCTURE

Most of the cooperating Nordic libraries are participants in FAO's AGRIS database. The well-known broad AGRIS subject categories were thus chosen as a first classification criteria of assigned resources. This brings for instance together the collections of veterinary medicine. The Agrovoc thesaurus of FAO is used for indexing resources in English. Additional indexing in a local Nordic language can be done. Subject indexing enables thesaurus-based searching and thus more relevant results to be retrieved in comparison to free text searching.

Each resource is also given a short description, both in English and it's local Nordic language. At present Danish and Finnish keywords are added to resources from these countries. The descriptions as well as the assigned subject terms are searchable and browsable. Searching support with a list of high frequency terms will possibly be added in the future.The system also allows searching on geographic areas e.g. the Nordic countries, and resource types.

Web guidelines have been produced by the Forestry Library of the University of Helsinki in order to support consistent practice and have been tested on a Nordic course for the cataloguers. ROADS has produced basic guidelines to assist in a shared approach to how data elements are described and which particular data elements are used.

FORM CRITERIA: USER INTERFACE

Much work has been put into user interface design by the Danish Veterinary and Agricultural Library. The interface has been tested and evaluated by at least university staff in Finland and the present interface with it's user support has turned out to be feasible.

Opinions on the cooperation

The Nordic cooperation, that started in December 1996 has resulted in a pilot subject information gateway NOVAGate, which from July 1998 will allow public access to quality-assessed Internet resources. The responsibility for different elements has at policy and project meetings been distributed between the libraries. The Agricultural library in Finland was the coordinator of the project in 1996 and 1997.

In 1998 the Swedish University of Agricultural Sciences library has that role as well as the responsibility for technical management and support. Denmark is responsible for the user interface and marketing, Finland has produced the Web guide and educates the cataloguers and Norway will evaluate the functioning service from the users point of view. The funds are distributed accordingly among the participants. All the libraries are involved in the production of the database.

The advantages of cooperation in this project are:
- a broader base of competence and thus a fruitful educational experience for every participant and an advantage for carrying out the project
- economic savings, in this case e.g.on equipment and technical management
- the achievement of a service with a wider base of resources that are locally quality controlled
- inspiring and educational experiences of cooperation in a multicultural, multilingual setting
- a common Nordic effort makes a greater impact internationally

The disadvantages of cooperation in this project has been:
- cultural and language differences requires understanding, patience and good planning, which means more meetings, more staff time and costly travels
- network cooperation, a first experience to this extent for the participants, requires stringent procedures for decision making before it becomes an advantage
- decision-making is often based on compromises
- progress is dependent on the performance of every participant

From the users point of view a collection of Nordic resources will hopefully strengthen the purpose of the NOVA university, which is closer contacts between teachers and students and common research projects, possibly also within an EU framework.

International cooperation

A cross-searching demonstrator, allowing people to cross-search a number of subject based gateways is available for exploration. Duplication of resources will naturally be the case if several gateways in the same subject area are cross-searched, if each country has not systematically catalogued only their own resources. Even overlapping will be found in subject areas that covers the same resources to some extent e.g. SOSIG and OMNI. These could either be left in or the results could be amalgamated and presented as one hit under one title or URL, but with the individual descriptions, or include only the resource with the longest description or let the user decide from which gateway she preferes the description, if there are duplicate resources.

Common guidelines for resource selection criteria and cataloguing rules on how to write descriptions and classify and index the resources would result in a cross search that will contain links to resources of a differing minimum quality as well as resource descriptions that are somewhat inconsistent in the way they are written. But the links would have been chosen locally, which guarantees some kind of maintenance and qulity. Thus cross-searching seems to be a good and also rational solution.

CITATION ANALYSIS OF THE VETERINARY LITERATURE: A TOOL TO UNDERSTANDING SCIENTIFIC COMMUNICATION

Tom Roper
ROYAL COLLEGE OF VETERINARY SURGEONS WELLCOME LIBRARY, LONDON, UK

Introduction

In this paper I shall report some results of a citation analysis of the veterinary literature carried out at the Royal College of Veterinary Surgeons Wellcome Library, and outline some directions in which further work could go. The RCVS Wellcome Library is the major British information service serving the practising veterinarian. All of the 18,000 members of the Royal College in the UK and abroad may use our services, and we also serve veterinary nurses, and other para-veterinary professionals. Increasingly we are also becoming the focus for enquiries on animal health matters from owners and the general public.

By way of background, perhaps I should explain how the idea for this analysis came about: I am a recent recruit to the ranks of veterinary information workers, having succeeded Benita Horder as Librarian at the RCVS eighteen months ago. In coming to a new subject field and literature, I realised that citation analysis was potentially a useful tool to help me to orientate myself on the map of animal health information. I was also interested, coming from a human health information background, in the interface between animal health and human health information issues, and the cross over in the use of the general biomedical literature by veterinarians. The issue of bovine spongiform encephalopathy (BSE) has focussed British minds quite sharply on these issues.

I performed a literature search on Library and Information Science Abstracts, (LISA), Library Literature, CAB Abstracts and MEDLINE and found that there was little published work on citation analysis of the purely veterinary literature that I could refer to, so I would have to do it myself. There have been 3 papers, as far as I could trace; one by Udofia[1], which concentrated on citation analysis as a tool to journal selection and deselection decisions, another by White[2], looking at the frequency of citations in the Consultant database and a study by Cho[3] which looks at citation characteristics based on articles in Advances in Veterinary Science and Comparative Medicine. At a more general level the recent project in the USA in of the Task Force on Bibliographic Access for the Allied Health Literature[4] has been an interesting attempt to map the literature of an important field and there is an extremely thorough review of the issues in Osareh.[5,6]

I approach citation analysis from a different perspective to that of Ulrich Korwitz (pp. 107-110). However, like him, and I hope without repeating any of the excellent critique of citation analysis he made, I wish to start with some caveats about the limitations of the technique.

Citation analysis

The first question I think we have to ask is whether or not the act of citation, of referring to previously published work in a list of references at the end of a scientific paper, actually tells us something. It is of course true that in many cases citation takes place to acknowledge intellectual debt, and can show us the trails of theoretical developments; we would need to distinguish between some of the different reasons for citation of another's work: support, homage, criticism. It may even be rash to assume that a cited item has in fact actually been used before it is cited. But equally, citation can and does take place for less noble reasons: a junior researcher may feel obliged to cite work by his or her supervisor, whether or not he or she considers that work important or correct. Citation may take place in order to question the validity and conclusions of earlier work. Some important articles may be ignored and not cited: groundbreaking work may take some time to find general acceptance in the biomedical community.

Some other problems of the method were well outlined by Ulrich Korwitz (pp. 107-110): the problems of self-citation and the citation ring, some of the shortcomings of Science Citation Index in taking account of non-journal literature, the bias towards English language, and US journals, and so on.

METHODS

Because of these reservations I determined, rather than using Science Citation Index, to start from scratch. I looked at a sample of articles in the Veterinary Records and the Journal of the American Veterinary Medical Association (JAVMA) for one month in 1995 and May of 1998. Only major scientific papers were included: case reports, editorials and letters were excluded. A total of 776 references from 38 articles, a sample of 5% of the total annual output of these two journals were analysed and the results entered into a Microsoft Excel spreadsheet. Citations were divided into citations of journal articles, citations of monographs, citations of conference proceedings, citations of these, and citations of electronic resources, by which I mean databases, web sites and electronic journals.

RESULTS AND ANALYSIS

The distribution of types of material does not change greatly from 1995 to 1998. Eighty per cent of the materials cited are journal articles, followed by monographs, conference proceedings, and theses. Electronic sources were only cited once and I shall discuss this further later. The half-life of the journals cited was ten years.

Using the Veterinary Medical Libraries Section of the Medical Library Association's Core list of veterinary journals, I analysed the extent to which authors cited materials from the veterinary literature or from the wider biomedical literature. The results suggest that veterinary medicine and surgery are not self-contained fields, but draw upon the wider bio-medical literature extensively.

Cited journals were predominantly English language, followed by German and French. The most cited journal was JAVMA (6.1%) followed by Veterinary Record (5.9%) and then the American Journal of Veterinary Research (3.7%).

Discussion

I must confess I was surprised at some of the findings. Much of what I found fits the known picture of veterinary information: the importance of conference proceedings, of theses, the grey literauture was already known, albeit instictively. But the low level of citation of electronic resources surprised me. We do not yet know much about the information-seeking behaviour of veterinarians, but we can suggest some tentative answers. It may be that while veterinary authors do use electronic sources, they do not cite them, either through ignorance of the conventions for citing such material. The frequent cries for help one encounters on Internet mailing lists ("I have a user who wants to know how to cite a URL according to Vancouver") lend support to this hypothesis. It may also be that they are simply not yet using electronic information sources to any great extent. It is certainly true that compared to human medicine, veterinary journal publishers have been slow to take advantage of the new opportunities offered in the global networked environment.

We need to know more: in particular, some analysis on historical lines would be useful, to determine how the patterns of citation have changed, to understand what we can extrapolate for the future.

The extent to which veterinary authors cite the non-veterinary literature is significant. At the most basic level, it has implications for the journals of holdings of veterinary information services, and demonstrates the necessity for cooperation between veterinary information services and our medical colleagues. Bibliometrics is, at bottom, bean counting. But I believe that it can, if used with discretion, offers some insights into the relationships between human and animal health.

As the United Kingdom considers, as a result of the Selborne report into veterinary research funding, how best to develop a strategy for veterinary research, the importance of the information that underpins that research, its accessibility and its dissemination, are crucial. And at the centre of that stands the veterinary librarian or information officer.

References

[1] Udofia UI. Selecting veterinary medical periodicals through citation analysis. Libr Rev 1997;46:105

[2] White ME. An analysis of journal citation frequency in the Consultant data base for computer assisted diagnosis. J Am Vet Med Assoc 1987;190:1098-1101

[3] Cho YJ. Citation characteristics of periodical literature in veterinary science. Am J Vet Res 1977;38:131-33

[4] Schloman BF. Mapping the literature of allied health: project overview. Bull Med Libr Assoc 1997;85:271-277

[5] Osareh F. Bibliometrics, citation analysis and co-citation analysis: a review of literature I. Libri 1996;46:149-58

[6] Osareh F. Bibliometrics, citation analysis and co-citation analysis: a review of literature II. Libri 1996;46:271-25

EUROPEAN VETERINARY DISSERTATION PROJECT

Gerdien de Jonge, Theo Elsinghorst
[1]Faculty of Veterinary Medicine, Library, University of Utrecht; [2]Euroscience, Bilthoven, The Netherlands

Short history

In May 1989 the first proposal for the European Veterinary Dissertation Service (EVDS) was done at the General Assembly of the European Association of Establishments for Veterinary Education (EAEVE) in Brussels. Some discussion at the Assembly and by correspondence led to a revised proposal, done at the Assembly of the EAEVE in Brescia, May 1990 by prof.dr. S.G. van den Bergh, dean of the Faculty of Veterinary Medicine in Utrecht.

After the approval of the EVDS on the Assembly in Brescia, questionnaires were sent to the participants of the General Assembly of EAEVE in Brescia. In December 1990 fourteen institutes had sent their answers. They were all enthousiastic about the project and intended to participate.

The first issue of the Current Bibliography of European Veterinary Dissertations (CBEVD) was published in spring 1992 by Euroscience in cooperation with the Library of the Faculty of Veterinary Medicine in Utrecht, with a foreword of professor B. Toma, president of the EAEVE. Since then the journal has been published bimonthly and several new participants joined the project.
Also some problems were discussed, for instance about:
a. copyright rules, in particular in the United Kingdom
b. imbedding the project in the Library Programme of the European Community
c. broadening the scope to "Information network in veterinary medicine"
d. different dissertation-types based on different degrees

Ad a. The copyright problems could be solved partly by sending just the bibliographic data, preferably with abstract, which is done by some participating establishments.

Ad b and c. To broaden a project is not always suitable for the realization of certain purposes. In the case of the EVD-project the realization of a smaller project was choosen. In 1996 the discussion has been started about the accessibility of the CBEVD on Internet.

Ad d. It was choosen to involve different levels, although restricted to postgraduate level, of dissertations or theses. The participating establishments themselves may decide which dissertations will be sent to be indexed in the EVD-database.

Table 1. Faculties participating in the EVD-project per 1-1-1998 (N = 33)

COUNTRY	CITY	NAME OF THE FACULTY
Austria	Vienna	University of Veterinary Medicine, Vienna
Belgium	Ghent	Faculty of Veterinary Medicine, University of Ghent
	Liège	College of Veterinary Medicine, University of Liège
Denmark	Copenhagen	The Royal Veterinary and Agricultural University, Copenhagen
Finland	Helsinki	College of Veterinary Medicine, Helsinki
France	Alfort	National Veterinary School of Alfort
	Lyon	National School of Veterinary Science, Lyon
	Nantes	National School of Veterinary Science, Nantes
	Toulouse	National Veterinary School of Toulouse
Germany	Berlin	Faculty of Veterinary Medicine, Free University Berlin
	Giessen	Faculty of Veterinary Medicine, Justus-Liebig-University of Giessen
	Hannover	Hannover School of Veterinary Medicine
	Leipzig	Faculty of Veterinary Medicine, University of Leipzig
	München	Veterinary Faculty of München
Greece	Thessaloniki	Veterinary Faculty Thessaloniki
Hungary	Budapest	University of Veterinary Science, Budapest
Ireland	Dublin	Faculty of Veterinary Medicine, University College Dublin
Netherlands	Utrecht	Faculty of Veterinary Medicine, Utrecht University
Norway	Oslo	Norwegian College of Veterinary Medicine, Oslo
Poland	Warsaw	Faculty of Veterinary Medicine, Warsaw Agricultural University
Portugal	Lisboa	Faculty of Veterinary Medicine Lisboa
	Vila Real	University of Trás-os-Montes and Alto Douro
Slovenia	Ljubljana	Veterinary Faculty Ljubljana
Spain	Barcelona	Faculty of Veterinary Medicine, University of Barcelona
	Córdoba	Veterinary Faculty of Córdoba
	Murcia	Veterinary Faculty of Murcia
	Zaragoza	Veterinary Faculty, University of Zaragoza
Sweden	Uppsala	Faculty of Veterinary Medicine, Swedish University of Agricultural Science
Switzerland	Bern	Faculty of Veterinary Medicine, University of Berne
	Zürich	Faculty of Veterinary Medicine, University of Zürich
Turkey	Konya	Faculty of Veterinary Medicine, University of Selçuk
United Kingdom	Cambridge	School of Veterinary Medicine, University of Cambridge
	Edinburgh	Faculty of Veterinary Medicine, University of Edinburgh

Situation now

Per 1-1-1998, 33 European veterinary faculties participated in the project, 25 by sending the whole dissertations and 8 by sending bibliographic data, mostly including abstracts. For a list of participating faculties see Table 1.

The total number of dissertations indexed in volumes 1-7 (1992-1997) of the Current Bibliography of European Veterinary Dissertations (CBEVD) is 7105.

At the end of 1998, the printed CBEVD will be continued as an electronic edition, on diskette or on CD-ROM. The choice between diskette and CD-ROM depends on the size of the file. The electronic edition not only contains the dissertations indexed after ceasing the printed CBEVD, but also the dissertations indexed in the CBEVD 1992-1997. Of the dissertations before 1998 only the bibliographic data and the index terms are given, not the table of contents or the abstract. From theses of 1998 onwards, the table of contents or the abstract is given as well.

The European Veterinary Dissertations on diskette or on CD-ROM will be updated bimonthly. Each update contains the whole file. The software used for compiling the EVD-file is ProCite, a storage and retrieval system produced by Personal Bibliographic Software, Ann Arbor, U.S.A.

Possibilities for cooperation

In the last six years the possibilities of producing and disseminating information have been changed tremendously. The purpose of the European Veterinary Dissertation Service is still the same as in 1990, but some of the means to realize and continue are changed. The purpose of the EVD-project may be formulated as follows:

Building one and best European Veterinary Dissertation site with reliable bibliographic data, accessible by Internet using common Web-browsers, and with relevant links to other available sources.

To realize this purpose the cooperation and the coordination on European level shoul be intensified, as we see that some possible participants are not joining the project. As we agree about the sense of the project and as the project is approved by the EAEVE, we should feel responsible to fill in the gaps as good and soon as possible.

A working group on the European Veterinary Dissertation project was set up in July 1997. The members are from France, Germany, Hungary, Netherlands and Sweden. This group has communicated mostly about local developments until now. To initiate further developments in this project we must formulate and discuss the problems why there are still some gaps and try to find solutions on the level which is possible (e.g. local or European).

More countries should participate in this discussion. By setting up a discussion list with the EVD project as main item might be a start to more cooperation in veterinary information services on European level. The coordination should be done at the Faculty of Veterinary Medicine in Utrecht.

Perspectives for the future

As far as full-text dissertations are available on Internet, links to these sites will be built in the EVD-database. At this moment most dissertations are only available in print and probably this will be so for at least 5 to 10 years or even much longer. It depends on the developments of: copyright rules, searching possibilities, reliability of the Internet, long-term preservation of and accessibility to the data, quality of data transmission.

The discussion about copyright is now broadened to printed and digital information sources. On the level of the European Union discussions about common rules are going on. Hopefully the experts in jurisprudence will influence this process in a satisfactory way for all the European Community members and the educational and scientific communities in particular.

The searching possibilities are improved by the development of intelligent searching programmes. The Utrecht University is testing searching programmes for selecting items on a specialized and personal subject area, not only on demand, but even by announcing. To get the right information on your desk, it is still needed that this information is structured: good structured databases are necessary to be able to make satisfying and reliable personal selections.

The long-term preservation techniques of digital information are being tested and the costs will be compared with the printed version (paper or microfiches).

The reliability of the Internet has to be proved in the future, at this moment it is sufficient for not urgently needed information. The quality of data transmission will get better and the printing techniques of local computer systems will compete with those of the printing offices.

WORLD WIDE ACCESS

The information technology gives us the possiblities to realize access from every place on the world, provided that the basic infrastructure and computer supplies are available. By joining the general accepted standard systems and programmes the EVD-database can be set up for world wide access. The Library of the Faculty of Veterinary Medicine of Utrecht will open its homepage in 1998 in collaboration with the PREX-organization, a specialized online information service at the Utrecht University.

SOLVING THE INFORMATION NEEDS OF VETERINARIANS IN AUSTRIA

Doris Reinitzer
VETERINÄRMEDIZINISCHE UNIVERSITÄT WIEN, VIENNA, AUSTRIA

The veterinary library

The Library of the Vienna University of Veterinary Medicine serves as a specialized referral center for applied veterinary science and in several areas of basic medical research. To fulfill our role as a current and comprehensive information center, continuous development and upgrading of the library's network is necessary.

Since 1990 the library has been using BIBOS, the library automation system of the Austrian Academic Library Network. The network is comprised of 22 Austrian libraries, including 18 universities. The OPAC, containing over one million titles, can be reached via **http://bibopac.univie.ac.at**. The most important current priority is the replacement of BIBOS within this year. At the beginning of 1999 we will begin using ALEPH integrated library system (Ex Libris Ltd.). For this reason we will also change our internal network structure from Novell to Windows NT. ALEPH is a generalized, fully integrated system, based on parameter tables for on-site tailoring of the system to our library's specific applications. An Austrian working group was established with one or two staff of each library to implement and adapt the system. For this reason one of our staff got special training in ALEPH and attended also a basic informatic course. Then she will be our teacher to use this system. We will replace the old system during the short winter university holidays to avoid a longer closing period as necessary. At the loan desk the loan module of the Allegro library automation system (aLF) is now in use. To maintain the loaning the loan module aLF will be used since the other system works well.

Available databases

Patron services would be enhanced by increasing the number of databases available and improving accessibility to the databases. Similar to other university libraries in Austria, the Library of the Vienna University of Veterinary Medicine used to offer only locally mounted databases. In 1996, the Central Library of Medicine, which is located in the most important hospital in Vienna, began using SilverPlatter's Electronic Reference Library Technology (ERL). The advantages of incorporating this technology are the unique user interface, the TCP/IP protocol which allows immediate access from a number of different platforms (Windows, Macintosh, etc.), and the client/server architecture with its inherent division of labour and reduction of network traffic. This networking solution led to the idea of sharing electronic resources among several Austrian libraries. In 1997 the Central Library of Medicine and the Veterinary Library, both in Vienna and the University Library of Graz, established a consortial arrangement to use a central server (SUN Ultra2) and a choice of six databases. Every library can access the databases they need and pay for what they use. We cannot offer more databases because of budget constrains. We join the consortium with Current Contents/5 Sci. Ed. and the complete MEDLINE Advanced database (1966 to the present). Now our users can simultaneously search these two databases in addition to our local CD-ROM drives under the unique user interface WinSPIRS or MacSPIRS. The statistics immediately showed an increased usage for all databases in all participating libraries. The current monthly usage level at our university averages about 2000 hours per month. With more than 1000 hours usage per month MEDLINE Advanced running on SilverPlatter's SPIRS is the most frequently used database within the consortium. We recommend MEDLINE especially for retrospective searches, e.g. for theses. We can only speculate that, with the user friendly software and free Internet access, PubMed will be popular and have widespread use. During the workshops held to help users select the most appropriate databases, we are seeing information-seeking behavioural changes. The retrieval interface of Current Contents on Diskette was not user friendly. When asked about their preference on search software, all of the patrons preferred SPIRS over Current Contents on Diskette. The use of Current Contents increased rapidly. Before faculties also tend to use the print format rather than change to the electronic format.

At the present time, our library users have access to thirteen bibliographic databases. Four of these databases are permanently accessible via the University's local area network (LAN). National databases, like the Austrian drug compendium, or full-text "scripts" for students are also accessible via the LAN. Distance learning through computer-modem interactions is not commonplace yet, but some "what's your diagnosis pages", radiographic images or bulletin boards are now available. I suppose that in the future solo practice veterinarians will seek distance continuing education for practical reasons. More and more rural practitoners are using e-mail to contact us. For long time we used to send books by post and they never had to come to Vienna to use our services. So we have a lot of questions on how to use the Internet, how to subscribe to databases or online journals. Sometimes our customers are disappointed that the commercial virtual library is more expensive as they expect. New users find the Web sometimes frustrating and confusing lists of search results bring them back to the library. Using our catalog, free access to PubMed or other trial access to databases, customers will go back on line again. But cyber-marketing overwhelms on-line users and even librarians have to struggle to be up to date. So we are in an excellenty position to analyze trends in the information field for our users and to do user education.

Instruction, training, support

The one semester lecture: "Introduction to scientific information, information retrieval and bibliography" taught by a library staff, trained in librarianship and veterinary medicine, is a free elective course in the curriculum. It is limited to 54 participants each semester and is always overbooked. Now we prefer postgraduates for doctoral studies leading to the degree of Doctor of Veterinary Medicine, because the examination of this course is accepted as lecture during the 4 semesters' doctoral studies. The number of students enrolling on the Doctoral course of studies is high and is rising: 274 veterinarians received the approval of their thesis during the last two years. Because so many undergraduates are on the waiting list for this lecture, we offer other courses for students. Or short hands-on courses are held to demonstrate our new resources. Weekly or on demand we offer additionally short courses (3 hours) in database searching. The library not only serves the university and veterinarians, but is open also to the the general public, so human doctors, breeders, pet-owners or other people looking for information attend our courses and can borrow books.

Especially for our students learning from the key textbooks written in German in the curriculum, starting scientific reading of English journals is not easy. They don't like to learn also "librarian English". Even if you always get a self-explanatory help screen to the databases or viving the WWW, a lot of our users want us to help read the English text. At the beginning I have to explain in German language, and step by step we enter the cyber-space with a search engine. But also the real library is frequently used each year. In 1997, 33.000 books were borrowed, 3400 document delivery requests received, and interlibrary loan has increased. It should not surprise that people like to visit us and are impressed by the buildings and equipment now available at the Veterinary University of Vienna. The facilities are among the very best in Europe.[1]

The feed-back of our participants indicate that as additional databases and Internet resources become accessible on the end-user's desktop computer, the academic librarian's role in providing training and support to these users will change accordingly.

Reference

[1] Olensky G, Stein S. Die neue Universitätsbibliothek der Veterinärmedizinischen Universität Wien. Ein Jahrhundertbauwerk wurde fertiggestellt. ABI-Technik 1997;17:19-26

VETERINARY PRACTITIONERS' ACCESS TO AND USE OF MODERN INFORMATION

Hans Kuiper, Gerdien B. de Jonge
[1] Laboratory of Animal Science; [2]Library, Faculty of Veterinary Medicine, Utrecht University, Utrecht, NL

Abstract

Many Dutch veterinary practioners are using computers for the management of their daily practice. The first management computer programs (in the eigthies) were dedicated to patient and financial administration. At that time the practioners were using mainly more or less traditional methods for keeping up-to-date with scientific developments: a personal library with journals and (hand)books, organizing journal circulating-systems, following post academic courses, going to meetings *et cetera*.

The library of the Faculty of Veterinary Medicine in Utrecht (the one and only in the Netherlands) was at that time steadily keeping up with the new developments of information retrieval systems: automation of the catalogue, buying new types of sources as CD-ROMs, offering online search facilities. As these new facilities were mostly still only locally useable within the university and rather difficult and/or expensive in use, they were not very well accessable for the veterinary practitioner or other interested people form outside the university.

Technical advancements (software and hardware) made the veterinary practioners slowly more aware of the accessability of new information sources. At the Faculty of Veterinary Medicine a small host-organisation, called PREX, was being set up in 1990, allowing veterinarians and others access to the CAB-database and other major biomedical databases. PREX operates on an annual subscription base and is for most practitioners an affordable accession to many information sources.

Courses were setup by the Dutch Post Academic Education Foundation to teach the basics on literature searching to veterinary practitioners. These courses were given by PREX and the veterinary library.

The consequences of the new developments on information technologies for PREX and the veterinary library were discussed. Several new digital databases are becoming available for keeping up-to-date with veterinary developments or getting access primary information, for instance on drug use (formularies) and animal diets. Some statistics of the use of these databases was presented. Internet as an information source is becoming more and more important. The number of home pages of Dutch veterinary practices is increasing, showing the involvement of the Dutch veterinary community with Internet. The expectations of the role of the Faculty of Veterinary Medicine, especially of the library and PREX, as information suppliers for the veterinary practioners was discussed.

THE VETERINARY LIBRARIAN AS KEEPER OF THE VETERINARY DOCUMENTARY HERITAGE

A.A.H.M. (Guus) Mathijsen
RETIRED LIBRARIAN, FACULTY OF VETERINARY MEDICINE, UTRECHT UNIVERSITY, UTRECHT, NL

Librarianship and the history of (veterinary) medicine

In earlier times it was taken for granted that a librarian was an historian or someone with knowledge in cultural history or book history. This applied especially to libraries for the humanities, but not exclusively. Also medical libraries were often headed by men who contributed to the field of medical history. I only have to mention the names of Fielding H. Garrison (1870-1935), librarian at the forerunner of the National Library of Medicine in Bethesda, Maryland, the Surgeon General's Library, who - next to his work at the first *Index Medicus* - wrote, among others, the standardwork *An introduction to the history of medicine*, or that of an other army surgeon John Shaw Billings (1838-1913), the originator of *Index Medicus,* who later founded the New York Public Library. In France we had Charles Wickersheimer (1880-1965), librarian of the Université de Strassbourg, author of *La médecine et les médecins en France à l'époque de la Renaissance*, and in Paris the three generations Hahn, librarians of the Faculté de Médecine, that had the largest medical library in the world before the rise of the Library of the Surgeon General in Washington; by their publications many treasures in their custody were disclosed. As examples in England I would like to mention Leslie T. Morton, librarian of the National Institute of Medical Research, whose *Annotated checklist of texts illustrating the history of medicine* has to be under reach of hands of every medical and veterinary librarian, and next to him Frederick Poynter (1908-), who was the librarian of the Wellcome Institute, and who is mainly known for his bibliographic work, amongst others for compiling the intricate bibliography of the most prolific 17th century English veterinary author Gervaise Markham.

WHAT ABOUT VETERINARY LIBRARIANS IN THIS RESPECT?

Of course the number of veterinary librarians is much smaller than that of medical librarians, but more importantly, the staffs are smaller so that it was often not possible to give attention to other matters than the daily routines. The only exceptions I know of are to be found in the German-speaking area, corresponding with the region where veterinary history is cultivated more intensively than in other parts of the world. The names that come to mind are those of the former librarian of the Veterinary School in Vienna, Oskar Ritter von Troll-Obergfell, who compiled

Ergänzungen und Berichtigungen zum Biographisch-literarischen Lexikon der Tierärzte aller Zeiten und Länder von Georg Wilhelm Schrader und Eduard Hering, published in a series of issues of *Beiträge zur Geschichte der Veterinärmedizin* between 1939 and 1945. Further the former librarian of the Veterinary Faculty in Bern, who was also the professor of veterinary parasitology, Bernard Hörning, and the former librarian of the Veterinary School in Hannover, Klaus Baresel. Both of them published bio/bibliographical studies. A man still active in the field of veterinary history is our former colleague in Kopenhagen, Ivan Katic, who after being pensioned as research librarian continues to teach veterinary history, to take care of the local Veterinary Museum and to edit *Historia Medicinae Veterinariae*, founded by him in 1976. Also Linda Warden of the Royal Veterinary College and Pelle Räf of the Skara Library are very much engaged in historical research. I cite these names only to demonstrate that the combination of medical or veterinary librarianship and activities in the field of medical or veterinary history are not exceptional at all. But, alas, they are not the rule either. The daily workload and the great efforts needed to face the rapid changes in the information landscape often prevent giving attention to matters of the past, how interesting they may be. It is also true that most of our patrons ask only very recent information, so that there is hardly an incentive to devote much time to investigate the older parts of the collection, to search the offers made in antiquarian or auction catalogues in order to supplement the own collection, to study the scope and coverage of special bibliographies that may be of use only incidentally, or to read much of the large supply of books and articles on the history of the biomedical sciences.

The question I want to lay before you is, whether this pragmatical attitude is to be regarded as the highest wisdom. In my opinion it is not. The reason behind springs from the idea of the librarian as an intermediary. Not only as an intermediary between the demands of patrons with specific subject questions and the databases that are the most likely to provide the answers, not only as intermediary between the booksellers or publishers and the needs of the community to serve, but also as intermediary between the past and the future.

The tasks to accomplish in bridging the past the and the future enclose two fields of activities: one directed to the collections of the older library materials, and the other directed to the users of the library.

With regard to the older library materials we are the temporary keepers of a heritage entrusted to our care for the period of time we are in office; then this heritage has to be passed on to our successors, well preserved and possibly enriched. In the most literal way we serve tradition; the word "tradition" is derived from the Latin "tradere" meaning: to transmit, to pass on.

During the last twenty years or so the problems connected with the keeping of the vulnerable printed materials are a main topic in the library world. Very costly solutions to prevent further crumbling of the paper, in use since the middle of the 19th century are proposed, but by lack of finances, generally, not more could be done than the creation of optimal conditions in the stacks or prevention of further decay by binding or storing in acid-free boxes. For veterinary medicine and allied sciences the situation is the more critical because the great bulk of its literature was published after 1850, precisely in the period of the bad quality paper. Furthermore the financing bodies of most veterinary libraries will turn a deaf ear to this kind of problems, as not many users are interested in the fate of old books and periodicals. And the programmes planned by organisations as the *European Commission on Preservation and Access (ECPA)* are directed to national or large research libraries. But these will concentrate their efforts to preserve the national literary production. This could mean that a veterinary historian of the future wanting to read the original papers of the first bacteriologists has to ask a copy from *Recueil Vétérinmaire* in the Bibliothèque de France or from *Berliner tierärztliche Wochenschrift* in the Deutsche Bibliothek! An alternative could be found in making accessible by computer the complete texts of the whole veterinary literature of the 19th century. But which organisation will take care? It is only to be hoped that it will not be too late at the time that the veterinary collections will be at their turn to be included in national de-acidification programmes. This is the more to be feared because they often belong to autonomous establishments of relativily small size as for instance the libraries of the Écoles Nationales Vétérinaires. For the libraries of Veterinary Faculties it is sometimes suggested that they should transfer their older materials to the central university library, because there conservation specialists are to be found, or there the environmental conditions would be better. In order to push of the problem, a Faculty Board could be inclined to this solution. I do not like this solution.

I believe that the primary and secondary sources have to be present in the same library. The fact that this condition cannot anymore be fulfilled for modern literature does not mean that this ideal has to be abandoned for the literature from the pre-World War II period, when the citations were not yet scatterd over so many journals. The knowledge of the primary and secondary sources, that is of the older publications and of the bibliographical and historiographical works, have to be concentrated in one hand, that of the veterinary librarian. Only then, the chance is given that the interested user can be served best. It has also to be remarked that the impediments to reach the wanted publications increase with the size of a library. By burying a historical veterinary collection in a university library the use of it will be still less than it is now. We must see to it that we do not make it too cumbersome for our users to check a reference in a periodical from the 19th century or to search illustrations from an old book.

However, this does not mean that books and periodicals that are not frequently consulted must be kept in open access. To protect them against unnecessary and unprofessional handling they have to be stored separated from the living collection in stacks in an optimal climate in order to preserve them. That is, indeed, the preferred method applied in most of the larger veterinary libraries now, as I was able to observe in Kopenhagen, Vienna, Hannover, Madrid and of course, also here in Utrecht; in Alfort only the very large old book collection is separated from the rest, but, alas, quite unaccessible.

A beautiful display of 5000 imprints from before 1850 is to be found in Budapest, housed in a stylish room and arranged according to the original classification. The collection contains among others 203 works collected by the founder of veterinary education in Hungary, prof. Sandor Tolnay. The reconstruction of this socalled *"Magyara-Kossa special historical collection"* very well illustrates what can be done by a veterinary library that understands its cultural role.

In this context mention is to be made of the *Comben-collection*, since 1987 incorporated in the Science Museum Library's Rare Book Collection in London; this collection was not formed over a long period of time in the framework of an establishment for veterinary education, but during the lifetime of a veterinarian, Norman Comben of Berkhamsted, England, who with much bibliographical knowledge and great zeal collected some 900 printed books and pamphlets, mainly illustrating the veterinary developments in the United Kingdom. It is well described in a published catalogue. It is meant as a research collection, and, therefore, contains "a substantial set of reference works and other secondary material, in particular bibliographies, catalogues, histories and biographies" (HMV, 18 (1993), p. 48).

A comparable collection, that illustrates mainly the much later developments in the United States, was brought together by prof. J. Fred Smithcors, "the dean of American veterinary historians", who donated this library to Washington State University. He compiled also a nicely produced catalogue under the title *Five centuries of veterinary medicine* (1997), that describes 1729 printed works and 26 archival entities.

The three mentioned special collections are all well catalogued, be it that the catalogue of the historical collection in Budapest is produced only by multiplying the catalogue cards on loose leaves (six on each leaf).

Disclosure

That brings me to the vexed question of the disclosure of the treasures, still hidden in the libraries of veterinary schools. Although more and more catalogues are already accessible through the Internet, most of them are far from complete with regard to the older parts of the collections.

For the cause of historical research, it would be of considerable interest to monitor the state of affairs of retrospective cataloguing in each European country and the degree of access to the several automated catalogues of the libraries with important collections of veterinary historical holdings. It would be very desirable to have a common database of all veterinary imprints of the 16th till the 19th century, like such a database is available for medical history at NLM or at the Wellcome Institute, in electronic as well as in printed form. An analogous facility for veterinary history could be achieved only by cooperation.

The Veterinary Library Group of EAHIL could perform a wonderful task to further this cause, starting with a report on the state of affairs of retrospective cataloging and discussing the possibility to set up a central catalogue for the pre-1900 imprints.

Preservation and access

Another sphere of activities by which the veterinary librarian can contribute to the cause of veterinary history is not so much connected with materials, but with human beings as professors, students, historians or their associations. The library has to supply them and to teach them. This task is especially important if the school or faculty does not have a special institute or chair for the history of veterinary medicine. In those cases only the library will be the place where people can orient themselves on historical matters. But, then, veterinary history has to be included in the collection development profile. As the literary production in the field is quite modest, the budget will not be burdened too much. The few periodicals, that exist[1] are cheap; the dissertations devoted to historical subjects can be obtained by exchange and the number of monographs, Festschriften, bibliographies, biographies, symposium proceedings or exhibition catalogs, generally, will, generally, not surpass the number of twenty per year, half of them belonging to the socalled grey literature.

Nevertheless, the situation is not as bright as might be expected. In an investigation, undertaken last year by prof. Schäffer (the professor for veterinary history at the Veterinary College of Hannover) one of the questions was: "Does your veterinary school library have a collection of books or a section dedicated to veterinary history?". Of the 90 answers received 37 were negative. It must be admitted that the question may have lead to some ambiguity, because some deans may have interpreted it as asking after the availability of an old book collection, whereas others may have interpreted the question as asking after the availability of a collection of historiographical materials. The negative answers came for a large part fom non-European schools; but even in Europe 9 of 48 schools reported negatively. And from 23 European schools no answer was received.

The lack of good historical resources is the more serious as regular courses in the history of veterinary medicine are presented only in a minority of the schools. Only twelve veterinary schools in the world have funded positions to teach history; half of them only on a part-time basis. There are ten more schools where the teaching is done by volunteers and in 17 cases some history education is provided in the framework of other courses, as pathology or microbiology. Only in Germany, Poland, Romania and Turkey the course is required; in the other countries, also here in Utrecht, it is optional. So, many establishments of veterinary education seem to consider history teaching as a posteriority. Some deans excused themselves pointing to the overburdened curriculum, others to the lack of funds to hire appropriate persons to teach a course or to set up a library with the necessary reference materials.

If you will agree with me that an academic library has the task to be as an encyclopaedia and to offer its users the full spectrum of the documents belonging to the disciplne it serves, then, in the first place, the generalities, including the history of the subject, have to be taken care of. The least we can do is to expose our users to the sources: by regular exhibitions of historical documents and by a proper arrangement on the shelves of historiographical documents.

A next step is to introduce potential users to these sources. Leading them to the items present, is a form of teaching. It must not be too difficult to direct the attention from the current literature to the literature of the immediate past and from there to its authors or to the circumstances in which the research was done, that means to the historical context.

Apart from the fact that each topic needs an introduction that reflects the work done earlier, each academically trained person has to develop a sense for the time dimension of his science, and he has to develop an understanding for the gradual growth of his discipline and his profession. This surely applies to the veterinarian whose forebearers had to fight so long before being allowed to enter academia.

The laws of causality, that are at the heart of the natural sciences, are to be supplemented by an understanding of another type of causality that lies in the succession of events that have led to the actual state of the art. In this view the library can make up for the holes in many programmes of veterinary education of today. It has to be admitted that in our pragmatic era students are often more inclined to obtain fast results or in winning study-points than in an understanding of much of the backgrounds; also it has to be admitted that most students are only willing to devote their attention to other matters than those that are strictly prescribed, if the value of this intellectual exercise is impressed on them by a parent or a teacher. If that turns out to be the case and they are sent to the library, are we then properly equiped to guide them? Not only with the reference materials I discussed earlier, but also with the knowledge to conduct them on the paths to follow? For that goal the librarian has to find time and energy to orient him- or herself on each of the topics brought forward. The usual catalogues and the databases, consulted for topics of actual research questions more often than not let us down in case of questions in the field of veterinary history. It must be noticed that the tools necessary for veterinary historical research are quite underdeveloped. Our two biographical dictionaries date from the

19th century and we have nothing comparable to the *Bibliography of the History of Medicine* (HISTLINE of NLM).

In order to further the case of veterinary history the World Association for the History of Veterinary Medicine has undertaken to set up a project to compile an *International Dictionary of Veterinary Biography*. Also preparations are made now, to make available on the Internet a database containing references to publications of relevance to the history of veterinary medicine. This database, compiled with the help of PROCITE, contains now nearly 7000 references, with indexes of persons, subjects, time periods and geographical areas. The non-English titles are translated in English. The intention is to present a research tool as comprehensive as possible, covering all types of the secondary literature: books, book chapters, periodical articles and dissertations from all countries and all times. You will understand that the completion of such a work will keep a person still busy for some time!

Most of you will have received recently a questionnaire asking for your cooperation in the setup of the *Dictionary of Veterinary Biography*. This questionnaire is sent worldwide to National Veterinary Associations, National Societies for the History of Veterinary Medicine and Veterinary Museums; and to all European Establishments of Veterinary Education and Veterinary Libraries, all together 311 addresses. It is intended, in the first place, to probe the interest for this project, and also to get an idea of the number of biographies to be written and an indication of possible authors. In a second phase a possible sponsor and publisher will be approached. I hope that all of you will give your support to this project that can bring forth not only a monument for all the people who helped to build the veterinary sciences what they are today, but also a new mighty work of reference.

It will be evident that I hope that all veterinary librarians will give their support to the cause of veterinary history. This can be done in various ways: by giving care to the resources under your guard, by guiding the library users to these resources, by cooperation with the veterinary history society in your country, with the curators of veterinary museums or the keepers of the archives in your neighbourhood, and by seeing to it that your library will be an associate member of the World Association for the History of Veterinary Medicine.

Notes

[1] ARGOS, Australian Veterinary History Record, Årbok: Norske Veterinærhistorisk Selskap, Dansk Veterinærhistorisk Årbog, Historia Medicinae Veterinariae, Japanese Journal of Veterinary History, Veterinärhistoriska Museet Skara Meddelande, Veterinary Heritage, Veterinary History

Chapter 8: MEDICAL SCHOOL AND UNIVERSITY LIBRARIES

Introduction

The papers brought together in this chapter are related to the state of the art and developments in academic libraries more or less involved in medical or pharmaceutical education. Some colleagues describe the role of their library in general; others give more detailed reports about the impact of changes in the curriculum on library services. Problem based learning (PBL) might, according to the editor's opinion, as well be named library based learning. The experiences show that it is impossible to perform a PBL program without the involvement and particpation of the library.

Another important development, i.e. that of evidence based medicine (EBM), is also reflected in medical education and the library's role. The methods vary, but the role of sound, high quality and ready available information both in PBL and EBM is obvious. For some the computer assisted learning (CAL) might seem a solution to get around the library. But our colleagues from the University of London, Susan Gove and Jean Yeoh report that the library is well suited to host the CAL facilities and will offer a 'natural habitat' of all kinds of learning material, where a whole range of individual study methods can be offered to the students.

Other papers in these proceedings related to education and therefore rather important for librarians working in academic medical institutions, are: the paper of Urquhart and Davies (Chpt. 9 p. 173) and the papers of Massiter and Urquhart, Faraino and Vieira, Simpson et al., Wickman, and Brice and Tomlin in chapter 10: "User education and user needs" (from p. 183).

LES AVANTAGES ET LES MENACES: LA RESTRUCTURATION DE LA BIBLIOTHÈQUE MÉDICALE UNIVERSITAIRE

Anna Maria Uryga
UNIVERSITÉ JAGELLONNE, COLEGIUM MÉDICUM, BIBLIOTHÈQUE MÉDICALE, POLAND

Abstract

The Medical Library of Jagiellonian University in Cracow consists of the Central Library and 70 small libraries at different institutes and clinics. The distances between Central Library, university centre, and branch libraries differ from 10 to 20 km. and this is a main reason for library dysfunctioning. An attempt, undertaken in 1996, to restructure the old library system, led to certain solutions. The assessment of these improvements is subject of this presentation. Among the barriers for facilitating access to information sources the most important was and is lack of tele-communication infrastructure in the area where the Central Library is located. Waiting for optimal solution to this problem (fiberoptic cable) didn't slow down changes in the library services, an introduction of several technological improvements. Among these changes are: the development of Intranet, providing network services through other, co-operating with us institutions, (i.e. access to MEDLINE installed at the host of Institute of Physics), modernisation of the library rooms, changes in organisational structure and in human resources policy, specialisation of information services, and new projects aiming towards tightening the co-operation among librarians, doctors and pharmacists. These developments allow for considerable optimism when looking into the future of medical library services in Cracow.

Introduction

La Bibliothèque Médicale de l'Université Jagellonne (BMUJ) est la plus ancienne des bibliothèques de ce type en Pologne. L'unité organisationnelle indépendante des facultés de médecine et de pharmacie (Collegium Médicum), elle fait partie de labibliothèque nationale (Bibliothèque Jagellonne) dont les missions sont: le service, la pédagogie et la recherche. Depuis 1984, la Bibliothèque Médicale fonctionne dans un nouveau bâtiment, qui est éloigné d'environ 10-20 km du centre universitaire et du centre hospitalier universitaire. Le système d'information de cette bibliothèque, comprenant la bibliothèque centrale au tant que centre logistique et 70 unités associées dans le cadre du C.H.U., présente beaucoup d'éléments de dysfonctionnement.

Evaluation du projet de la restructuration

En considérant la distance qui sépare la bibliothèque de la vie universitaire et hospitalière, on peut constater que ce modèle concret exprime un besoin de devolopper l'idée de la bibliothèque virtuelle et sans limite à l'avenir. Les objectifs de la restructuration que nous avons définis en 1996 se réalisent sous la pression du temps et des moyens financiers. Un premier bilan indique les points positifs, les difficultes rencontrées et les prospectives.

LE TRAVAIL EN RESEAU

* l'optimisation de l'accès à l'information par la connexion par fibre optique de notre réseau local au réseau municipal (en conséquence, aux réseaux nationaux et à l'Internet) n'est pas atteint à l'heure actuelle.
* l'infrastructure téléinformatique et le NASK (Réseau de télécommunication pour l'enseignement et la recherche) ne sont pas developpés sur le terrain, où se trouve notre bibliothèque. La numérisation et la multiplication des réseaux ne sont pas considérées par les autorités universitaires et d'autres acteurs comme une entreprise commune et stratégique
* dans la situation, où le plan de l'informatisation du Collegium Médicum n'est pas vraiement défini (il n'y pas de la politique gestionnaire du réseau de campus et du centre de ressources informatiques), tous les besoins techniques et financiers de la bibliothèque médicale sont considérés comme peu importants par rapport aux dépenses lourdes du budget annuel de notre université
* tous les travaux liés à la conexion avec le système VTLS (Virginia Tech Library System) dont le server central se trouve dans la Bibliothèque Jagellonne (distance:16 km) et l'automatisation complète des tâches documentaires (surtout l'enregistrement éléctronique des cataloques) sont impossibles. Parmi les 12 grandes bibliothèques universitaires seulement la bibliothèque médicale ne peut pas participer activement dans le projet de l'informatisation piloté par le service interétablissement de coopération documentaire.

LES AUTRES FORMES TECHNIQUES À L'ACCES A L'INFORMATION

* le réseau local prévu pour les 70 postes est en cours d'installation. A l'heure actuelle sont à notre disposition: 20 ordinateurs, le server du réseau local équipé d'un processor Intel Pentium II avec la platforme Windows NT, 5 imprimantes et 2 modems.
* malgré tous les obstacles mentionnés ci-dessus, c'était bien sur l'initiation propre de la Bibliothèque Médicale et la première de ce type à Cracovie, que la base de donnés MEDLINE de système ERL (Silver Platter) a été mise en place en réseaux locaux de l'Université, via le server de l'Institut de la Physique
* la mise en place de quelques bases de données bibliographiques médicales polonaises et étrangères (Biblio, MEDLINE, Current Contents, International Pharmacetical Abstracts) et les bases multimédiales accessibles sur les CD-ROM dans l'atelier multimédia de la bibliothèque
* la modernisation avec la réorganisation des salles de lecture s'est trouvée dans le projet financé par la Fondation pour le Développement de la Science Polonaises en 1997. Grâce à ces moyens financiers nous avons obtenu un nouveau rayonage en raison de la présentation des collections en libre-accès, une salle de consultation de bases de données, un système d'observation des collections et le système anti-vol.

Tous les travaux qui ont été entreprises par ce projet nous ont permis d'économiser l'espace de la bibliothèque et de réstructurer les activités du personnel par l'exploitation appropriée des locaux.

LA STRUCTURE ORGANISATIONNELLE ET LA POLITIQUE D'EMPLOI

* d'après l'estimation des besoins quantitaifs et qualitatifs, la nouvelle structure d'organisation s'inscrit dans la logique du projet d'automatisation de la bibliothèque. Nous avons défini toutes les tâches correspondantes aux missions des 9 départements. Dans ce contexte nous avons prévu aussi la formation des documentalistes s'occupant de l'acquisition électronique, du catalogage dans le format USMARC du VTLS et de l'indexation adaptée au RAMEAU et au système d'information médicale. Cette formation était possible grâce à la coopération pilotée par le service interétablissement de coopération documentaire
* le plan d'emploi a permis de hiérarchiser la pyramide d'âges à savoir d'augmenter le nombre d'employés (12 personnes) dans la tranche d'âge 20-35 et de renforcer les qualifications professionnelles du personnel.

L'ORGANISATION DES SERVICES D'INFORMATION ET LA DOCUMENTATION SPECIALISÉE

* la recherche documentaire informatisée pour les étudiants et les professionels de la santé avec l'aide du personnel des documentalistes specialisés en nouvelles techniques d'information et de recherche
* la préparation des outils d'informations sur l'Internet médical et les abonements des journaux accessibles en version imprimée/ou on-line dans le système d'organisation de notre bibliothèque et 70 unités (les bibliothèques d'établissements)
* le renforcement des services des prêts locaux, des prêts entre-bibliothèques et des prêts interétrangers de même qu'une meilleure circulation des documents entre toutes les établissements
* suite aux efforts de formation des utilisateurs à la recherche documentaire nous réalisons les cours pour les praticiens préparant leurs thèses de doctorat. Les séminaires et les ateliers basés sur les consultations des bases de données comprennent 10 heurs.
* nous avons commencé la préparation d'ouvrages et de périodiques pour leurs presentation en libre-accès et leurs évaluation qualificative et quantitative. Nous voudrions renforcer certains secteurs de différents domaines et aider les bibliothèques d'établissements à se spécialiser. Pour ce faire, nous avons adapté le plan de classements de NLM (National Library of Medicine) aux besoins de nos collections et aux conditions polonaises. L'accès-libre, la présentation de toutes les collections récentes, l'installation d'un atelier multimédia en rapport avec les nouvelles techniques de réproduction et de traitement de l'image permettront d'augmenter l'attractivité des services d'information et la fréquentation des usagers.

LES PROSPECTIVES

* dans le but de la création d'un club de l'Internet pour le professionel de la santé nous avons envisagé la coopération très proche avec une maison d'édition 'Medycyna Praktyczna' Ce nouveau projet est financé par la Fondation S. Batory (Open Society Fund) et il nous permet d'organiser les cours de formation dans le domaine de l'Internet médical.

* l'autre projet commun avec la Fondation de la Santé Publique et la Pharmacie Hospitalière du C.H.U concerne la création d'un nouveau outil accesible dans l'Internet: "la base de données question-réponse sur les medicaments". Il sera basé sur les documents et les réferences distribuées par l'intermédiaire de notre bibliothèque. Dans ce deuxième projet, dont l'idée de même que le budget a trouvé l'acceptation de la part de la Fondation S. Batory, participent activement les pharmaciens hospitaliers ainsi que les médecins.

Conclusions

AU PLAN CONCRÈTE

La constitution d'un système des bibliothèques d'établissements avec bibliothèque centrale par la fusion et la réorganisation des collections et des services sur l'ensemble des locaux anciens et nouveaux nous permettra d'intensifier le rôle du coordinateur du service commun. Cette nouvelle entité, résolument axée sur la rapidité et l'accès libre à l'information et aux documents, est ouvert au public. En ce qui concerne la distance entre la bibliothèque et les usagers de l'information, dans le proche avenir, il faudra trouver les modes de financement des investissements pour que ce projet soit realisé avec utilisation de plusieurs outils informatiques.

Les changements progressifs des formes d'organisation du travail, la formation et l'amélioration des capacités du personnel, l'exploitation et le développement des talents: tout ceci devrait viser à retenir un plan garantissant la stabilité et la satisfaction professionnele de l'équipe de la bibliothèque. Dans l'exercise de la fonction du directeur de la bibliothèque il faut être toujours attaché à gérer le personel comprenant toutes catégories professionnelles de manière à optimiser les services rendus au public. En effet, dans un contexte souvant peu favorable tant au niveau des moyens en personnel que budgétaires, le directeur devrait avoir la conviction que la motivation et la dynamisation de l'équipe sur des objectifs clairement définis sera la seule solution pour accompagner l'évolution de l'environnement universitaire et documentaire.

Une étape importante pour la Bibliothèque est celle de l'informatisation de la gestion et des catalogues. Cette mutation implique une formation et une adaptation plus ou moins rapides du personnel ainsi qu'une analyse approfondie du fonctionnement des services en vue de leur rationalisation. Par ailleurs, l'explosion de la demande dans le domaine de la recherche documentaire informatisée impose un changement radical des pratiques documentaires traditionnelles. Cependant, la multiplication des bases de données et la diffusion de l'information par l'Internet induit la nécessité de généraliser la formation des utilisateurs à l'interrogation par le biais de differénts moyens d'information.

AU PLAN GENERAL

Le développement des réseaux en Pologne, notamment de l'Internet, a connu un essor considérable ces dernières années[1]. Il concerne presque tous les domaines de la vie social. Malheureusement, l'Internet n'a toutefois pas progressé de la même manière dans tous les secteurs. Le développement des réseaux dans les bibliothèques de santé dispose malgré tout de certains atouts pour une progression rapide. Le premier en est une grande motivation: l'absence quasi complète de possibilités de connexion aux réseaux (aux réseaux régionaux, nationaux et internationaux) sous l'ancien régime a crée une énorme soif d'information et de communication. Le second est une grande capacité d'absorption: il existe un grand nombre de spécialistes ayant une préparation théorique et pratique suffisante pour intégrer très rapidement les rangs des professionels de l'information médicale et de l'Internet médico-pharmaceutique. Le seul obstacle qui nous reste souvent à franchir est la barrière linguistique. On peut constater que beaucoup reste à faire pour que les modes de fonctionnement des centres de documentation dans le domaine de la santé ainsi que la densité de l'Internet dans notre pays se rapproche de celle de l'Europe occidentale. Mais, grâce au potentiel local, à la cooperation entre les institutions au niveau national, à l'aide internationale et à la nature même de l'Internet, les chances de réussite sont grandes.

Bibliographie

[1] Sterba M. L'Internet dans les pays de l'Europe de l'Est. Dans: L'Internet professionnel. Témoignages, expériences, conseils pratiques de la communauté enseignement et recherche. Paris: CNRS Editons, 1995

NEW CHALLENGES AND ROLES FOR LIBRARY STAFF IN RESPONSE TO CHANGES IN THE BIOMEDICAL CURRICULA IN U.K. UNIVERSITIES

Michelle Wake, Linda Lisgarten
LIBRARY AND INFORMATION SERVICE, SCHOOL OF PHARMACY, UNIVERSITY OF LONDON, LONDON, UK

The school of pharmacy and it's library

The Library at the School of Pharmacy serves an independent biomedical college of the University of London. Two undergraduate courses are taught at the School and postgraduate courses are also provided for. Research is also undertaken on the highest level.

The Library, which serves approximately 900 users, is part of a converged Information Service, which is headed by the Chief Librarian. However, the Computer and Multimedia Units are unable to give the Library a high level of support. The Library itself is small in size having been built to serve only 200 students and staff. The Library has now been extended three times however it is still way below any U.K. Government recommendations for study space and shelving.

Like many medical libraries, we have been in the forefront of utilising new technology. Many of our everyday procedures are computerised and we have a host of PCs. However, before the major changes to the curriculum in 1996 the pace of life was a little slower!

The case examined in this paper is an example of how the introduction of problem based learning (PBL) affects the library and how libraries tight for spaces and with even tighter budgets can cope.

The change to PBL

However, in the past 2 years there have been changes in the content and execution of the undergraduate courses at the School and this has had a profound effect on the Library, with two major curriculum reviews having been implemented. The biggest impact on the Library so far has been a change to teaching methods which are similar to problem based learning.

Medical schools have been at the forefront of this method since the 1960s.[1] In the U.K. we have taken a little longer than some to introduce the method. In 1989 one of The School's departments experimented with PBL and declared it a success.[2] The University of Manchester, in 1994, became the first British medical school to use PBL as its main learning method[2] and it is now used to some degree in medical schools in Glasgow, Liverpool and elsewhere.[1] After positive reports from medical schools and with encouragement from the RPSGB and the GMC[4,5] the use of PBL was extended at the School of Pharmacy in 1996.

The problem

At the School we experienced changes very similar to those reported in the majority of PBL libraries.[6] There has been a great increase in the use of printed stock, electronic databases are accessed more, videos are played to destruction, photocopiers are put on overdrive, CAL (computer assisted learning) packages are devoured and interlibrary loans have risen dramatically. It is true that all students use these methods of learning, but we have found that PBL students not only use them more intensively but also present us with more complex enquiries.

These changes have put pressure on library staff time and the library staff themselves need to learn new skills to keep up with the new technologies and to take on a para-academic role. At the School we have always had a "teaching" role. However, our teaching wasn't fully integrated into the curriculum.

In the autumn term of 1996 we were suddenly swamped by first years needing to use the library in an advanced fashion. We quickly realised that they needed to have the skills that we had traditionally associated with final year undergraduates or even postgraduates. The academics involved with teaching hadn't realised how big our role would be.

The biggest change in library use has been caused by group study. As Jennifer Blake has said, PBL students "travel in packs".[7] However, we still have users who need to work alone and want the Library to remain quiet. The layout and size of our library doesn't help. It wasn't built for group study. Desks are next to the walls and noise travels from one area of the library to another.

Of course for some of the problems exacerbated by PBL, such as inadequate seating space and funding, there are textbook recommendations. However, the internal politics of the College have meant that we cannot always do what the textbooks recommend.

The solution?

We began by reviewing the literature on PBL and contacted the teaching staff to find out exactly what the new curriculum involved and sat down to analyze how it would probably affect us. We then attempted to convince them that we had a vital role to play.

As a result of these contacts we were able to have some influence and make suggestions. For instance, we created a new short loan "Teaching Collection" of textbooks with funds from the College's Teaching Budget, i.e. extra to the library budget. This has proved to be a great success with the inevitable result that our issue desk transactions went up even more! However, this alone gave us good grounds to ask for another member of library staff.

We are also trying to encourage the academics to produce lists of textbooks that they recommend students to purchase to ease demand on the library's collections.

We are trying very hard to maintain a dialogue with all our users and although library staff are on various committees, we have found that informal discussions are often the most productive. However, we are seeing less of the academic staff in the library because of the electronic networking of information and because of the noise levels. Recognising this long distance relationship, we've set up an e-mail suggestions box, we post information onto our Web site and send out newsletters.

It was obvious early on that we had to re-think how we trained undergraduates. For our own sanity we knew we had to teach them in time tabled groups. It also had to be relevant to their course work and be taught when they needed it. So, we began teaching first years just after they have been given their first assignment. We lean this training heavily towards solving that assignment and incorporate question sheets on library skills. However, because of a shortage of library staff time and a packed timetable we only have the students for a half day so we can really only skim the surface of what they will eventually need.

The question sheets that we set for the students have been useful, in that we can see where the students have problems. It's made us think about how we explain things, and has prompted us to re-design the layout of the library stock into a more simple format. For example we have tried to combine our different reference sections into one. This re-arrangement of stock was made easier by the fact that the library had a small extension built in the Summer of 1996 which gave us more shelf space and also provided us with extra seating and computer sockets. To help cope with the increased demand for our PCs, we brought in a reservation system.

We are still struggling with the noise issue. We initially felt that the library should be maintained as a quiet area. Our first idea was to allow Teaching Collection books to be taken out of the library. However, it is obvious to us that the noise problem is not going to go away and it's true that students prefer to work in the library where they can be close to a range of sources. To find out what all members of the College think we have sent out a questionnaire. But ultimately we will always have to organise study areas outside the library as we only have 70 seats.

So we have tried to maximise as efficiently as we can our own resources and to redirect funding to the undergraduates as fairly as we can without harming the researchers. But we are a small library and we can't meet the needs of our users all the time. So we do rely on interlibrary co-operation.

The future

Although the merits of PBL compared to traditional methods are part of a continued debate PBL appears to have many benefits to students including effective development of self-directing learning skills.[8] With this in mind it is probable that the use of PBL will increase.

Our PBL students do use the library differently to those using traditional methods and we are increasingly going to have to take this into account. In the future we aim to make information skills teaching an integral part of the curriculum, something that has been achieved by the University of Manchester,[9] so that students are highly motivated and can see how it can help with their course work and future profession. We need to constantly review user needs and find time to have training ourselves. We also hope to be able to network more of our database services to ease space problems.

Benefits to the library / Conclusion

I hope this paper has not given the impression that problem based learning is just one big problem for libraries. There have been some aspects to it. PBL's encouragement of independent learning gives libraries an increased role in higher education. The

Library becomes essential to the success of the undergraduate courses. It's encouraged us to review our services to make sure we are providing our users with what they want and what they need. It's improved our contacts with the academics, made us more proactive and raised our profile within the College. It's also made our jobs more interesting - busier, but definitely more interesting!

References

[1] Bligh J. Problem based, small group learning: an idea whose time has come. Br Med J 1995;311:342-343

[2] Buckton G, Bates IP. A problem-based learning approach to pharmaceutical education. Int Pharm J 1991;5:7-13

[3] O'Neill PA. [letter]. Br Med J 1995;311:1643

[4] Council of the Royal Pharmaceutical Society. Approval of four-year degree courses from 1997. Pharm J 1995;254:504-509

[5] General Medical Council. Tomorrow's doctors. Report of the Education Committee. London: GMC, 1993

[6] Rankin JA. Problem-based learning and libraries: a survey of the literature. Health Libr Rev 1996;13:33-42

[7] Blake J. Library resources for problem-based learning: the program perspective. Comp Meth Progr Biomed 1994;44:167-173

[8] Donner RS, Bickley H. Problem based learning: an assessment of its feasibility and cost. Hum Pathol 1990;21:881-885

[9] Ferguson V. Planning and providing a course of problem-based library skills for medical and dental undergraduates: the first year. Health Libr Rev 1996;13:43-47

INTRODUCING EVIDENCE BASED PRACTICE: THE LIBRARY'S ROLE IN TEACHING ABOUT CRITICAL INFORMATION TOOLS

Keir Reavie
VERA P. SCHIFFMAN MEDICAL LIBRARY, WAYNE STATE UNIVERSITY,. DETROIT, USA

Introduction

The introduction of evidence based practice to medical students is spreading rapidly in medical education. In the majority of cases, this education begins in Residency programs,[1-3] where the student, for the first time, is required to access and use the medical literature. It has been shown however, that there is a dramatic effect on the efficiency and quality of a student's future clinical performance if exposed to evidence based practice earlier, in an undergraduate curriculum.[4] At the Wayne State University (WSU) School of Medicine the student is introduced to evidence based concepts in medical practice in a mandatory two and a half week first-year course, well before they will encounter real-life clinical situations. The earlier exposure to evidence based practice can alleviate many of the problems encountered in introducing students to these concepts later in their education.

The Shiffman Medical Library at WSU plays an integral part in the mandatory first year evidence-based medicine course. The Library first became involved in the class in the Fall semester of 1996. In the Fall of 1997 the course changed significantly, and the Library became more heavily involved in the teaching process. The library moved from discussing and demonstrating the access and use of essential evidence based practice resources, presented in a single lecture, to being involved in a lecture, demonstrations, hands-on training, and one-on-one assistance in the library, directed toward the completion of a required assignment.

Methods

In the first lecture, students receive an assignment that presents a series of specific questions, each of which are best answered by different information sources: 1) A recent textbook of internal medicine, such as Harrison's Principle's of Internal Medicine; 2) The journal literature, accessed by searching the MEDLINE database, and; 3) A structured review, found in publications like the ACP Journal Club. The assignment focused on diagnostic and therapeutic questions about a patient with congestive heart failure. Students were required to answer clinical questions, and briefly discuss the resources they used to answer them. The assignment is not marked, but must be completed. It is discussed amongst students and medical faculty in group settings at the end of the course. The assignment provided significant detail on how to access and use the resources needed to answer the questions.

The large size of the first year class at WSU (over 250 students) posed some unique teaching problems for the library. To prepare students for completing the assignment, optional hands-on training sessions, facilitated by librarians, were held within the library's computer labs. Ten 1 hour sessions with an upper limit of 25 students per session, were scheduled to accommodate the possible attendance of the 262 registered students. Expectations for the number of actual participants were far lower. These sessions consisted of a demonstration on accessing and using key health sciences information resources within the library and on the Internet, as well as hands-on time, in which the students could work on their assignment and ask any questions of the attending librarians. The training provided students with the background to locate a book in the library, and to use MEDLINE and Internet resources. Librarians were also available in the library for the duration of the course to provide personal assistance to students.

The library also created a World Wide Web resource that contained the assignment and direct links to the Internet resources needed for its completion. The inclusion of this online resource is particularly important because of the enormity of the first-year class. Not all students would be able to attend the hands-on training, and many students prefer to learn certain concepts via the computer. Students could also ask questions regarding the material directly from the resource using an electronic mail link.

Toward the end of the course, a team composed of a librarian and a physician presented a lecture that included a demonstration of information resources available for evidence based practice. The lecture discussed how the medical literature works; from basic research, to clinical trials, to reviews and meta-analyses, to becoming standard knowledge in practice guidelines and textbooks. The lecture concluded with a demonstration on how to access the different kinds of literature in the library and on the Internet.

Attendance at the optional hands-on training and the frequency of access to the web resource was used to elucidate the students preferences for learning this material; either in a one-on-one session, through group training, or web-based learning on their own time. The course has been part of the curriculum for only two years, and data on learning preferences will provide important information for its future structure.

Results

Attempting to assist the 262 first-year students with the exercises posed a major problem. There was no way to focus the needed attention on individual students, or to provide small group learning sessions. Because of the short time-frame for the course (two and a half weeks), student assistance had to be squeezed into a short time-frame as well. Only 12 students in total attended the scheduled hands-on straining, or 4.6 percent of the entire class. As well, only 38 students, or 14.5 percent of the class, asked a librarian for individual assistance with the assignment. In contrast, 98 percent of the class handed in a completed assignment. Follow-up discussions between students and faculty indicated that the students had a good grasp of what was required to complete the assignment. The results show that students were able to develop at least a basic understanding of the important tools for accessing evidence based practice materials without much help.

The small group of students that requested assistance had fairly standard problems with the assignment: How to access and use the Internet, and: how to access and search MEDLINE. They did not seem to grasp the complexity of searching the MEDLINE database well. These were people that had little or no experience in using computers, or the Internet. As well, the web resource was not used. It is a reasonable assumption that students with Internet experience could simply access the resources by using the Internet addresses provided in the assignment handouts, rather than using the web resource as a guide.

An unforeseen problem with the scheduling of the hands-on sessions was an anatomy exam that fell near the end of the course. This may be one indicator of the small turnout at the sessions. It was highly unlikely that students would tackle the assignment until the last minute, after the exam. Time is always a problem in medical education and practice, particularly when having to access and evaluate the evidence in addition to regular clinical tasks.[5] However, since a large number of students completed the assignment, the objective of exposing them to the important resources, and in not having them spend too much time learning to be the most efficient online searcher, met with reasonable success. Hopefully, with early exposure to evidence based concepts, student's searching efficiency can be developed throughout their education.

Conclusions

There was much to be learned from this first attempt to expose medical students to accessing and using medical literature early in their undergraduate medical education. It would appear that many of the incoming students already have some understanding of the Internet and using computers to access information, and even in searching MEDLINE.

Students rated the lectures and demonstrations highly in the course evaluations. They found them useful and insightful, and as such, they will be used again this year. Fewer hands-on sessions will be scheduled for this year's class. However, the librarians will continue to be prepared to provide personal assistance, since there appears to be a greater preference for this mode of learning with students that do require help.

The first-year evidence based medicine class has exposed students to the access and use of medical literature, but over time they will have to be continually exposed, enabling them to become more efficient in retrieving vital clinical information, and to overcome the time constraint problems associated with using the evidence. Future steps in this educational process will be to involve the library in further training of students as they enter the clinical years of their education, and as they graduate and move into Residency programs.

References

[1] Evidence-Based Medicine Working Group. Evidence-Based Medicine. A New Approach to Teaching the Practice of Medicine. JAMA 1992;268:2420-2425

[2] Chessare JB. Teaching Clinical Decision-making to Pediatric Residents in an Era of Managed Care. Pediatrics 1998;101:762-767

[3] Grimes DA. Introducing Evidence-based Medicine into a Department of Obstetrics and Gynecology. Obstet Gynecol 1995;86:451-457

[4] Shin JH, Haynes RB, Johnston ME. Effect of Problem-based, Self-directed Undergraduate Education on Life-long Learning. Can Med Assoc J 1993;148:969-976

[5] Sackett DL. ...so little time, and... Evidence-Based Med 1997;2:39

RECALL: RETRIEVING AND EVALUATING CAL IN LIBRARIES

Susan Gove, Jean Yeoh
St George's Hospital Medical School, University of London, London, UK

Abstract

This paper examined a project which places libraries at the centre of a programme to promote CAL (Computer Assitsed Learning) packages to teaching staff and explore the role of libraries in curriculum and learning processes. CAL programmes will be evaluated in terms of quality and use and made available to students and staff in the library environment. There are increasing numbers of computer assisted learning programs and multimedia packages available in medicine, dentistry, pharmacy, nursing, radiography and allied health. Other relevant materials for students of medicine and health care include generic programs on study skills and research.

As the central resources area the library already provides a 'one stop shop' for learning, with students able to move easily between different types of learning activity, and where resources in different formats complement each other in the learning process. Many CAL programmes are ideally suited to independent individualised learning and libraries are uniquely placed within academic institutions to offer a supportive environment where students are able to adopt learning methods and learning style of choice.

NLM FREE MEDLINE IN THE BIOMEDICAL LIBRARIES OF PADUA UNIVERSITY

Luciano Galfano, Elisabetta Marinoni, Pierangela Mazzon, Donata Pieri, Roberta Sato
UNIVERSITÀ DEGLI STUDI DI PADOVA, ITALY

PubMed, Grateful Med, ERL: a comparison

The recent decision of the National Library of Medicine of Bethesda (NLM) to allow all Internet users access to the PubMed database[1] (has stimulated our Libraries (the Vallisneri Biomedical Library, the Library of Department of Pharmacology and the Library of Institute of Hygiene) to make a comparison between the MEDLINE free-use and the product available in the local Padua University network (Silver Platter MEDLINE Advanced).

In our University, MEDLINE and other biomedical databases are ERL (Electronic Reference Library) compliant and they can be accessed through the World Wide Web browsers too, without having to install special software and set up formal workstations. The common access software for various databases allows not only ease and speed of access but also gives priority to locally installed databases.

However, at the beginning an intensive personnel training program was necessary to understand the characteristics of the different databases, in order to exploit the potentiality of the software to the full. The training program (which still continues) involves both the users and the librarians of the various University structures.

On the other hand, some of the free MEDLINE[2] has come over as extremely user-friendly, even suitable for first time MEDLINE users. In this respect, PubMed (in its recently modified versions, Basic and Advanced Search mode) is a valuable source of bibliographic updating, given that even basic citation information becomes available before it are included in MEDLINE (PreMEDLINE). Available records go back to 1964-1965. This service can therefore be used to update bibliographic searches, available thanks to our local databases or to recuperate MEDLINE records not present in these. PubMed supplies links with other databases (DNA/protein sequences and 3-D structure data) and links with Web sites for full-text articles from journals, sometimes even available without password. After making a search, PubMed links up to other pertinent records, retrieved by the system with a complex relational algorithm. The Basic Search mode version of PubMed presents the option "Clinical Queries" (for searching subjects with a strictly clinical background) and also the option "Citation Matcher" which gives an easy and rapid check of bibliographic citations, together with a link to PubMed Advanced Search mode.

For those who are used to consulting the thesaurus directly, PubMed may have some limitations. However, in the latest version of PubMed an attempt to overcome this limitation is made with the option "Thesaurus browser". This option allows the MeSH thesaurus to be browsed, choosing the MeSH terms and transferring them to the search in PubMed Advanced Search (very suitable for complex searches).

In any case, there is also the free MEDLINE of the NLM, Internet Grateful MEDLINE (IGM), whose thesaurus contains also a link up to the Online Images web page available in History of Medicine databases. IGM can link up to other NLM free databases: AIDSLINE, AIDSDRUGS etc.

One limitation in using free MEDLINE is derived from Internet access in some periods of the day and during long link ups (especially for IGM) but above all in the long waits to obtain the record display and their abstracts (a problem that will be resolved thanks to future developments foreseen by NLM for PubMed.[3]

Conclusion

A comparative evaluation shows that the MEDLINE free version is, by now, consolidated and no less efficient and reliable than the proprietary version.

However, the proprietary product is still preferable when there is a vast and articulate academic community with a relevant number of connected WAN databases. In fact, it is extremely convenient for the academic researcher to be able to use the same software to consult with several databases, even at the same time.

References

[1] PubMed. <http://www.nlm.nih.gov/databases/freemedl.html>
[2] Anagnostelis B, et al. Evaluation criteria for different versions of the same database: a comparison of MEDLINE services available via the World Wide Web. <http://omni.ac.uk/agec/iolim97>
[3] PubMed News. <http://www4.ncbi.nlm.nih.gov/PubMed/news.html>

THE INFORMATION SERVICES OF THE CENTRAL LIBRARY OF THE SEMMELWEIS UNIVERSITY OF MEDICINE

Judit Szabó Szávay, Ildikó Rédei
CENTRAL LIBRARY OF THE SEMMELWEIS UNIVERSITY OF MEDICINE, BUDAPEST, HUNGARY

Information sources and data at the HELP DESK

TRADITIONAL SERVICES

Reference collection (dictionaires, almanacs, directories, registers)
Periodicals/journals lists (national and local)
Databases (books and journal bibliographies e.g.: National Periodical Database on CD-ROM 1981-1993, Hungarian Books Database on CD-ROM 1976-1991, Hungarian Medical Dissertation Database, Periodical List of the Semmelweis Medical University; commercial databases e.g.: Ulrich's Plus, Books in Print, Springer)
Integrated library system: HORIZON - OPAC

INFORMATION SOURCES IN THE ELECTRONIC LIBRARY CAMPUS-WIDE NETWORK

- CD-ROM

Bibliographic databases: ERL MEDLINE on Silver Platter, ERL International Pharmaceutical Abstracts, Science Citation Index, Current Contents Life Sciences, Current Contents Clinical Medicine
Full text databases: MEDLINE + OVID Biomedical Collections, MICROMEDEX CCIS, + Quality Assurance In Education
Educational and training programs

- Internet possibilities

The poster illustrated how the library serves the readers.

References

[1] Annual report of the Central Library of the Semmelweis University of Medicine 1990-1997. Budapest. 1991-1998. 8 pp.

Chapter 9: NURSING LIBRARIES

Editorial comment

The number of librarians specialized in nursing is rather small, probably because in many institutions the nursing collection is either part of the medical library or even not existing. It depends on the system and organization of higher education, whether there are specialized, more or less independent nursing schools with a specialized library, or that nursing education is an in-service training in hospitals or is part of a larger institute for all kinds of tertiary education.

The developments in nursing and nursing education are nonetheless of high relevance and very important for the services of both nursing and hospital libraries. Also in this area of health care a strong movement towards quality management and standards in professionalism is noticed. Professional development depends in the first place on professional bodies and organizations, on registration and certification of the profession and specific education. But to the heart of professionalism belongs a knowledge base, a cumulation of experience and knowledge, theory and practice, broad together along lines of critical and systematic procedures and evaluations, i.e. the professional literature found in libraries and documentation centres. The nursing libraries are essential elements to growth and further development of the nursing profession.

If it is not the nursing profession that seeks cooperation with the library, than librarians or the medical library professional bodies have to consider whether or not to take the initiative for cooperation and to offer support. In many countries the nursing education and profession is still on its way to grow and rise to academic levels. Scientific communication and publishing is not yet a self-evident part of nursing practice. The support of librarianship in the process of professionalization of nurses could turn out to be beneficial to both parties and could add to the image and self-esteem of both nurses and librarians.

USER EDUCATION STRATEGIES FOR SUPPORTING EVIDENCE-BASED NURSING PRACTICE: THE EVINCE PROJECT

Christine J. Urquhart, Rebecca Davies
DEPARTMENT OF INFORMATION AND LIBRARY STUDIES, UNIVERSITY OF WALES, ABERYSTWYTH, WALES, UK

EVINCE

The EVINCE (Establishing the Value of Information to Nursing Continuing Education) project, funded by the British Library Research and Innovation Centre had two aims: 1) to establish the value of information provided by library and information services to nursing knowledge and competence; and 2) to devise quality assurance guidelines for library services to nursing staff. The project lasted 12 months (1 November 1995 to 31 October 1996). The survey covered nurses and midwives (nursing professionals is the term used in this paper). Full results are found in the report[1] with main findings also available in.[2]

Nursing and midwifery staff account for a large proportion of National Health Service (NHS) staff and most UK nursing staff are still based in hospitals, though some work in the private sector. Post-registration nursing education has to cater for health professionals who may have several career breaks for family reasons. In the UK, library and information service provision for nursing professionals has been affected by the move of pre-registration nursing education into higher education. Libraries for nursing professionals are now more likely to be concentrated at higher education sites, and less likely to be in or near hospitals. More hospital libraries are now multidisciplinary, offering access to resources to all staff although their specialised nursing collections may be limited. Efforts are being made to meet the need for better library services for nursing professionals, but more co-operation between higher education and the NHS is required.[3]

SURVEYS

In the EVINCE project, nursing professionals using the library and information services of a variety of organisations (national services, higher education and/or NHS funded services) were asked to assess the value to their present and future competence of information obtained from various types of information request. Thirteen services were studied, with a response rate of 40% (311/776 requests - inter-library loan, CD-ROM (end-user) search or mediated search by library staff).

The information service users were also asked about the purposes of their information request, the background to the request and their attitudes towards information seeking. To set those assessments in context, a random sample of 210 nursing professionals was surveyed to help determine the general patterns of information need and use among the total population, not merely the library and information service users. A critical incident technique was used in this second survey. Five sites were surveyed with overall response 52%: (434/840 questionnaires, with 78% of individuals surveyed replying at least once to the series of four questionnaires).

Follow-up interviews with 106 individuals provided details of: specific examples of the areas of competence affected; information-seeking strategies and skills among nursing professionals; effect of information supply on nursing practice. Later surveys of another 16 library sites provided details of the actual use of library services by nursing and midwifery staff. User profiles were constructed from the available data (which varied considerably).

RESULTS

Results indicated that information provided did or would contribute to improved nursing competence, with 96% of the respondents indicating that one or more categories of competence would be improved. EVINCE showed how libraries could enhance support for evidence-based nursing practice. For example, nursing professionals valued the information highly particularly when on an educational course. There is a need for closer liaison with nursing educators and opinion leaders, active encouragement of the publication of nursing research, and better management information to support claims for extra resources (staff and materials).

User education

In the interviews vignettes were used to explore the information seeking strategies that might be used by the respondents for an information problem. A range of vignettes was devised, and the interviewer picked one appropriate to the clinical experience of the interviewee. Responses were analysed to determine level of confidence in information seeking, awareness and personal knowledge of sources that could be used, strategies for finding information and reliance on colleagues and personal contacts. The method was based on a previous small-scale study.[4]

The majority of interviewees were able to make constructive suggestions about sources of information that could be tried. A small minority indicated that they would not know how or where to start (apart from asking their line manager). Around 60% would probably use two or fewer sources of information to solve the problem, though this depended on the vignette used. Sometimes there might be a definite strategy outlined. However, the sequencing strategy (knowing which sources to try first and why these sources might be productive) was significantly more likely to be associated with the 40% of respondents who used more than two sources of information. Further analysis yielded the following categories:
25% are confident information seekers (experts, with strategy and knowledge of sources)
15% knowledgeably use a limited number of sources (narrowly focused)
15% know sources but are less sure about strategies (aware)
25% have some knowledge of sources and information skills (novices)
20% have limited knowledge of sources and information skills (dependent)

Approaches taken to solve the vignette problem varied, but many strategies combined the formal literature search with consultation with colleagues or the use of personal contacts. A combination approach of formal and informal sources was popular.

Implications for user education

Information professionals need to be aware of the information 'gatekeepers' among their nursing staff. These are the people other nurses will consult for advice and expert opinion. The 'expert' information users will be amenable to courses on critical appraisal of the research literature. The 'dependent' and 'novice' groups need instruction in the types and quality of sources available and need to acquire confidence in information retrieval. The middle group, those not experts, but more knowledgeable than novices, need to be carefully assessed for information skills training.

USER EDUCATION FOR NURSES

The researcher on the EVINCE project, Rebecca Davies, was on secondment from University of Wales Swansea. On return, she has continued to develop user education programmes in line with EVINCE findings. EVINCE found minimal use of the Internet and a later Swansea study found that 50% of qualified nurses on post-basic courses did not use the CD-ROM or online catalogue. Developments at Swansea include construction of profiles of the different categories of student. These profiles are used to develop specific teaching plans for each category of student. These profiles also aid other library staff helping the nursing and midwifery students, whose needs differ from those of higher education students. Analysis of management information revealed that some services were not being used as much as expected, and these sources and services were highlighted in a guide to services. Library guides are often discarded by users, but this library guide contains a guide to referencing which the post-registration students will have to consult regularly, and will therefore be reminded of the electronic sources they should learn to use (CD-ROM, Internet).

Teaching sessions can be informal but structured. One approach is for students to work on a topic, evaluating information sources for themselves and reflecting on the approaches they took in a 'reflective practice' essay.[5] This appears to be more successful than the formal library tour at induction. At Swansea groups of around four post-registration nursing students assess a CD-ROM resource (CINAHL, MEDLINE or British Nursing Index) and then explain to the other groups how to use the resource and why it might be useful. Analysis of the comments revealed the following evaluation criteria: relevance of information found, ease of use, currency and potential costs. Promotion of journals is managed in a similar manner, with students asked to assess for themselves a journal's audience, the type of contributors, and how the articles could be used (for assignments, evidence for practice etc.). All teaching sessions are evaluated.

Conclusion

The EVINCE recommendations included a strategy for user education covering registration, tours, printed (and electronic) support materials (user guides), direction to self-study tutorial material and formal education sessions (one to one, or group). Evaluation, such as that used in Swansea, is essential, and may require a variety of methods.[6]

References

[1] Davies R, Urquhart CJ, Smith J, Massiter C, Hepworth JB. Establishing the value of information to nursing continuing education: report of the EVINCE project (British Library Research and Innovation Report 44). Boston Spa, Wetherby, West Yorkshire LS23 7BQ: British Library Document Supply Centre (British Thesis Service), 1997

[2] Urquhart C, Davies R. EVINCE: the value of information in developing nursing knowledge. Health Libr Rev 1997;14:61-72

[3] Capel S, Banwell L, Walton G. Library and information services to support the education and development of nurses. Health Libr Rev 1991;14:233-246

[4] Urquhart C, Crane S. Nurses' information-seeking skills and perceptions of information sources: assessment using vignettes. J Inf Sci 1994;20:237-246

[5] Martin S. Reflections on a user education session with nurses. Health Libr Rev 1998;15:111-116

[6] Fox LM, Richter JM, White NE. A multidimensional evaluation of a nursing information-literacy program. Bull Med Libr Assoc 1996;84:182-190

INFORMATION SEEKING FROM THE WORK PLACE: HOW NURSES SEEK AND USE NETWORKED INFORMATION SOURCES

Olof Sundin, Harriet Berthold
THE BORAS UNIVERSITY COLLEGE OF HEALTH SCIENCES, BORAS, SWEDEN

Introduction

The present study focuses on the nurse's role as seeker and provider of information to patients and their families. The specific aim is to study nurses' information behaviour after a short user education programme and improved access to networked information channels and sources.

The present study is inter-linked with the Swedish participation in a European nursing-led project called ACTION (Assisting Carers using Telematics Interventions to meet Older Person's Needs) which emphasises the role of the nurse as information provider to old patients and their family carers. The settings for this study are four health care units in a middle-sized town in Sweden. One unit is a nursing home and the other three units perform either hospital care, community care, or primary care. Only the hospital department has direct access to a medical/nursing library. The ACTION-project, however, supports all four sites with newly developed web-based information sources, new channels for information-seeking, and education as to how to use these as part of daily work routines. In total, there are about 600 health care workers in the four units and among these 86 are registered nurses. Although all 600 are involved in the project, this paper deals only with the nurses.

The study is divided into four parts:
- *a literature study* to obtain background knowledge for use in a theoretical reference base.
- *a questionnaire* that explores and describes information behaviour of the nurses in the participating health care units before the user education programme and the installation of new information sources/channels.
- *a user education programme*, containing eight sessions of three hours each, for 32 participants who are to act as "gatekeepers" at the participating sites.
- *a follow up* when a number of nurses are to be interviewed and observed.

Results

This paper presents the findings of the first three parts, which were carried out during the spring of 1998. The questionnaire had a response rate of 83% for the registered nurses and was analysed using SPSS. The mean age of the respondents was 45 years and 94% where women. Although the sample used in the questionnaire study is by no means random, the results are assumed to indicate the situation in similar health care units throughout Sweden. Complementary qualitative data was collected during the user education programme by an observer in the tutor-led discussions.

QUESTIONNAIRE

Previous education: 79% of the nurses reported having received an introduction to library use during their education, 34% reported an introduction to database searching, and 13% an introduction in how to use the World Wide Web for information retrieval.

Information-seeking situations: 53% of the nurses reported seeking information related to patient specific problems at least once a week and 54% in order to keep up to date within their profession. Only 23% of the nurses reported that they sought information related to patient education at least once a week.

Frequency: While 33% of the nurses had, or thought they had, access to the WWW from their workplace, only 7% reported that they used it for finding knowledge-based information sources at least once a month. Similarly 13% had access to reference databases but only 4% reported that they used such databases at least once a month. There were no significant differences in the frequency of use between those who had previous education in how to use databases or WWW and those who had no such education. In comparison 67% of the nurses reported that they used colleagues as a knowledge source on a daily basis.

Attitudes: The nurses did not feel that they had sufficient knowledge and experience in areas of concern. Instead, 81% disagreed with the statement "I already have enough knowledge and experience" concerning the need for seeking additional information in their job. Oral sources of information were preferred. Only 16% disagreed with the statement "I prefer to ask colleagues/other health care workers". The participants in the user education sessions frequently discussed the time factor and only 26% disagreed with the statement "I have seldom time to seek information.

Attitudes towards evidence-based care was positive with 68% reporting that access to evidence-based medicine could support them in their work and 52% reporting that access to evidence-based nursing could support them in their work.

USER EDUCATION PROGRAMME

The ACTION-project is developing web-based patient information to fill a need for easily accessible and quality assured tertiary information in the area of nursing interventions such as incontinence, stroke & feeding and transfer. As part of the ACTION-project, new multimedia computers with videoconference possibilities and Internet access were installed at the workplaces of the participating health care units.

The educational programme introduced:
- the basis of information technology
- an overview of the Internet
- the different information sources in the ACTION-system
- basic information-seeking skills

- how to use the web for retrieving knowledge-based information (full-text resources as well as bibliographical databases)
- quality aspects of health information on the web
- the function of the videoconferencing system

All sessions included a lot of practical exercises with a focus on patient education in the framework of the ACTION-project even though this knowledge can obviously be used in other information-seeking situations. The participants were given information-seeking tasks to solve and issue to discuss at their own workplaces between sessions in order to bridge the distance between educational activities and clinical work. An example of such a discussion topic is: "In what way do you think increased information access among patients and their families will increase demands on the professional carers?"

Discussion and conclusions

According to both the nursing and LIS literature, nurses have a limited tradition of reading as a source of new knowledge, and scientific results are used only to a minor extent.[1,2] Nurses are rare users of hospital libraries[3] and are, in general, heavily dependent upon oral informal information sources.[4] Studies have also shown that access to and knowledge of networked information channels can have an impact on nurses' information-seeking behaviour.[5,6] The present study confirms these results in general, but emphasises that the need for, and use of, written information is not static. The information needs of a profession is here viewed as a social construction and can as such be developed given the right circumstances. This study shows that the majority of the nurses participating in the study carried out different kinds of information-seeking activities every week, but even though attitudes towards external knowledge resources and evidence-based care were positive, the use of information technology to support these activities was very infrequent.

The frequency of information-seeking in relation to patient education was low before the user education programme started. More than a third of the respondents had been trained in information seeking using databases or WWW during their nursing education or continuing education, but that fact did not seem to have influenced the frequency of information-seeking. The present study suggests a closer relationship between education in information-seeking and clinical practice. The user education programme tried to make use of the positive attitudes towards seeking and using external information. Good examples of available information sources/channels and possible scenarios as to when they could be used were provided in order to create an information need.

WWW, both as a channel and a source for information, has proven to be an important potential resource for a better relationship between clinical work and the use of knowledge-based information, both concerning information-seeking in general and information-seeking related to patient education in particular, given that the users have access, proper training, and view information-seeking and use as a part of their job routines. How to retrieve and provide information is an important issue among nurses as well as information professionals. An important experience drawn from this study is the advantage of collaboration between information professionals, nursing professionals, and technicians to create better conditions for information-seeking from the workplace.

References

[1] Wakeham M. Nurses - their information needs and use of libraries: the views of some librarians. Health Libr Rev 1993;10:85-94
[2] Luker KA, Kenrick M. An exploratory study of the sources of influence on the clinical decisions of community nurses. J Adv Nurs 1992;17:457-466
[3] King DN. The contribution of hospital library information service to clinical care: a study in eight hospitals. Bull Med Libr Ass 1987;75:291-301
[4] Urquhart C, Crane S. Nurses' information-seeking skills and perceptions of information sources: assessment using vignettes. J Inf Sci 1994;20:237-246
[5] Farmer J, Richardson A. Information for trained nurses in remote areas: do electronically networked resources provide an answer? Health Libr Rev 1997;14:97-103
[6] Royle JA, Blythe J, Potvin C, Oolup P, Chan IM. Literature search and retrieval in the workplace. Comput Nurs 1995;13:25-31

EARLY LIBRARIES FOR NURSES: THE EVIDENCE

Linda Parr
CITY UNIVERSITY LIBRARY, LONDON, UK

The introduction of formal nurse training in England in the late nineteenth century and the emergence of nursing as a profession resulted in the publication of nursing literature and the formation of libraries for nurses. Libraries were attached to training schools and societies.

The historical record is incomplete, for although there were numerous hospitals and nursing schools, the pattern of health care provision has changed and due to administrative reorganisations, not all records have survived or are easy to locate. The larger well known libraries tend to be better documented, but they were not necessarily typical nursing libraries. Nursing journals, however, include references to and news about books and libraries and so are a valuable source of information.

Nurses read medical textbooks and early textbooks for nurses were written by both doctors and nurses. Professional journals provided a forum for discussion on all aspects of nursing. There was also a strong recreational element in nursing libraries. Library catalogues and lists of books in nursing journals give an indication of what was being published and which books nurses were reading. The book catalogue at the Midwives' Institute and Trained Nurses' Club in 1893 covered a number of subjects.[1] The library was professional with books on nursing and midwifery with a strong medical element whereas the library catalogue of the Royal British Nurses' Association of 1896 provides a contrast as most books were fiction.[2] One opinion expressed in the *Nursing Record* 19 January 1893 by Lina Mollett was that the nurses' library should not be too exclusively professional and scientific and should have variety as nurses had the varied tastes, character and interests of the ordinary nineteenth century woman.[3]

Libraries for nurses at this time lacked professional librarians, nevertheless library administration was planned in detail as exemplified in the rules of the library of the Royal British Nurses' Association in 1898.[4]

References

[1] Catalogus of books at Midwives' Institute and Trained Nurses' Club. Nursing Notes 1893 1 Nov;6(pt 171):151-2

[2] Library catalogue. Nurses' Journal 1896:(2)23-30

[3] Mollett L. The nurses' library. Nurs Rec 1893 19 Jan:42

[4] The library. Nurses' Journal 1898;8(3):40

INFORMATION FOR NURSES IN ITALY: IS THERE ANY NEWS?

Rosamaria Rotolo
BIBLIOTECA POLO DIDATTICO DI VIALBA, UNIVERSITÀ DI MILANO, MILANO, ITALY

Introduction

A re-organization has been recently introduced in Italian nursing schools. At the end of the courses they have been allowed to confer a degree equivalent to a three-year university level; applicants must have a high school diploma. This paper offers a survey of Italian sources dedicated to nursing science and discusses how University and hospital libraries can cooperate with nursing libraries in order to support student nurses during their theoretical studies and the training period and satisfy employed nurses' requests of up-to-date information.

Discussion

Unfortunately, there is a lack of nursing libraries in Italy and most Italian medical libraries are seldom attended by nurses so they are not yet equipped for nurses specific needs and can supply limited in-house literature. Furthermore these users require suggestions in the use of bibliographical sources, and assistance for the use of computerized systems and show a limited knowledge of English language so it is often unuseful to refer to data-bases like MEDLINE or CINAHL on CD-ROM or through the Internet.

Conclusions

A cooperation between both medical and nursing school libraries in the North of Italy has been recently promoted by the library where I work in order to built a printed catalogue of specialistic journals and to exchange documents. It is also aspected to transfer data on the University of Milano Internet site so that private users too could have access to documents available in Italy, expecially to those written in Italian. The first results of our project were presented.

Chapter 10: USER EDUCATION & USER NEEDS

Introduction

It is hard to imagine that libraries could exist without users; it is therefore unthinkable that a library's aims and scopes would not include a statement about *supporting it's users*. To know your users' information needs is the first commandment for a librarian. The new thing about users' information needs is the introduction of information technology and, as a consequence, the changing information habits. The many changes cannot be followed and implemented all at the same time, choices have to be made and priorities set. User surveys will ever be needed to be able to make the right choice in changing the library and the library services.

Librarians are aware of the changing environment, not the least by the speed of developments in information technology, and therefor they are more than anybody else convinced of the need to educate their users in order to benefit most of the services of the library. The following papers describe projects undertaken either to investigate the information needs or to promote a better usage of existing library services.

The educational role of libraries, being public, governmental, industrial or academic, does not differ in essence of curricular activities of libraries in higher education. Therefore chapter 8 "Medical school and university libraries" (p. 153) as well as chapter 9 "Nursing libraries" (p. 171) and chapter 7 "Veterinary libraries" (p. 129) are of interest to every reader who wants to know more about user needs.

THE PROVISION OF INFORMATION FOR R&D UNITS AT THE COUNTY COUNCILS IN SWEDEN

Lotta Haglund
SPRI LIBRARY AND RESEARCH REPORT BANK, STOCKHOLM, SWEDEN

Introduction

In Sweden, as in most European countries, research is mostly carried out at traditional institutions; universities. Research within the county councils has mainly been medical research carried out by physicians. From the beginning of the 1980s many of the Swedish county councils have started research and development units with the aim to work with questions related to everything except medical research, concerning the county council. Their work includes for example; epidemiology, health care provision and organisation. The traditional research institutions usually have access to a library in their institution, a university library with all the services that such can provide. Researchers working in universities also were among the first to have access to the Internet.

The purpose of the study was to get answers on the following questions: How does the researcher working at a R&D unit in a county council manage his information needs? How do they search, and for what? Do they have their own library, big or small? Do they have access to the Internet and to databases? These were some of the questions I sought to find an answer to in this study. I also wanted to see if there was any differences or similarities in information seeking habits between researchers working at universities and those working at the R&D units.

Literature study

A literature study was done to provide a base for comparison. I decided to concentrate on the Swedish literature on the subject even though most of the literature to be found describes American settings, because it would be hard to compare the American experiences with Swedish circumstances. Since I had an idea that the researchers working at the R&D units would have information seeking habits similar to researchers in the social sciences I also read two studies from other countries dealing with this group, one British and one from the Netherlands.

Conclusions drawn from the literature are that social scientists:

- use more monographs and less scientific journals than for example researchers within the sciences. This means that they rely on 'older' material.
- do not 'like' large libraries because they are hard to use for browsing stacks;

- use informal sources in search of current information;
- use different types of research reports (unpublished grey material);
- feel they lack sufficient time for information searching;
- do not like to delegate their information searching to anyone, neither a librarian, nor anyone else, and would never delegate the selection of information;
- find information technology hard and they are in great need of training in that area;
- when using libraries, order a special title and seldom attempt broader subject searches.

Study results

In January 1997 a questionnaire with eighteen questions regarding information seeking habits were sent out to 149 researchers at 28 Swedish R&D units. After two months and one reminder 123 people had answered the questionnaire, a total of 83%.

The results of the questionnaire showed that this group of researchers relied rather heavily on libraries for their provision of information. The most used library was often a hospital library. The explanation for this is probably that the units have their offices in a hospital or in the vicinity of a hospital. Fifteen per cent used university libraries and 8% used national libraries such as Spri Library and Research Report Bank. I could draw no conclusions regarding the use of these large libraries, they were not more utilised by the units in the same geographical area. The researchers seem to use the nearest library within the right subject area regardless of distance. Only 7% never used libraries at all. The most frequently asked service in the library was to request an inter library loan (84%) and to recieve help with database searches (54%).

When it comes to the use of different sources of information the majority (42%) read 4-6 scientific journals and they had access to them by subscription, either directly to themselves or to the workplace, by membership in an association, or they read them in the library. Books they either borrow from a library or buy out of their research budget.

When they search for literature many of them (68%) make broader searches by subject, contrary to what the literature study showed. Only 25% answered that they wanted a special title.

Asked how many and which databases within their subject area they knew about, 70% answered they know of 1-6 different databases, but 27% had no knowledge at all about relevant databases. A total of 42 national and international databases was listed, with MEDLINE on top of the list. When asked if, and how, they had access to the databases and to the Internet, the results show that databases are available both on their own computer and in the library, that a lot of them are connected to an Intranet and therefore have access to databases on CD-ROM and almost 80% have access to the Internet.

In the literature study most authors agreed that to delegate information searching and selection of information was unthinkable. In my study only 26% said no to delegation of information searching but 65% said no to the thought of delegating the selection of relevant material. Of those who thought it possible to delegate searching 50% preferred to delegate searching to a librarian and 22% to a colleague or assistant. Delegation of the selection of material to a librarian said 13% was possible, and to an assistant 19%.

When asked to list their most important sources from 1 to 5, scientific journals were placed as number one by 41%, at second place came books (17%), at third place research reports (15%), at fourth and fifth place came informal sources within (12%) and outside the organisation (10%).

Finally they were asked if they were satisfied with how their information needs were met, and what kind of services they thought were missing. Only 6% answered that their information needs were met poorly or badly. In their comments they showed a lot of satisfaction with their local library and its service. On the other hand the list of what they wanted to improve was diverse. Many emphasised instruction on how to conduct database searches, and how to find useful things on the Internet etc. What many of them lacked when it came to their information needs was time, time, time ...

Conclusion

Contrary to the literature on the subject the population in my study relies heavily on library services, and they have great confidence in librarians as professionals. They also know a lot about different databases, and often use them themselves, as well as the Internet. They express lack of time and too little knowledge as major problems limiting their use of all the resources they have access to.

Compared with the researchers described in the literature my population does not use informal sources very much, and when asked to rank information sources according to importance they prefer journals and other formal sources.

On the matter of delegation of information searching my results also differ from those in the literature. As many as 75% would like to delegate the actual searching to either a colleague or a librarian, and more than 35% were positive to the thought of delegating the selection of interesting documents from the search to someone else!

My results show that the researchers working at the county councils are satisfied with how their information needs are met, but of course there is room for improvements. There are quite a lot of differences between researchers working at universities and my population working at county councils, regarding information seeking habits. I can see several explanations for this; the group studied in my paper is very heterogeneous and it is therefore hard to compare with any other group of researchers; secondly the literature used in the literature study was not very recent which reduced it's relevance to today's circumstances. There is one single factor that has had such a big impact in recent years that it makes everything written a couple of years back seem very old-fashioned - and that is, of course, the rapid growth of information technology and the Internet.

Finally, I would like to remind you, that even though researchers have access to all the relevant sources of information, they still need someone to help them! They do not have the time or the knowledge themselves to find all the information they need. And the someone to help them is likely to be a librarian!

INFORMATION SERVICES FOR VOCATIONAL TRAINEES: SUPPORT FOR EVIDENCE BASED PRACTICE IN TRAINING FOR PRIMARY CARE

Catherine Massiter, Christine Urquhart
DEPT. OF INFORMATION AND LIBRARY STUDIES, UNIVERSITY OF WALES, ABERYSTWYTH, UK

Introduction

Evidence based clinical practice has been defined as "the conscientious, explicit, and judicious use of current best evidence in making decisions about the care of individual patients".[1] Information services supporting evidence based medicine need to facilitate access to the evidence, and provide training in the information retrieval skills required for on-line, Internet and CD-ROM sources.

The Value Project looked at patterns of information need and use among hospital medical staff and GPs.[2] It noted that while Senior House Officers (SHOs - hospital-based junior doctors, including some who will be training for general practice) recognise the need for up-to-date information for patient care, and ascribe great clinical value to information obtained from the information services available in medical libraries, they are among the groups of medical staff least likely to make use of use such services. For those who are training for general practice this raises particular issues as they may later find themselves among those GPs who find it difficult to get access to the evidence needed to support their practice.[3]

USE OF INFORMATION BY SHOs AND GPs

Findings from the Value Project indicated that for SHOs personal education and patient care were the prime reasons for seeking information, and these purposes are often closely linked. Sources used are often those most easily to hand such as textbooks or colleagues. Awareness and use of MEDLINE and other on-line sources appeared low.

A similar pattern emerged for the GPs who were surveyed. Patient care was a frequent stimulus for searching out information but personal education needs and updating were also important. Reference books and colleagues were again among the most frequent sources consulted. Use of MEDLINE appeared limited except perhaps for special pieces of research such as audit projects.

DELIVERY OF INFORMATION SUPPORTING CLINICAL EFFECTIVENESS

The primary sources of research information are the journals, but this information also comes packaged and reviewed in secondary publications on clinical evidence (e.g. guidelines on clinical effectiveness, the Cochrane Library, the ACP Journal Club, etc.). The bibliographic databases such as MEDLINE are available in several electronic formats, with MEDLINE now available in various free versions on the Internet. The quantity of clinical information available is immense and its quality often uncertain. However formats such as systematic reviews, critical abstracts,[4] guidelines, etc. can offer reliable and concise information and such resources can be made available either on local intranets or more widely via the Internet. A few of the information services studied in the Value project offered current awareness services tailored to the needs of groups such as SHOs. These appeared popular and effective in encouraging use of other information services.

A survey undertaken as part of the GIVTS project shows that clinical decision making and evidence based care are important issues for junior doctors, both hospital and general practice based, who are training for primary care. However, many of them recognise a problem in locating and identifying the best external clinical evidence. Evidence based medicine can be seen as time-consuming and unconnected with the demands of immediate patient care,[5] at least in the particular circumstances in which the trainees find themselves working. There is a general reluctance, particularly among SHOs, to make use of IT based sources of information and knowledge and use of the Internet as a source of medical information is very low.

If GP trainees are to be encouraged to seek the up-to-date information necessary for effective clinical decision making, they need support both in information retrieval and in appraising the information found. Although most of them will have learnt the basics of MEDLINE searching at medical school many of those interviewed for the GIVTS project expressed a wish for further training in computer skills generally, including the use of MEDLINE and the Internet.

The main educational motivation for many GP trainees is (understandably) the scheme of assessment during training. Support in critical appraisal of the information provided by services should fit in well with the audit project work that is a compulsory part of this assessment.

INFORMATION PROVISION FOR GENERAL PRACTICE

The Value project audit phase showed that formal information service provision for GPs was extremely uneven. In some areas of the UK one medical staff library user in six might be a GP while in others GP use was virtually negligible. Within present resource constraints improved provision is only possible by better targeting of services, and more effective use of telematics.

Formerly a junior doctor would have to come to the library to read the journals or do a search of MEDLINE on CD-ROM. Now, increasingly, MEDLINE and other resources are available via local networks. In addition these resources, together with a great mass of other information, are now available on the Internet, allowing doctors to carry out much of their research at home. Junior doctors need to become adept in the use of intranets and the Internet, particularly if patients themselves are better informed about their treatment through use of the Internet.

Aims and objectives of GIVTS

The aims and objectives of the current research project Getting Information to Vocational Trainees (GIVTS, running from mid January 1997 till mid January 1999) focus on the evaluation of the effectiveness of targeted information services to GP trainees throughout the three year training period. Twelve sites have been selected in England and Wales of which 6 are designated as test and 6 as control sites. The aim at the test sites is to provide relevant information at, or near the point of care, and to encourage GP trainees to make more active use of services which supply the evidence and guidelines required for patient care.

THE PHASES OF THE STUDY ARE:

Baseline study of information service delivery and trainees' uptake of information and educational services, to establish the factors which will affect choice of control and test sites, and implementation of services.

The baseline study began with interviews with librarians and GP Course Organisers at all the selected sites. This was followed by visits to training sessions at all sites, where there was an opportunity for discussion of information needs with individual GP trainees. Telephone interviews have been carried out with 100 trainees, 50 from test and 50 from control sites, building up a more detailed picture of knowledge and use of information resources and information skills.

Main phase study, in which around 50 vocational trainees in the test sites will be provided with the specialist service. The assessment of the service will include measurement of the uptake of information services and qualitative assessment of the effectiveness of the services. Control sites provide a basis for comparison.

For this phase, around 50 trainees at test sites have been provided with the results of a mediated literature search on a topic of their choice. The searches covered not only MEDLINE (using both CD-ROM and the Internet) but also the Cochrane Library and a range of Internet sites offering evidence based clinical information. It is hoped that questionnaires testing reactions to the results of these searches will build up a picture of the types and formats of information which may best meet user needs. A seminar has been held involving librarians from the test sites to co-ordinate further training particularly in the use of Internet resources, and packs will be prepared to support the use of these resources.

Evaluation phase study which will assess the longer term effect of the specific clinical educational intervention.

For the evaluation we hope to have access to audit projects completed by GP trainees at both test and control sites which should provide a basis for investigating and evaluating any differences in the use made of the various resources.

Conclusion

The Value project results and the preliminary indications from GIVTS emphasise the importance of understanding the particular needs of individual user groups such as GP trainees. Support and training needs to be directed at enabling appropriate use of information resources supporting evidence based medicine in primary care.

Acknowledgements

We thank the British Library Research and Innovation Centre for funding the GIVTS and Value projects, and Postgraduate Deans for contributing funds to the Value project.

References

[1] Sackett DL, Rosenberg WMC, Muir Gray JA, Haynes RB, Richardson WS. Evidence based medicine: what it is and what it isn't. BMJ 1996;312:71-72
[2] Urquhart CJ, Hepworth JB. The value to clinical decision making of information supplied by NHS library and information services. Boston Spa, Wetherby: British Library Document Supply Centre, 1995; British Library R&D Report 6205
[3] Felton T, Lister G. Consider the evidence: the NHS on the move towards evidence based medicine. Uxbridge: Coopers & Lybrand, 1996
[4] Hayward RSA, Wilson MC, Tunis SR, Bass EB, Rubin HR, Haynes RB. More informative abstracts of articles describing clinical practice guidelines. Ann Intern Med 1993;118:731-737
[5] Rosenberg W, Donald A. Evidence based medicine: an approach to clinical problem solving. BMJ 1996;310:1122-1126

LIBRARIAN INSTRUCTORS/PHYSICIAN SEARCHERS: CHANGING NEEDS--CHANGING ROLES

Richard L. Faraino, Dorice L. Vieira
EHRMAN MEDICAL LIBRARY, NEW YORK UNIVERSITY SCHOOL OF MEDICINE, NEW YORK, N.Y., USA

Introduction

Both the librarian and physician are confronted with changing needs and roles. The environment of clinical medicine poses many teaching challenges for medical librarians. Quality end-user searching of the medical literature is of major concern for the physician. They must perform searches within the time constraints of the clinic or are more apt to be searching when the need for expertise is most acute and while little assistance is available. Three significant events have been a catalyst for prompting the physician to become a better searcher of biomedical information: (1) the impact of managed care, seeing more patients in less time; (2) the impact of the world wide web, for information access, interchange and instruction; and (3) the rise of evidence-based medicine; the acknowledgment of the need for objective evidence from the literature to complement education, experience and expert opinion.

The dynamics of the world wide web provide a link between the physician and the librarian. There are issues of how physicians are trained as literature searchers, how they can apply these skills effectively, will they keep up with re-training, and how do they evaluate the tools they select for consultation.

The impact of the librarian can be quite profound. Librarians must be a constant voice in advocating the provision of "quality" services rather than taking the passive stance. Medical librarians have traditionally taken such courses as medical terminology, searching the medical literature, and the like, but now must focus on higher learning, teaching alongside faculty in small group sessions, and taking advantage of opportunities to get involved in evidence-based medicine. Continuing education for librarians includes, but is not limited to, learning epidemiological concepts and developing appropriate teaching strategies for adult learners.

This paper is a report on a project in progress. While the conclusions are some time away, this interim report highlights significant findings for medical librarians. This paper is also a call for participation in a multicenter study to evaluate a new tool for instruction. We designed a start-to-finish flow chart which summarizes each step the physician should take and what possible steps may be followed to refine patient-care searches based on the varying criteria found at each step. Because a flow chart follows a hierarchy from start to finish, it is more dynamic than traditional handouts and guides that serve as reference pieces. It is easily reproduced for electronic and print access and can be kept by the computer, on a wall, or in a pocket and is available whenever the need is present. With access to the world wide web links can be placed on the flow chart providing flexibility and interactivity to match the instructional pace of the physician.

Background

Information Express was a six month pilot project which coordinated library instruction and services with a residency training program at Gouverneur Hospital's department of medicine. Gouverneur Hospital has an affiliation with New York University Medical Center, is located in a different part of the city and serves a large outpatient population. The pilot project involved 23 residents and students, 10 preceptors and approximately 12 attendings. From the library, three educational services instructors and the document delivery department where involved. During the program period, from January through June, library faculty held instructional sessions several times per month for 1 to 2 hours on site. The objective of the project was to educate the clinicians in the basic principles of evidence-based medicine as it pertains to the literature. Physicians were to identify clinical questions based on their patients and apply informatics skills toward resolving those questions. They were instructed in the use of MEDLINE, MedCAT (the library's OPAC) and other electronic sources such as Harrison's Textbook of Internal Medicine, Scientific American Medicine, and the Cochrane Library. All participants were given passwords for searching six databases by remote access from the medical library . The instructional sessions given by the librarians were originally intended for the ten preceptors. The preceptors working closely with the residents and students would in turn instruct them on how to effectively search the databases. Once participants performed a search they could then fax an article request to our document delivery department. We agreed to fax their articles to them within 24 hours of receipt of their request. The goal was to have clinicians define a clinical question, efficiently search the literature and receive the information they need as expeditiously as possible.

Interim findings

By mutual agreement the project was not completed in accordance with the original design. Although formal pre-assessment forms were distributed to all participants and post-assessments were planned, the clinical faculty informally evaluated the project at weekly meetings. This timely approach allowed for anecdotal data collection and commentary while the length of the project left open the possibility for adhoc changes. At about halfway through the project the clinical coordinators decided to change its fundamental structure. Instead of having the preceptors train the residents and students in searching the literature, it was decided that it would be more effective to have the librarians present to instruct both groups for the more complex questions that arise during clinic hours. It was efficient for the preceptors to give basic lessons in literature searching but the clinical scenario seemed to require the librarians expertise. The new model had the librarian present during the preceptor sessions. The preceptor would guide the resident in the specifics of the patient's case while the librarian would help to define clinical questions appropriate for a literature search. The librarian would further guide the resident in choosing the most appropriate resource to search and help to develop the strategies. The preceptor and the resident would analyze the search results amid other existing evidence for decision-making.

This fundamental change moved the librarian from a secondary role as instructor to active participant in residency training and the patient care team. From the sessions that were conducted in this way we were able to identify the clinicians needs, the librarian's strengths and opportunities for improvement.

Librarian strengths
- Clinical Question To Search Strategy
- Comprehensive Strategies
- Knowledge Of Subject Headings/Vocabulary Systems
- Knowledge Of Appropriate Resources:
- MEDLINE Is Not Always The Best Resource
- "Filters" For Publication Types: Therapy; Prognosis; Diagnosis; Etiology

Clinician needs
- Defining the clinical question
- A comprehensive understanding of resources (more than MEDLINE)
- MEDLINE: subject headings, text words, explode, boolean, limits (applying filters)

Opportunities for librarians
- Attend clinics, grand rounds, journal clubs
- Stimulates understanding, appreciation, team setting
- Continuing education: courses in epidemiology, microbiology, adult learning
- Data collection & analysis: utilizing technology for distance education

Restrictions
- Availability is limited to relatively few hours per day: not economically feasible to staff all clinical departments

Potential solutions
- Librarians as part of the clinical team when possible
- Develop "filters"
- Design a flow chart
- Internet for distance education

Next step
- Flow chart
- Design an evaluation tool
- Recreate in print & web-based formats
- Implement study

Summary

Changes in medical practice, medical education and information technology have affected change for both librarians and physicians. This evolving environment offers the librarian the opportunity to become an asset to the patient care team and to develop new methods for instruction. As librarians integrate into the environment of medicine, the greater their expertise is understood.

DISTANCE LEARNING FOR RESPIRATORY REGISTRARS VIA THE INTERNET

Andy Simpson, Mike Roberts, Anne Weist*
*MEDICAL EDUCATION CENTRE, WHIPPS CROSS HOSPITAL, LEYSTONE, LONDON, UK

Background

The introduction of the Specialist Registrar (SpR) grade in Britain has meant a more structured training programme for senior postgraduate doctors. Responsibility for Respiratory Medicine training in the North Thames (East) area has been devolved to the local British Thoracic Society training committee. A major part of their training programme is the monthly study days. It is the study day that is being supported by distance learning over the Internet.

The project is being funded by the Postgraduate Dean, North Thames and the Forest Group of Hospitals Education and Research Trust.

SPECIALIST REGISTRARS IN THE AREA

North Thames (East) is a geographically wide area covering the North East of London and stretching out as far as Southend and Colchester. It currently has 38 SpRs in Respiratory Medicine on 16 different sites. The study days allow about 25 of them to meet on any one occasion, but it is never the same 25. So, one of the main aims of the project is to enhance the communication, interaction and participation in the learning process between study days. It also aims to reinforce learning and provide relevant preparatory exercises with feedback from Tutors. Unlike many other Internet learning sites[1] it has restricted access and is maintained by a core team of three on a limited budget.

Of the 38 SpRs only those 10 with research posts in University Departments have access to the British academic network (JANET), the rest are reliant on commercial Internet Providers. At the start of the project only 11 respondents to our survey had ever used the Internet of whom 9 had access to the Internet either at home or at work. None were young enough to have benefited from computer training as part of the medical undergraduate curriculum. Thus there were a potential 27 SpRs who might need considerable support with using the Internet and who would also need access. The Coordinator sought the support of her fellow Library and Information Professionals because she knew that they all had Internet access and were committed to cooperative/ reciprocal working. They agreed to support the project. On the University Medical School Hospital sites it was impossible to use the academic access points so local arrangements were made. On the one site where there was no Library a standalone connection was funded. In the future the Britain's National Health Service Network will mean that access is not a problem but, in the interim, such contingency measures will have to be employed.

Phase One March 1997 to December 1997

Andy Simpson created the WEB pages from the materials provided by study day organisers and the SpRs themselves and designed the project logo. An introductory training day was arranged for the Librarians in March 1997. All of them were already experienced users of the Internet so what we were initially getting across were the aims of the project, and an indication of how we hoped they might be achieved. The Librarians were keen to support the project recognising that it was making them more active partners in the education process.

As the pages were all web based and it was extremely easy to navigate between them but access was somewhat complicated by the need to use passwords. In all 24 SpRs were introduced to the project during a study day. Those who did not attend were told about it by letter and were promised support from librarians locally. The uptake was patchy. Although 75% of SpRs used it during the 5 months of the first phase as a percentage of total activity 30% took place in June, 28% in July, 11% in August, 23% in October and 4% in November. The need for local support from Librarians was all the more keen because most SpRs waited before attempting to use the system, arrived in the Library without their personal instructions and had little idea of how to log on. Once they did log on the complaint was that the system was too slow.

Phase two from December 1997 to March 1998

NETTSpRite: the North Thames East Thoracic Society Specialist Registrar Internet Training Environment. It was accepted that the system was too slow and difficult to maintain. The solution was to use a commercial conferencing system called FirstClass. This meant new training needs on top the existing ones. Again the support of the local librarians was engaged. This time they had to load new software locally and support those who wished to use FirstClass from their home PCs. Having anticipated some of the problems that they might encounter largely by looking at her own difficulties, the Coordinator was able to write a concise set of instructions. These were tested by her librarian colleagues before being given to the SpRs. Setting up the correct software parameters in *FirstClass* was one thing but actually using it was another. So again the Coordinator drew up a set of instructions.

It is clear that instructions alone are not enough and some SpRs requested more 'hands on' training so the Coordinator ran 4 small group sessions with no more than 4 SpRs at any one time. These introduced them to the new FirstClass system which could be likened to an email intranet environment with a closed user group. It is arranged in a hierarchy with the desktop being the top level. From there 4 folder icons will take you to: personal mail, conferences, news or help. The conferences icon links to the study day support pages. These contain multiple choice questions on previous study days, case histories written by the SpRs themselves, an x-ray quiz, and discussion topics. Images can be quickly downloaded on to screen for viewing and can be then be minimised alongside quiz questions. Alternatively, they can downloaded on to disk or printed out. The quality is generally good and where those setting the questions can be involved in setting up the pages the results are better. Any text which users of the system add can be pasted from their wordprocessors straight into *FirstClass* and then amended using the edit function to change the font size and colour. There is also an Internet link folder from which SpRs can leave the *FirstClass* pages and go straight to the Internet. Indeed any message sent to the system using a URL will automatically be recognised and changed into a hot link. In addition there are icons which link to archive months, technical support, information on the project. The SpRs have enjoyed the facility for real time chat in training and a virtual study is planned for August 1998.

Findings

All librarian trainers have been surprised by the range of ability amongst the SpRs and by the variations in IT confidence. Our findings seem to back up the research on librarians which suggests that for some the barrier may be "a fear that one does not have the technical competence" and a fear of "losing face online".[2] Where SpRs are both lacking in experience and IT confidence, the facilitator has to provide a high level of support in a non threatening way. In the small group sessions, this has proved possible but it takes time. Between sixty and ninety minutes is necessary for those with little computer experience to learn their way around *FirstClass*, and more importantly feel confident. This is an essential time commitment which is difficult to arrange in the busy schedule of doctors and facilitators.

Having to change to the *FirstClass* system has not been easy for the SpRs or the Librarians and the Project team have had to provide a great deal of telephone support. The system itself is not intuitive and there are some problems with navigating between screens that users will continue to encounter. It is, however, faster to use, easier to maintain and the early indications suggest more SpRs are logging on more regularly so perhaps we are beginning to see a culture change.

References

[1] Dark GG. Learning on the Internet. Br J Hosp Med 1997;58:572-4

[2] Johnson DT, Sievert MC, Hartman T, Patrick T. Constructs for investigating lack of persistence in experimental distance education: a study of health science librarians. In: Layzell U, Ward P, Weingard P. Human development competancies for the twenty-first century. Munchen: KG Saur 1997:49-59

END-USER EDUCATION AT THE KAROLINSKA INSTITUTE LIBRARY IN SWEDEN

Christine Wickman
KAROLINSKA INSTITUTE LIBRARY, STOCKHOLM, SWEDEN

Introduction

The Karolinska Institute is the only medical university in Sweden with focus on health care with 7,000 students in basic curricula and about 2,000 graduate students. The Karolinska Institute Library is the Swedish National Resource Library in Medicine and the largest biomedical library in Sweden. The Library runs courses for undergraduate students, for graduate students and participants in continuing education courses. Our education program includes courses on a national basis, courses in cooperation with other organizations as well as tailor-made courses.

In the early nineties PBL (Problem-based Learning) was introduced in the basic curriculum for future physicians. The library was rebuilt to house group rooms and a computer room for project work, tutor-lead discussions and individual work.

Courses in information retrieval

When we started courses in information retrieval for students we had to bear in mind that the average student of the first term has a limited knowledge of medical terminology. This combined with English language problems complicates how to formulate search questions and how to evaluate search results.

Twice a term 120 first-term students in medicine come to the library. They receive one hour for library instruction and an introduction to the library catalog and two hours for literature searching in MEDLINE. These same students come back in their third term, when the course focus on how to access various kinds of information in databases, library catalogs and on the Web.

When is teaching information retrieval most successful and when are students most motivated? When they need information, of course! Therefore students come to the library's course when they are working on a specific project. Our courses are curriculum-integrated and compulsory for first term students. The course in literature searching in MEDLINE includes an introduction to the content and structure of MEDLINE and MeSH as well as practical exercises on the students' project topics. We try to offer individual searching as far as possible. We don't have examination at the end of the course, but the results of literature searching have to be included in the written project report.

After our introduction most of the students are capable of using computers for information retrieval. It also decreases the number of requests for help from staff at the reception counter.

To run our curriculum-integrated courses requires positive cooperation between the library and the teaching staff of the Institute as well as the administration of the basic curriculum. Course secretaries play a key roll. There are committees for planning each term of the basic curriculum in medicine. Our library is represented in the committee for term 1 and 3.

Experiences

We have learned that it is important to achieve an understanding for our specific competence. Try to meet the students several times. Teaching large student groups each term demands resources in time and personnel.

The aim of our courses for graduate students at the Karolinska Institute is to develop and increase information literacy and to provide a comprehensive knowledge of biomedical databases and resources on the Internet and Web. For many graduate students this course will be the first one in information retrieval. They are highly motivated to learn how to use databases, library catalogs and the Web for information searching in their own research areas. Information on reference handling, impact factors and criteria for evaluation of information in general, is included in the course. We run 12 courses each year. These 2-day courses are given in Swedish and English. The importance of the Library's competence in teaching how to search biomedical information resources is underlined by the fact that our course is praised as very useful by the graduate students themselves. From this year onwards, graduate students registered from 1 July onwards, will have to take a compulsory basic course which is five weeks long in which our library's course is included!

User-friendly search-programs and the search facilities of the Web make it much easier for end-users to search information. But end-users need guidance in how to find what they are looking for, how search programs work and how to use help functions. They need facts about different information resources. To apply for a course and to get that introduction is often much better and quicker. To do practical exercises, to put questions and get answers immediately is appreciated. We use the Web site of our library as a starting point for searching information. This makes it possible to integrate internal and external information in our courses.

Information professionals are needed as teachers, as structurers and guides. With our professional competence we can teach end-users where they can find the information they are looking for!

TUITION OF THE FINAL USER OF BIOMEDICAL DATABANKS: EXPERIENCE IN A DOCUMENTATION SERVICE

Andrea Zeccato, Cesare Carrà, Gabriella Gabutti, Carmine Tinelli, Catherine Klersy, Moreno Curti
[1 2 3 6]SCIENTIFIC DIRECTION LIBRARY; [4 5]EPIDEMIOLOGY SERVICE, IRCCS POLICLINICO SAN MATTEO, PAVIA,ITALY

Background

The Documentation Service (SDS) of San Matteo's Scientific Library in Pavia has been already offering for the last few years the access to international databanks for retrieval of biomedical scientific documentation. At that purpose consultant librarians have always been at researcher's disposal. The informatic development of the site, the setup and spread of the Intranet, the implementation of client/server services, and so on, has favored the increase in the number of distant acces sites to databanks. However, in order to make final users self-sufficient in performing bibliographic searches and thus to assign them an individual access password, we felt a tuition course being recommended. These course should have the following requirements: 1) to be clear and comprehensive; 2) to be concise; 3) to be operative; 4) to hand out teaching material. Starting January 1996 up to June 1997, 40 tuition sessions have been performed with 255 participating users (6-7 persons/session). In the same time period databanks interrogation sessions were 5247; 62% were performed by users qualified to the course, while 38% by the Scientific Library's consultant librarians.

Object

In order to further assess the success of the tuition in terms of the obtained results (efficacy of searches and results quality), the authors have set up a questionnaire, constructed following the different points raised during the course, to be administered to the password owners for databanks consulting. The purpose is to quantify, after a certain time lap, the appropriateness of databanks searching, based on the strategies taught during the course. Data quantifying the use of databanks will be compared between users having and having not attended the course (control group). Controls have already developed information skills by themselves.

Methods

The questionnaire proposed 17 questions, most of which with "closed-answers". Moreover, some "control-questions", requiring an articulated answer, have been inserted with the aim to verify the outcome of the previous questions. To give a weight to the different questions, scores were assigned in relation to the importance within the questionnaire. Particular attention was given to the quality and quantity of the results, the correct use of free-words or key-words and refining tools offered by the searching system, the preservation and utilisation of the results.

Conclusions

The number of subjects contacted was 108; 72 (77.7%) fulfilled the questionnaire and 18 among these were from the control group (Table 1). The first outcome from the questionnaire examination is that the answers of the course attendants are mostly correct and therefore there are no substantial differences with the control group. If we look at the total score of weighted questions, we observe an almost equal mean value, with a standard deviation of 15.15 for the course attendants and 19.10 for the other ones (Table 2). This shows that the efficiacy of the queries and the quality of the retrieves obtained do not present significant variations when comparing the control and the attendants group. As from the data concerning the total score of the weighted questions, even from the results of the single questions no relevant difference can be noticed: in fact, there is always a lack of significance by comparing the two groups, with the exception of the question about the use of the utility "restriction of years search" ($p<0.0333$).

The examination of the results allow us to state that the course attendance not only produced a substantial increase in the number of search sessions, but also provided to the users the necessary and sufficient knowledge for document searching in the principal scientific databanks. Since the control group users have been admitted to databanks use on the basis of the knowledge of the databanks working modalities and tools, it is possible to affirm that the course attendance provided to the searches, until then depending on the librarians work, an acceptable level of autonomy in query performing.

Table 1

QUESTIONNAIRES	*returned*	*not ret.*	*TOTAL*
course attendance	18	10	28
control group	54	26	80
TOTAL	72	36	108

Table 2

	nr	*Mean*	*S.D.*
course attendance	54	59.4	15.15
control group	18	58.04	19.10

ASSESSMENT OF INFORMATION NEEDS IN PUBLIC HEALTH IN GERMANY: RESULTS OF A NATIONWIDE SURVEY

Anke Scheiber, Rüdiger Schneemann, R. Wischer
[1]FACHHOCHSCHULE MAGDEBURG, FACHBEREICH SOZIAL- UND GESUNDHEITSWESEN, MAGDEBURG; [2]TECHNICAL UNIVERSITY BERLIN, INSTITUTE FOR HEALTH SCIENCES, BERLIN, GERMANY

Abstract

Since Public Health in Germany is a new multidisciplinary area, there is no well established informational infrastructure to offer researchers, as well as other experts, an overview of current research activities and recently published literature. Therefore, a preliminary study is assessing the informational needs in public health research and practice. A survey about the experience with online databases and demands for specific information resources was conducted in order to analyse the extent of problems experienced with information retrieval. The main conclusions of the survey findings are: (a) there is a serious demand for information filtering and information supply in Public Health in Germany, (b) some of the "missed" databases do already exist, but are obviously not well known or accessible, thus indicating a need of promoting information resources and (c) although some of the respondents have had access to the Internet, only very few of them are using email or the world wide web to find and exchange information.

Full text of this article was published on 11 February 1998 on the Internet in: Information Research 1998;3(3)
URL: <http://www.shef.ac.uk/~is/publications/infres/paper43.html>

Information Research: an electronic journal, is published four times a year by the Department of Information Studies, University of Sheffield.
ISSN 1368-1613

USING HUMAN AND ELECTRONIC NETWORKS TO SUPPORT END-USER TRAINING IN FINDING THE EVIDENCE

Anne Brice, Andre Tomlin
HEALTH CARE LIBRARIES UNIT, JOHN RADCLIFFE HOSPITAL, OXFORD, UK

Introduction

A range of workshops, designed to help health practitioners improve their ability to find evidence systematically about clinical effectiveness, has been developed by the Critical Appraisal Skills Programme (CASP) and librarians from the Health Libraries and Information Network in the Anglia and Oxford health region.[1]

The CASP Finding the Evidence Workshop (CASPfew) aims to provide participants with an awareness of available sources, and to help them develop skills in searching effectively for evidence relating to their own information needs. The workshops use a range of problem-based and hands-on activities, and have attracted a wide variety of health professionals.

Implementation of the CASPfew programme has encouraged users to structure their information-seeking behaviour and therefore has led to greater user-empowerment. Users have also become more aware of their need for information skills training, the changing role of information professionals and the impact of the electronic library.

The CASPfew Process

The initial workshops were led by a small team of librarians from the network, and followed the cascade model of delivery adopted by the critical appraisal skills programme. As library staff became familiar with the teaching content and methods, it was envisaged that responsibility for organising and running workshops would then devolve to a local level.

In order to aid this process a comprehensive Workshop Organiser was produced. This formed a key educational support tool, and contained sample programmes, demonstrations and teaching notes, both in paper and electronic format. This tool, it was hoped, would allow the structure and content of each workshop to be tailored for different audiences.

There were, however, a number of problems in this process. Firstly, the materials became quickly out of date, and the existing format of paper file and diskette did not provide an effective and efficient mechanism for gathering feedback, developing the teaching material, and disseminating changes back to network members. Secondly, unlike the critical appraisal workshops, local libraries were already offering user education in information skills, and careful consideration needed to be given to how the programme would integrate with existing work.

The questions that needed to be addressed could be summarised as:
- how to meet demand for more workshops, both regional and local
- how to make the most of resources and materials developed centrally in order to maintain quality and reduce duplication of effort
- how to promote and support implementation and ownership of local programmes
- how to provide training in appropriate skills for librarians to support workshop delivery
- how to feedback local experiences and expertise into further development
- how to evaluate the impact of training programmes on end-users
- how to serve the needs of users unable to attend workshop events

After discussion with some of the original members of the CASPfew team, it was clear that a strategic approach was required to further development and implementation. It was agreed that this strategy would aim to:
- further develop centralised resources at a regional level using a CASPfew web site to maximise access and reduce duplication of effort
- provide training and support in new teaching, learning and facilitation skills
- monitor the quality of the materials used in training programmes
- carry out impact evaluation of training programmes and methods
- enable local librarians to offer cross-organisational and multi-disciplinary training, and to share subject and training expertise

In summary our task was to balance centralised development and the maintenance of quality while at the same time empowering library staff and encouraging local ownership. We were also keen to exploit the potential of the Health Care Libraries Unit web site, and to ensure that our electronic network complemented our existing human network of contacts and expertise, thereby developing a two-tier approach - the human and electronic network.

The CASPfew Strategy

The elements of the CASPfew strategy consist of:

The Regional CASPfew Team is responsible for areas of work that benefit from centralisation, and help to reduce duplication of effort. This work includes developing regional strategies, updating materials, developing toolkits and web resources, organising training, undertaking impact evaluations, and liaising with other health professionals at a regional level.

Local CASPfew Teams have been formed to develop local strategies, deliver local workshops, liaise with local CASP teams, share expertise and training opportunities, and to feedback into regional development. They are also in a crucial position to liaise and set up alliances with other health professionals in order to make sure that information skills training is incorporated in the local multi-disciplinary training agenda.

The CASPfew Web Site development is at the centre of the strategy. The pages are designed to provide background and contact information on CASPfew, and to enable the development and dissemination of high quality workshop and teaching materials to local teams. At the heart of the web site is the CASPfew Toolkit. This contains hints and tips on workshop planning, teaching materials including scenarios, activities and handouts, sample forms and questionnaires, and slide presentations. The materials can be viewed via a browser or downloaded for local adaptation and use. In this way the quality, relevance and effectiveness of materials can be monitored, while encouraging use, feedback and further development. We have found that once local teams have been established, they gain in confidence and skills, and both teams and individuals have the potential to gain encouragement and recognition from sharing their work. In addition the health libraries network as a whole is strengthened, and benefits from the promotion of a collaborative, resource-sharing culture.

Training the Trainers. In order to deliver high-quality end-user training, librarians need to be provided with high quality professional development. Librarians in the Oxford region have access to a planned professional development programme organised by the Health Care Libraries Unit. A highly successful Librarian of the 21st Century Programme[2,3] has provided a foundation for developing new roles and skills, such as in teaching and learning, facilitation skills, new technology, marketing and change management. The original CASPfew Training the Trainers workshop has been redesigned to complement the regional Professional Development programme.

The new Training the Trainers workshop looks at the skills and planning involved in organising successful Finding the Evidence events. Topics covered include the background and structure of CASPfew; workshop planning and content; teaching methods and evaluation; and using the CASPfew Toolkit. The workshops are highly interactive, and use group work, scenarios and demonstrations to help people get more from organising events in their local settings.

Beyond the workshop - Distance Learning. There is now an increasing need to develop our teaching materials beyond the workshop. Limited accessibility, and the increase in demand for the skills required in an evidence-based culture have required CASP and CASPfew to investigate alternative training methods. Although the face-to-face and group work aspects of the CASP model are hard to replicate, the inherent difficulties in relying on workshop models to train large numbers of health professionals in finding, appraising and acting on evidence are obvious. A decision was therefore taken to investigate translating the teaching materials into a distance learning format, which could both meet a wide variety of needs, and take advantage of developments in technology. It is hoped that this will increase accessibility and extend support networks to those working in all areas of the health service, particularly those in primary and community care. Distance learning, by allowing learners to learn at their own pace, time, and level will help provide flexible training in appraisal and information skills to meet a wide range of learning styles and organisational requirements. Further integration with teaching and training networks can help to promote this. Two projects are now under way developing open learning and multiple-media products. Collaborative work is also being considered with the Centre for Evidence Based Medicine, and the Centre for Evidence Based Mental Health, in Oxford to investigate the development of web based teaching materials.

Conclusion

Our experience has shown that human networks can support the provision of high quality library and information services, and promote the development of new models of teaching information skills within an evidence-based framework. The existing human network within the Oxford region has been enhanced by the development of an electronic network that complements this expertise and supports the work of local staff. The Critical Appraisal Skills Programme Finding the Evidence Workshop strategy and programme will continue to work at a regional and local level in order to help librarians play a high-profile, pro-active role as mediators, educators and facilitators, helping their users to find the evidence.

References

[1] Palmer J. Where is the evidence? – teaching health professionals how to find the evidence. In: Bakker S (ed). Health information management: what strategies? Proceedings of the 5th European Conference of Medical and Health Libraries, Coimbra, 1996: Dordrecht: Kluwer, 1997:299-301

[2] Palmer J. Skills for a virtual future. Bibl Med Can 1997;19(2):62-65

[3] Palmer J, Streatfield D. Good diagnosis for the twenty-first century. Libr Assoc Rec 1995;97:153-154

Chapter 11: NATIONAL AND INTERNATIONAL COOPERATION

Editorial introduction

Cooperation and networking belong to the second nature of libraries. Whatever subject in librarianship is chosen as subject for discussion, sooner or later aspects related to interlibrary loan, union catalogues or controlled vocabularies, will come into focus. The emphasis that is placed by the publishing industry upon forming consortia in order to arrange large scale licence agreements fits rather well in the tradition of cooperation among libraries. To what extent the trust and mutual benefits - essential elements of cooperation - can survive alongside negotiations and licence agreements with commercial publishers, is soon to be discovered.

The reports in this chapter deal with different kinds of collaboration on different levels: Arlette Pailley-Katz reports on the project supported by the European Community to the benefit of the University of Tirana (Albania). Marian van Wegen reports about the collaboration of hospital librarians for whom cooperation was a neccesity not only to reach a common goal, but also to the benefit of all participants. Elisabeth Akre reports on the project funded by the Norwegian Government to realize a better information provision as part of the Plan for a National Network of Health. Interesting in this respect is the summary of the activities on a regional level in the UK, reported by Shane Godbolt. And from Italy there are three reports: Laura Cavazza describes the project of rationalization (deduplication) of library collections within one institute, Maurella Della Seta is involved in making an inventory of the many Internet sites and Elisabetta Marinoni reports on the sharing of bibliographic databases on the university computer network.

All presented projects of cooperation are part of the gradually changes taking place in (medical) librarianship caused by the tension between limited (local) resources, growing awareness of available information, increasing information needs, and the seducing glamour of very promising technological innovations. In chapter 12 more papers can be found on remote access and providing service over long distance.

EAST AND WEST: A COLLABORATION EXPERIENCE AMONGST BIO-MEDICAL UNIVERSITY LIBRARIES

Arlette Pailley-Katz, Elisabetta Marinoni
[1]Bibliothèque de l'Université Paris 7, Denis-Diderot, Paris, France; [2]Biblioteca Vallisneri, Complesso Biologico Interdipartmentale, Università di Padova, Italy

Introduction

The experience of European cooperation that we present today is located within the framework of the project TEMPUS PHARE (Trans-European Cooperation Scheme for Higher Education) developed by the Commission of the European Communities (General Direction XXII). These programs apply to the economic and social reorganisation of Central and Eastern European countries. They are built on the principle of a partnership between one of these countries and two European Convention countries. This specific project associates the University of Padua and the University of Paris 7 - Denis Diderot, and in particular, the Faculty of Medicine of Padua University, and the Lariboisere Saint Louis Faculty of Medicine, for the benefit of the University of Tirana (Albania). The initial project, named MEDALBA, carried out from 1993 to 1995, renewed the first years of medical studies.

The project

The project, called KLINIK-ALBA, and carried out in 1996-1998, concerns the modernisation of the Faculty of Medicine of the University of Tirana through:
- the reorganisation (and division) of clinical courses of medicine concerning about fifteen specialities;
- teacher training;
- the development of didactic laboratories, and finally
- the modernisation of the Faculty of Medicine library.

The total amount of the contract is ECU 381.550.
Understandably the modernisation of this library constitutes a strong basis of the project for two essential reasons:
- the reform of the medical studies requires the levelling of the structures and the documentary tools;
- the Tirana Faculty of Medicine library is the only medical library in Albania.

The A. Vallisneri Biomedical library of the University of Padua and the Lariboisiere Saint Louis Faculty of Medicine library of the University of Paris 7 were thus involved in the Tempus program, as consultants for the planning and the organisation, with Tirana, of a new library, according to European standards.

The program

The collaboration between the three libraries was discussed and conceived at preliminary work meetings, held in Padua and Paris, between the heads and the teams of the respective libraries and with the heads of the Tirana Faculty of Medicine. Accordingly, it was decided to proceed in two stages: (1) staff training of the Tirana Faculty of Medicine library; (2) development and the implementation of the project of reorganisation and modernisation of the Albanian medical library. This program was selected in order to allow the Albanian librarians reflection on the evolution of their professional practices and the design of the future medical library, so as to understand new working tools.

THE BIBLIOGRAPHIC-ECONOMIC TRAINING PROGRAM

In January 1997 two Albanian librarians began training at the Lariboisiere Saint Louis Faculty of Medicine library with a first session of updating and recycling of general knowledge in documentary techniques: this session comprised theoretical recalls, a practical training course and a visit to various libraries in Paris. The topics included: document classification, fund management, document processing, catalogues, reader classification, front office organisation, inter- library loans, specialised bibliographies.

From September 22 to October 10, 1997: two Albanian librarians came to the A. Vallisneri library of Padua, to follow a training course This enabled them to re-examine some of the topics previously presented in Paris in a new context (reader classification, services available, document supply service) and to examine the following topics in more detail: the library search computerised on CD and the local network and search on Internet. This session also included a visit to several libraries in Rome and also a training three-day course on "library users" (efficiency and effectiveness in resource and service management, quality assessment, statistics, reference service, marketing) Finally, an analysis of the organisation of the Tirana Faculty of Medicine library was carried out in order to optimise existing library space.

THE DEVELOPMENT OF THE PROJECT OF MODERNISATION AND REORGANISATION

The project of modernisation and reorganisation of the library the Faculty of Medicine of Tirana began, in fact, in May 1998, with a first mission going to Tirana, followed by a work meeting in Padua. This program made it possible to draw up an initial list of priorities (a visit to the library and to the Faculty, meetings with the Dean of the Faculty), and in particular to analyse the equipment and the computerisation of the library.

Comment on the situation and an initial plan
The first programming was elaborated taking into account the major aspects of the operation of a modern library: the work to be undertaken, the equipment and furnishings required including computers and written documents such as books and journals. The objectives of modernisation focused on the following:
* setting up of a free-access system through workspaces within documentary spaces;

* reorganisation and development of the computerised information retrieval system;
* bringing up to date the databases and developing the collections on various supports.

Comment on the plan suggested
The creation of a reading room of 120 m^2 completely furnished (shelves, worktables etc.); was resolved with a special supplementary grant from the Veneto Region. (The financing of this part of the program is not foreseen by the TEMPUS project)

The data-processing equipment: a computer and a printer for the reproduction of the cards in several specimens starting with CDS-ISIS software provided by UNESCO; a fax for inter-library lending and document delivery; a computer with CD and a printer for information retrieval. The library subscribes to MEDLINE CD thanks to the SOROS foundation. Internet search will be studied later on.

The priorities for setting up documents was given consideration and identified:
- essential textbooks: recent works will be chosen according to an agreed list of the teachers (great works in English, French manuals, Italian manuals...);
- reference books: dictionaries, Medical-Surgical Encyclopaedia...;
- journals: subscriptions to fundamental titles will be renewed to complement certain titles already allotted by the SOROS Foundation, in CDs (BMJ, Lancet, N Engl J Med).

The allowance for this program cannot exceed the library budget allocation as specified in the TEMPUS project i.e. ECU. 50.000 is available for 1998.

Results and near future

The result of these two years of work on the modernisation of the Medical Library of Tirana and the training of the Albanian librarians has been, in spite of the enormous difficulties encountered, very positive. This experience has allowed the Albanian colleagues to confront the situation of Tirana medical library with the organisation of two modern libraries, and therefore, has allowed them to plan radical changes for themselves. On the other hand, for the western librarians, this experience has permitted a very important moment reflection on the role of the librarian's mission (which does not only reside in the management of innovative technologies) but also has introduced them to the novelty that the Albanian colleagues teach daily.

Next year (1998-99), two visits are expected from the Albanian librarians in Paris and Padua. During there visits our colleagues will have the opportunity to check that the innovations introduced in Tirana have been implemented correctly. They will have, moreover, the opportunity to gain experience in the advanced techniques of information-retrieval, techniques which they could afterwards make use of in the libraries of their home-country.

AUTOMATION AND CENTRALISATION OF CATALOGUES OF HOSPITAL LIBRARIES: LEARNING FROM TOO MUCH SUCCESS

Marjan van Wegen
St Lucas Andreas Hospital, Amsterdam, NL

Background

In 1984, a number of small medical or hospital libraries initiated a project to reach a common goal: the automation of their local catalogues wich ultimately led to the building and maintaining of a central, on-line available, catalogue of all participating libraries. These libraries primarily wanted to join forces in order to improve efficiency and enhance the quality of their library services. However the project was very succesfull there are also a few problems.

Tasks of an average Dutch hospital library

A medical library in a hospital is mostly a one- or two- person library. A medical library in a hospital offers services for the medical profession in a hospital. It primarily serves clinical staff. Depending on a hospital's educational function, its library also serves medical students during their clinical training at the hospital. Larger hospitals, with about 500 beds, usually offer training schemes for medical specialisation. For the past few years, medical libraries have also been open to other hopital workers like nurses en paramedical workers.

The size of a medical library collection varies, ranging from 5000 to 10.000 titels. Medical journals are still the most important part of the collection.

There is a difference between the relatively small medical library in a hospital and the larger medical library in a university hospital. The group of library users in the regular hospital is smaller so the service in more personal.

Automation needs of an average Dutch hospital library

In the past decade medical libraries in hospitals have become more and more professional. An enormous flow of clinical sciences texts and an increasing demand for library services in hospitals have forced the small libraries to expand and adapt their organisation. About 15 years ago most of the libraries did not have a real automated system. Automating the organisation however, was very much needed.

In 1984, a medical librarian employed at a hospital in the mid-east of the Netherlands, appealed to fellow librarians in the periodical for medical librarians. The librarian wondered whether her collegues had any experience and expertise in automating their libraries, especially automating their card catalogue. She received a lot of response from fellow librarians who also needed information about this, but there was no medical library that had completed or even started automation. This librarian's appeal led to the formation of an national working group for the automation of medical libraries.

Start of collaboration in 1984

Its goal was to join forces and exchange ideas in order to design a system that would be usable for as many medical hospital libraries as possible. They decided to work with a sophisticated information storage and retrieval system for automating each catalogue. This system will also be a framework for automating the library's desk work. In 1986 this led to a new working group. Libraries participating in this group agreed on precise regulations with regard to the structure of the database and the storage of data. By the end of 1994 the group had more than 60 participants. To keep in contact the members of the group met twice a year.

The original reason or occasion for collaboration among the libraries was automation of the catalogues and automation of the administration of the library. But over the years this led to collaboration in more areas than just automation.

Other ways of collaborations led to:

* Creating a collective list of journal collections:
* Creation of a Dutch Thesaurus of 2000 medical reference terms
* Creation of a Dutch edition of the National Library of Medicine Classification
* Organizing meetings wich special themes

Forming a central catalogue system

The fast increasing number of participating medical libraries meant that a long cherised wish became feasible: the creation of a centralised catalogue.

After many researches the group decided to organize the centralization by PICA, a company specialised in automated library systems. Pica also maintains the Dutch National Central Catalague. It was in this time that the group has changed its name into "Working Group Central Catalogue Medical Libraries (CCZ).

Results

At the start of creating a central database there were -as agreed with Pica- 15 libraries who participated in the central database. In a very short time more and more libraries decided to join the database. There are now 60 libraries who participate in the system and the common catalogue contains 90.000 titles

Characteristic for the database is the comprehensive structure of the titles and different retrieval possibilities. Titles can be retrieved by the usual headings, such as author, title- words. But because the Dutch Medical thesaurus and the Dutch NLM-codes where created in the database it is possible to search on this special keys. Moreover, the catalogue of one library can be seperated from the rest and then looked through exclusively. When necessary, a library can exclude its own collection while searching through the catalogue system. A record also indicates in which library a title is available and under which shelf mark it can be found. Libraries still create and maintain their own catalogue seperately. Titles are catalogued in the general Dutch library system. These titles are downloaded from the general automated library catalogue to the separate medical library and incorporated in the medical catalogue.

ADVANTAGES OF THE CENTRAL CATALOGUE

* By common use of references and system-codes, a considerable amount of time could be saved in daily cataloguing work
* The users of an individual medical library now have a considerably larger collection at their disposal.
* Thanks to the Automation Project, any medical library that wants to automate now or wishes to extend their automated services can join an cooperative that has been tried and tested.

ORGANIZATIONAL DISADVANTAGES AND MISTAKES

Even though the automated centralised catalogue system for medical libraries had been achieved, not every hospital library could participate. For a few tiny medical libraries it was too expensive to join and pay the fixed price. To make things more complicated, these non-participating libraries could still participate in the working group that achieved and maintained the automated catalogue system. These small libraries did for instance participate in the shared list of medical journals, use the meanwhile developed thesaurus or NLM-codes. These 'poor' libraries also were wellcome to the meetings that were held twice a year.

Organization

The many activities of the working group led to extra management and organizational duties such as:

* Updating, printing and distribution of the journal lists, keyword lists, and NLM-codes
* Preparing and organizing the bi-annual meetings. This meant: finding a proper meeting place and coming up with a interesting theme to be discussed at the meeting.
* Maintaining the database itself and keeping in close contact and collaboration with automation company Pica.

These time and energy consuming activities have led to organizational problems. A number of the working group participants has recently reconsidered its goals. After some discussion and evaluation of the actual situation the working group has decided to reduce its activities to its original purpose: the automated central catalogue system. This means that the CCZ-Group only consist of participants in the central automated catalogue. All the other members are referred to the BMI as the activities as mentioned above, are delegated to this Dutch medical library organization. This also prevents further confusion about the fact the working group is a part of the BMI, and not -as some people still thought- an independent group.

Management

From 1998 on, the management and activities of the original working group will be co-ordinated by a so-called core group. This group consists of seven members from the larger working group. Each core group member has an organizational task.

Recommendations to fellow librarians. Learning from the mistakes

Looking back on 15 years of collaboration there will be the conclusion that you can achieve a lot by joining forces.

It is important that when you start collaborating in a project, that you have a clear goal and stick to it. It easily evolves into a larger and multi-purpose project. This ultimately can lead to a overgrowth in activities and becomes to big to manage and to expensive to organize permanently.

Another important recommendation is to look for an existent structure within which the collaboration project can operate. In this case it would have been better from the start that the working group should have operated within the structure of the Dutch medical library organization BMI. In the beginning the CCZ originally operated as a more independent group. This led to the inefficient situation that both BMI and the working group were simultaneously organizing theme meetings about more or less the same subjects.

Summary

The three basic questions for collaboration are:

a. What is the main purpose of our collaboration (a clear goal).
b. How to achieve this goal and keep this collaboration manageable.
c. How can we operate within an existing structure.

EQUAL ACCESS, SIMPLE ACCESS: CONSORTIA AGREEMENTS IN NORWAY

Elisabeth Akre
NORWEGIAN LIBRARY ASSOCIATION, SECTION FOR MEDICINE AND HEALTH, OSLO, NORWAY

Introduction and background

The library vision is that knowledge and information shall be easily accessible and to a high extent free to everyone. A major goal for libraries must be to contribute to equal and simple access to quality-controlled information sources. Consortia agreements are one way of obtaining this.

The Norwegian project "Consortia Agreements for the Health Sector" co-ordinated by RBT, the National Office for Research, Documentation, Academic and Special Libraries. The Norwegian Ministry of Health is a co-operative partner, and so is the Norwegian Library Association, Section for Medicine and Health, SMH.

Aims and goals

The Norwegian Ministry of Health through their “Plan for a National Network for Health”, to be ready by the year 2000, stated the goals of the project:
- access to quality-controlled medical information;
- the databases should contain relevant information for the user groups;
- access must be equal for all categories of health professionals;
- access should be effective both in terms of costs and in terms of time;
- life-long learning and continuous professional updating are national goals and the health sector focuses on knowledge-based-practice and sources of evidence-based-medicine. Access to digital information sources is part of this aspect.

RBT signed two licence agreements in 1995, one with the Institute for Scientific Information (ISI) and one with Online Computer Library Centre (OCLC). The databases covered by these agreements were partly relevant to health professions, but did not cover the field sufficiently.

The access was restricted to academic institutions, meaning that a medical student has access to information and knowledge in order to treat his “virtual patient”, while the physician working with the diagnosis and treatment of the real patient has not.

The project

The hospital librarians were alarmed by this fact on behalf of their users and turned to SMH for help. SMH requested RBT to contribute to consortia agreements for the health sector, covering health databases such as MEDLINE, EMBASE, CINAHL, Cochrane etc. with access for both academic and non-academic health institutions. RBT saw the needs for both a health database agreement and the need to include all categories of health professions and health institutions. A co-operative project between RBT and SMH was established.

In 1997 the products from the three producers Silver Platter, OCLC and OVID were tested. MEDLINE, CINAHL, EMBASE and BIOSIS were chosen as test databases. The testing and the evaluation should be made by user groups in non-academic institutions as well as by users in the academic sector, co-ordinated by the librarians of the institutions.The test results were somewhat difficult to systematize, partly due to technical problems during the test period.

After the trial in 1997, the focus has mainly been on analysing which groups of health institutions would be interested in joining a consortium agreement. RBT has already decided to start negotiations on behalf of the academic institutions and established this spring a reference group of interested parties from the non-academic institutions and a working group, which is looking into the contents of an agreement regarding the specific interests of the different non-academic user groups, and which institutions in this category should be included. The report of the working group will be ready in the autumn of 1998 and is meant to give input to the planned negotiations.

Issues to be resolved

SECURITY

Network security regulations in Norway does not allow sensitive information in a network with external access, particularly in the health sector. The technical solutions for firewalls available at the moment are so far not accepted. To have access to Internet a separate network has to be established. This is a question of economic priorities and health institution budgets are tight. The national plan for a health network will hopefully solve this problem. Lacking sufficient possibilities for accessing Internet has consequences for joining a consortia agreement.

ORGANISATIONAL PROBLEMS

The role of RBT is to co-ordinate and negotiate on behalf of groups of interested institutions. The academic institutions do not have security problems, the Internet connection has been established and they have already experienced the advantages of consortia agreements. As part of the Ministry of Education, Research and Church affairs RBT will enter into negotiations for the academic sector. Each institution will have to finance the participation from its own budget.

Non-academic health institutions belong to the Ministry of Health and are organised under three different authority levels: state, county and community. The Ministry can make a central decision on behalf of state institutions. Individually practising physicians can be covered this way.

The non-academic hospitals are administered on two levels, county and community, and it is difficult to identify a national authority which can speak for the hospitals as a group. This poses a real problem: access to information may be determined by a structural position rather than by the needs of access to the information.

An alternative solution is to co-ordinate and administrate by the five health regions of the country with access via regional hospital Intranets and the university clinic of the region as a database host.

TECHNICAL ISSUES

BIBSYS is a library and information system covering the academic institutions in Norway. The ISI databases are hosted by BIBSYS and accessible through their web interface, and are linked to the holdings in the BIBSYS database, making the national resources more visible and simplifying the interlibrary loan process.

Access to the services is based on IP-identification. Many non-academic health institutions access Internet via a modem. A solution must be found allowing access this way, e.g. a password solution.

Waiting for better Internet connection, there may be a need for interim solutions, such as combining CD-ROM-solutions with Internet admission.

CONTENT

Different health professions have different needs of information. One of the tasks of the working group is to analyse profiles of information needs for the different professions to set up a content profile for an agreement, combining general interests with specific interests, such as CINAHL for nurses.

PRICE

At this stage it is not possible to give an accurate estimate of what the institutions are willing to pay to join an agreement. But a subscription through a consortium agreement must offer more favourable prices than individual subscriptions.

TRAINING

Many health professionals in Norway, especially in the hospitals, are still unfamiliar with Internet and with document searching in online databases. This is due to a lack of appropriate equipment, a lack of access possibilities, and a lack of time. Internet access and search training are vital in order to get these categories of health professionals to use database searching in their professional updating. Libraries and librarians will be important partners in training programme, focusing on:

- attitudes to using knowledge based sources for clinical updating as well as for case documentation
- searching skills, applying both to technical aspects and to database content.

The Norwegian Nursing Association has made an application to integrate such training in the educational programme for nurses.

Concluding remarks

Why consortia agreements?
A better price for a better product.
Time saving by centralising of the updating and administrating of the services

Why pay for the information?
More and more health information seems to be available on the Internet at no cost. The NLM MEDLINE web site is perhaps the most outstanding example of a free source which is quality-controlled both regarding contents and search structure. So why bother to pay?

Accessing the information sources directly from his desk PC the user needs linking possibilities between reference databases and sources of full text. Consortia agreements can offer additional values, such as:
- access to several quality-controlled and evidence based information sources from one web site;
- one search language and one web interface;
- linking from reference databases to full text and vice versa;
- linking to interlibrary loan services and to document delivery services.

Where are we?
Equal access, simple access to health information - is it Utopia or can it become reality?

For the academic and some non-academic institutions a national health database agreement seems within reach. For other non-academic institutions, mainly the hospitals, the future is more uncertain due to:
- lack of technological infrastructure
- lack of an official "umbrella" which can speak for the group as a whole
- local lack of awareness of how important the quality-controlled Internet sources are for knowledge based professional updating.

The near future
RBT and SMH shall continue to work to achieve the goal:
- to build a bridge over the information gap between academic and non-academic health institutions;
- to make it possible for physicians and other therapists to build their patient's diagnosis and treatment on updated and evidence based knowledge.

The situation in Norway indicates that the way to achieve this may be the regional way via hospital intranets in the five health regions.

TOWARDS AN INTEGRATED POLICY OF ACQUISITIONS OF SERIALS IN THE LIBRARIES OF A HOSPITAL

Laura Cavazza, Leslie Locche
SOPRINTENDENZA PER I BENE LIBRARI E DOCUMENTARI, REGIONE EMILIA-ROMAGNA, BOLOGNA, ITALY

Introduction

There are 30 libraries at the Policlinico S.Orsola-Malpighi, 12 owned by Azienda Ospedaliera di Bologna (Bologna Health Unit of NHS) and 18 leading libraries of the medical faculties of the Universita di Bologna. The libraries, all located in adjoining premises, regularly publish their union catalogue of serials.

The research shown here (carried out by Biblioteca Centralizzata of the Azienda Ospedaliera di Bologna in collaboration with Soprintendenza per i beni librari e documentari-Regione Emilia-Romagna) was determined by the need to control the sums going into subscriptions; it aims at enhancing the quality of the titles, at brushing up the collections, at covering each discipline and at eliminating, wherever possible, any overlap between the collections of the two administrations.This is a first step to reach a coordinated programme of subscriptions and a minimum standard of service which could be the focus of a future agreement between the Azienda and the University.

Methodology

- the analysis is based upon the data published in the 1998 edition of the union catalogue;[1]
- the class of hematology was chosen and checked against the Brandon-Hill List,[2] the Abridged Index Medicus[3] and the Journal Citation Reports[4] (20% top relevant titles);
- high quality titles which are not present in the collections were indicated; duplicates were singled out;
- the number of titles of hematology was compared with the grand total listed in the Journal Citation Report in order to evaluate the ratio between quantity and quality.

Results

Figure 1 describes the data observed in the survey. Out of 1129 current titles 180 are to be found both at Azienda and at the University; the number of subscriptions is

1419. The 290 subscriptions, further duplicating the existing ones, were outlined: some subscriptions arrive to the libraries as a gift, 180 are common to both administrations, 19 at the Azienda, 91 at the University. A rough estimate of the expenditure for excess copies can be made.

Hematology was chosen as a sample category among the 61 classes covered by the union catalogue.The category was strechted to include three border-line titles. The qualitative analisys based upon the comparison between the existing titles and the relevant top 20% of the impact factor of the JCR titles showed that two high quality titles are not present in the union catalogue, whereas four titles are held by both organizations and three of them arrive by separate subscriptions in even more copies within the same University libraries (see figure 2).

Discussion and conclusions

The quantitative analysis of the collection, described by the union catalogue, outlined a situation with a high number of more than one subscription per title and duplicated titles which should be dealt with.

The qualitative analysis showed that, although the collections can rely upon good quality journals, there are many subscriptions in excess and that a very few high quality titles never entered the libraries.

The research methodology hit the mark: a joint study group will be suggested and the application of the same methodology to all the classes. The intended survey would then supply data to back future agreements between Azienda and University on the management of serial collections and minimum service standards in the library of the Policlinico.

References

[1] Azienda Ospedaliera di Bologna, Policlinico Sant'Orsola-Malpighi, Biblioteca Centralizzata. Catalogo dei periodici delle biblioteche dell'Azienda Ospedaliera di Bologna, Policlinico Sant'Orsola-Malpighi e dell'Universita' degli Studi di Bologna, Facolta' di Medicina e Chirurgia, Settore Sanitario del Sistema Bibliotecario d'Ateneo. Bologna: Azienda Ospedaliera di Bologna, Policlinico Sant'Orsola-Malpighi, 1998

[2] Brandon AN, Hill DR. Selected list of books and journals for the small medical library. Bull Med Libr Assoc 1997;85:111-35

[3] National Library of Medicine. List of journals indexed in Index Medicus, 1997. Bethesda: National Library of Medicine, 1997

[4] Institute for Scientific Information. Journal Citation Reports: a bibliometric analisys of science journals in the ISI database. Philadelphia: Institute for Scientific Information, 1996

The text of the paper was translated by Margherita Spinazzola.

Figure 1:
Data of the survey regarding journal subscriptions, titles and duplicates

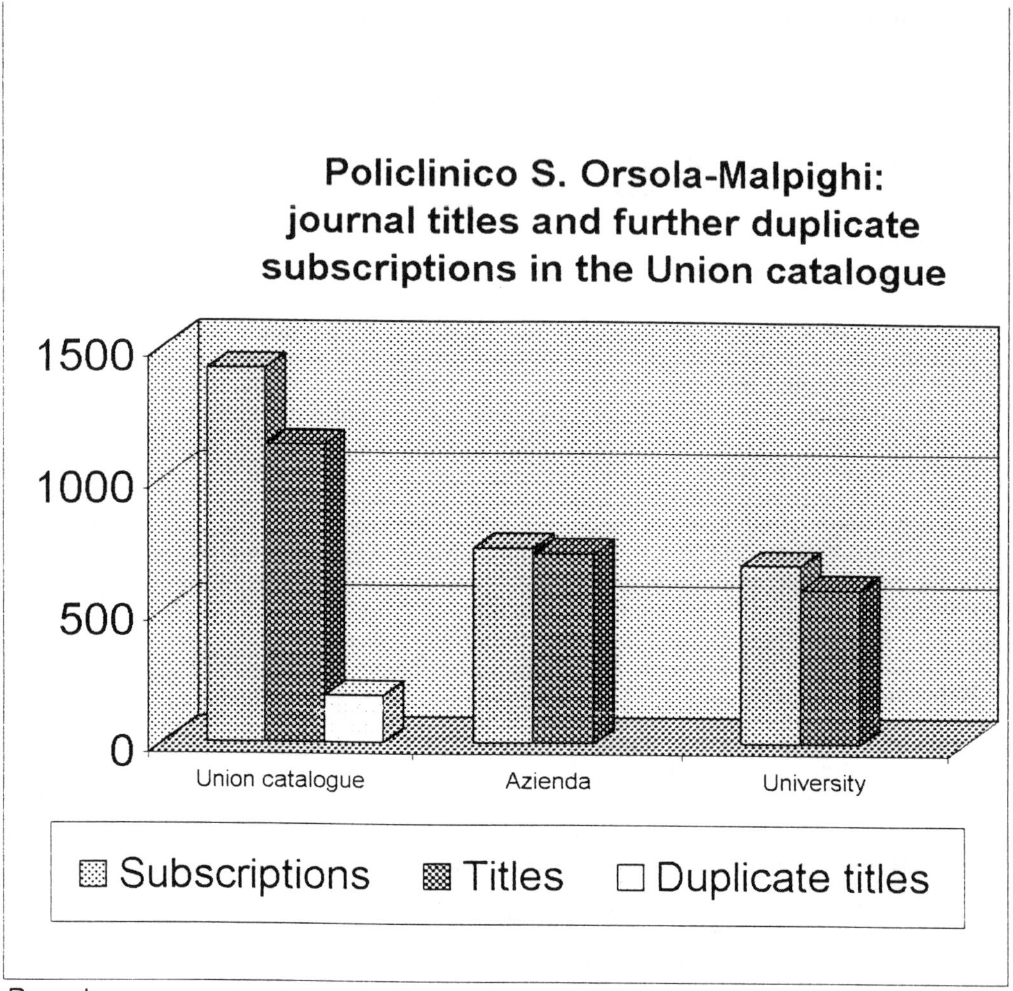

Remarks:

* Duplicate titles between Azienda and University:
  180 in the Union catalogue

* Further subscriptions of the same titles:
  290 in the union catalogue
  19 in the azienda catalogue
  91 in the university catalogue

Figure 2:
Analysis of the collection of hematology journals

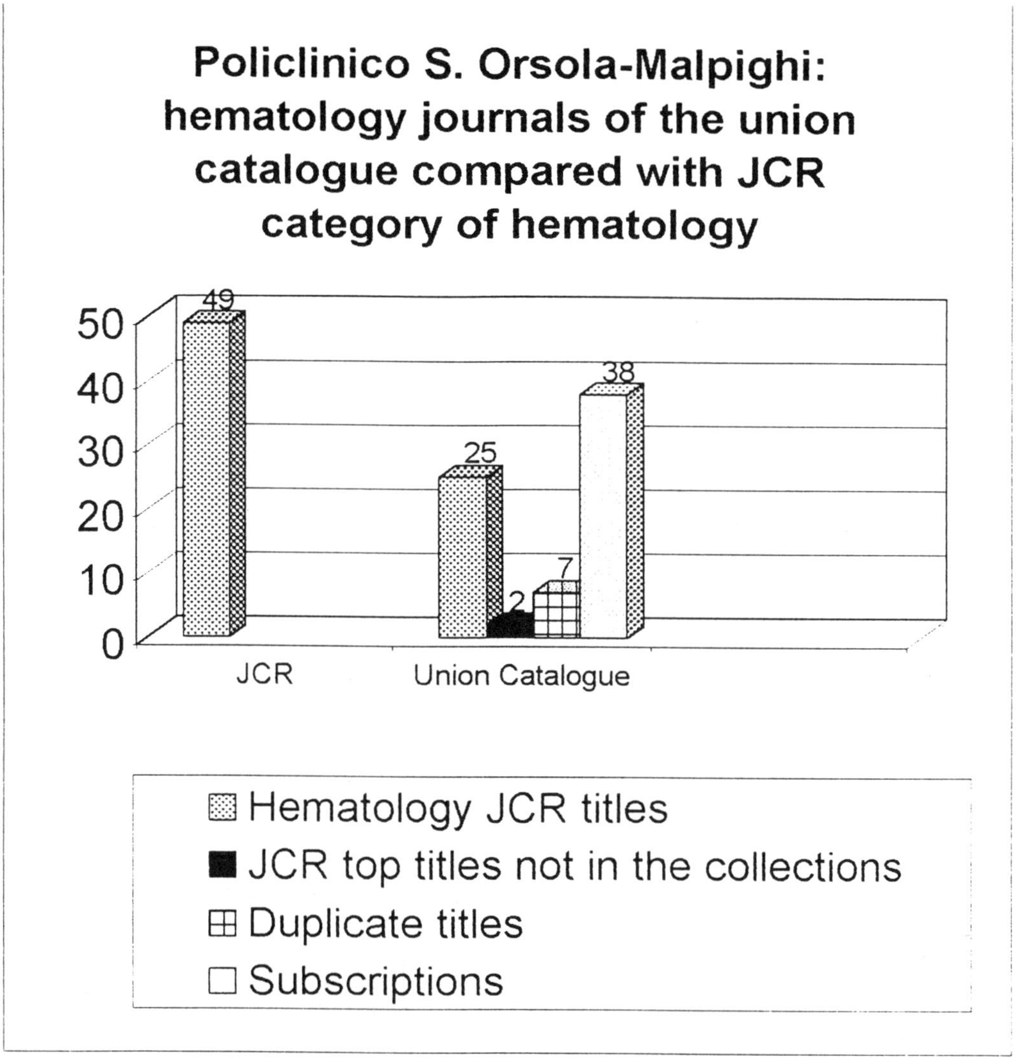

INDEXING ITALIAN BIOMEDICAL RESOURCES AVAILABLE ON THE INTERNET: A FIRST APPROACH

Maurella Della Seta, Antonietta Monaco, Adriana Dracos
ISTITUTO SUPERIORE DI SANITÀ, DOCUMENTATION SERVICE, ROME, ITALY

Project description

Widespreading biomedical information on the Internet has triggered new challenges for the information specialists and new roles have been identified: (1) developing and applying information filtering systems; (2) assisting users to manage the information overload through training and advice.[1,2]

End-users discovered the countless resources available on the Web and are exploring the net by the help of the evolution of searching tools: from the access to web pages by the identification of the specific address (URL), to subject searching by means of search engines, until the creation of metasites, which serve as pointers to several other web pages specialised in similar areas.[3] Organising and indexing Internet resources represent, therefore, a current issue of major concern. The purpose of this paper is to describe the preliminary experience of the authors in developing a tool providing access to carefully selected web pages. Our intention is to filter the information available to select the most useful and usable pages for Italian health professionals and health consumers.

As a first step, a survey has been performed with the purpose of identifying and assessing Italian biomedical resources on the Internet. Relevant web sites were located by search engines, employing Italian terms for health, medicine, physician and patient. Other useful tools were the Italian Web Pages (http://www.iwp.it) and the Italian General Subject Tree (http://www.mi.cnr.it/IGST/Medicina/), which are both directories of Italian web sites, arranged into broad categories without any attempt of selection or evaluation.

Microsoft Access 97 has been chosen for the organisation of data retrieved into a database. One of the reasons for this choice has been the possibility of converting data into HTML format. For each site a record has been provided, with the indication of the following fields: identification number, name of the resource, URL, audience to which the information is addressed, brief description including, if necessary, charging policy or restrictions to access, presence of links to other sites, evaluation, language or languages used, kind of authorship, MeSH headings and subheadings in Italian and in English.

Indexing of each site has been carried out in order to provide subject access to the selected resources. MeSH have been chosen thanks to their large acceptance by the scientific community and biomedical libraries users, within the scope of a project – the Italian translation of MeSH - which is being developed by our Institute.

Results and conclusions

Until now about 250 sites have been identified and analysed. Special attention was paid to the authorship, since clear and unambiguous responsibility for the site is an essential factor to be taken into consideration for the selection of the resource.[4] Responsible for the contents of the sites were: 27% charities or volunteers associations, 25% individual health professionals, 14% professional associations, 13% academic institutions or research institutes, 12% hospitals, 4% commercial firms, 4% governmental or regional organisations, 1% authors were not clearly indicated. Selection and evaluation of sites were also carried out according to the following criteria: accessibility and workability; accuracy of information provided; relevance, value and coverage of contents; currency of data; disclosure of web site ownership or of possible sponsors; readability of language used with regard to the expected audience; listing of references for all contents. For each selected site a score was assigned: very poor (no star); poor (one star); sufficient (two stars); good (three stars); excellent (four stars). Only sites scoring at least two stars or more have been included in the database. A deep analysis of the identified 250 sites, evidenced that only about one third of them owned the requirements necessary to be defined a quality resource.

Moreover, from the analysis of the web pages, it emerged that the focus of most sites was the management of widespread diseases. By the indexing process we are planning to disclose missing or only partially-covered health related areas: on the light of this experience, new concern on these topics may lead to initiatives, by public or private institutions, in order to fill possible information gaps in the biomedical field.

The preliminary results of our survey have outlined that Italian end-users have at their hand a broad range of resources, but health-related information should always be carefully checked and evaluated by information specialists in order to assure access to quality materials.

Further investigation is necessary in order to provide an exhaustive overview of the Italian resources on the Internet in the biomedical field. Future developments of our project contemplate access and indexing of a widest variety of sites, also through the collaboration of the whole Italian biomedical librarians community.

References

[1] Hopkins RL. Countering information overload: the role of the librarian. Ref Libr 1995;49/50:305-322

[2] Anagnostelis B, Cox J. Data on the Internet: Evaluating the quality or 'Less is more'. <http://www.omni.ac.uk/agec/ukolug.html>

[3] Marshall L. Health & medical industry research information on the World Wide Web: a metasite. Database 1997;20(2):57-60

[4] MacKay D, Sutton-Curr J. Hypertext links from HEBSWeb – a protocol to evaluate Internet resources. Health Libr Rev 1997;14:184-189

OPTIMISM FOR THE FUTURE: A REGIONAL HEALTH CARE LIBRARY AND INFORMATION SERVICE NETWORK

Shane Godbolt c.s.
REGIONAL LIBRARY & NORTH THAMES INFORMATION UNIT, THAMES POSTGRADUATE MEDICAL & DENTAL EDUCATION, UNIVERSITY OF LONDON, LONDON, UK

Summary

Public enterprises have become more like business. The management techniques of the business world have introduced all health service managers including librarians to the concepts of customers, quality assurance, monitoring, accountability and increasingly value for money. The NHS is a people processing organisation. Its purpose is output people transformed by its input or as stated in its planning guidances 'to secure through resources available the greatest possible improvement to the physical and mental health of the people of England'. Added value lies in the transformation of 'input' into 'output' and whether it represents good value for money is determined mostly by calculating the cost of transformation set against the notional costs and benefits of any alternative system.Librarians have to reposition themselves within their organisational frameworks and to understand the new contexts in which they are operating. The external environment is rapidly changing and increasingly sophisticated. Access to the knowledge base of health care is crucial for all health care professionals. Healthcare Librarians and Information Specialists have to be proactive in working to improve the provision and accessibility of high quality, appropriate and cost effective services which underpin clinical effectiveness and evidence-based health care. The Regional Library and Information Unit in North Thames works with over 200 information professional and front-line service staff with around 100 service points. The customer base covers a diverse range of professions and interests. The poster presentation outlined the opportunities offered to work with colleagues in a variety of library and educational structures as well as with health care professionals including consultants, training grade doctors, general practitioners, nurses, professions allied to medicine as well as senior managers and support staff in the regional office, in Trust and Health Authorities. The skills and knowledge of librarians and information specialists are valued by those struggling with the dilemma in information overload coupled with lack of ability and time to identify that which is relevant and specific to the purpose for which it is required. Business development and marketing strategies are needed to raise awareness of value of the service with policy makers and funders at the regional and local level. The approach to developing these strategies was presented.

SHARING THE RESOURCES: ON-LINE DATABASES AT THE UNIVERSITY

Elisabetta Marinoni, Pierangela Mazzon, Maurizio Tiziano Moretto, Donata Pieri, Roberta Sato, Maurizio Vedaldi
UNIVERSITÀ DEGLI STUDI DI PADOVA, PADOVA, ITALY

Since Spring 1996 the sharing of database resources by means of the University Computer Network has been successfully experimented at the University of Padua using Silver Platter Electronic Reference Library (ERL) technology. Prior to this, several databases such as MEDLINE and Current Contents had already been set up in the scientific libraries of our university (9 copies of MEDLINE, 5 copies of Current Contents) and these were available on a CD support running many different software programs. However, this resulted in bad resources allocation, not always justified by the number of searches, together with correspondingly high costs. Moreover, training proved difficult because of the heterogeneous and uncoordinated software packages used by various libraries.

The possibility of sharing the online resources at the University of Padua by using a single networked platform seemed to be the ideal solution for obtaining a common method of access to the bibliographic databases and allowing all researchers access to a larger number of databases at lower total costs.

The network licence for 12 customers costs approximately a third of the total of the previous nine stand-alone versions. This choice has encouraged collaboration and integration of different human resources such as librarians and computer technicians involving not only testing friendly user interface but also the drawing-up of common instructions for end-users. These instructions had to be both simple and detailed allowing anyone access to the databases. Besides the standard mode of access personalised the installation of the 'client' software on each personal computer, the possibility to query databases via World Wide Web browsers was highly appreciated. In this sense the installation of specific programmes or 'dedicated' workstations has become redundant.

The experience, has been extremely positive and has increased the number of databases available to the entire University scientific community. Moreover, databases, particularly the biomedical ones, proofed to be useful for researchers in other fields such as life sciences. Vice versa the CAB Abstract database has also proved useful to public health physicians. Although the infrastructure is rather expensive the wide availability of information has amply justified the cost. The result of this experience and the consequent capillary spreading of scientific database use has been extremely positive.

We are grateful to Luca Ciano for his technical support.

Chapter 12: REMOTE ACCESS AND DOCUMENT SUPPLY

Editorial introduction

This chapter contains two papers form France, three from Italy, and also papers from the UK, Norway, Sweden, and Slovenia, all dealing with the distance between the user of information and the source of information. In traditional library services (from times before computers and fax machines were available) this meant document delivery either in its original form or as photocopies. Nowadays a range of technology is in use for requesting and delivering: electronic computer sytems, facsimile and electronic transmission, scanning and printing on demand. None of these technologies are fully and completely replacing the older technique: a mixture of technology is in use within the library.

The first two papers contain comparisons of document ordering and delivery: one focussing on systems and the other on performance and costs. The following papers discuss the possibilities for end-users to access information resources of the library or on the Internet by using computer technology. The paper of Ragnhild Lande presents an example of a university library that is able to expand its services over longer distances. The papers of Hélène Breul et al. and of Anamarija Rozic-Hristovski et al. discuss the available web-based information sources, either national resources or locally stored information sources.

The last paper reports about a European project making use of a combination of telecommunication channels in order to support family carers by delivering information at their homes.

These examples show the multitude of possibilities and the opportunities for library and information professionals to expand their services. Distance is no longer a real barrier to information; but not all barriers are yet broken down by technology: organisational changes, cooperation and political choices are necessary to bring boundary- and barrier-free information provision into reality.

L'ACCES AU DOCUMENT PRIMAIRE DANS LE DOMAINE BIOMEDICAL: UNE ENQUETE INTERNATIONALE

Laurent Ghirardi, Madeleine Wolff-Terroine
PEGASOS/ICC, PARIS, FRANCE

Summary

While it is easier to search databases, the access to original documents remains a problem for both end-users and information professionnals. The results (ordering and delivery methods, non-reception reasons, costs, delays) of a survey of document delivery services in Europe and North America, several thousands of document request with more than 20% in biomedical field, are presented. Some astonishing facts are highlighted, such as the length of delay or the prevailing use of mail.

Introduction

L'obtention du document primaire a toujours été un problème essentiel, tant pour les bibliothécaires et documentalistes que pour les utilisateurs finals. La réduction des budgets des bibliothèques conjuguée à l'augmentation du coût des abonnements ont aggravé la situation. EUSIDIC (European Association for Information Services) a donc décidé en 1995 d'entreprendre une enquête approfondie sur ce problème, enquête confiée aux associations nationales d'utilisateurs. C'est dans ce cadre que l'AFUSIE (Association française des utilisateurs de systèmes d'information électronique), après avoir mis au point une méthodologie, a réalisé l'ensemble de cette étude. Cette enquête, réitérée les années suivantes et qui a porté sur plus 13.000 documents a attiré l'intérêt des Etats-Unis; ils ont adopté le questionnaire établi et leurs résultats ont été analysés par l'équipe de l'AFUSIE, assurant ainsi l'homogénéité indispensable à toute comparaison ultérieure.

La communauté biomédicale est largement représentée dans cette enquête, puisqu'elle est à l'origine de 24,3% des demandes de documents en Europe et de 21% en Amérique du Nord (NA). Il était donc intéressant d'étudier si une certaine spécificité caractérisait ce domaine et si des différences Europe/NA pouvaient être décelées.

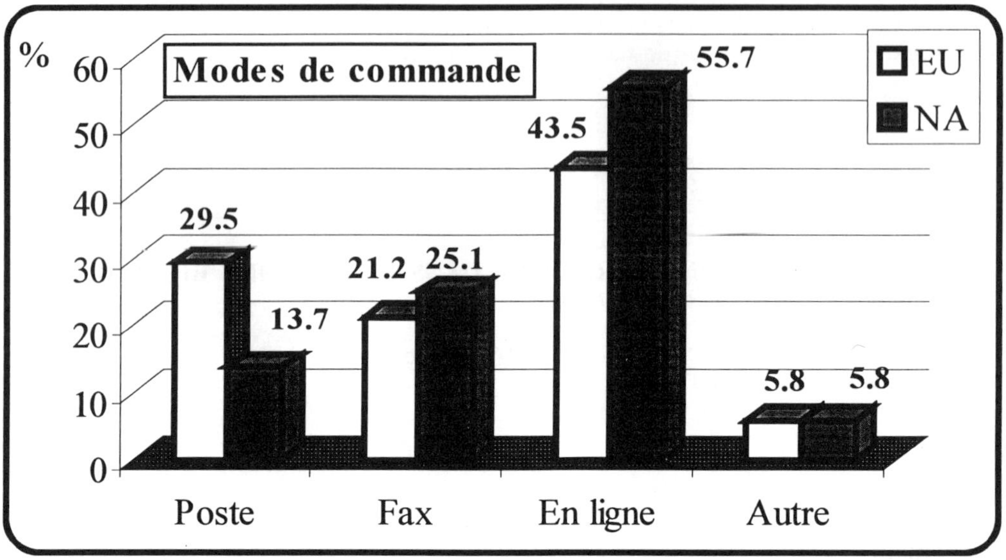

Figure 1 : Modes de commande des documents

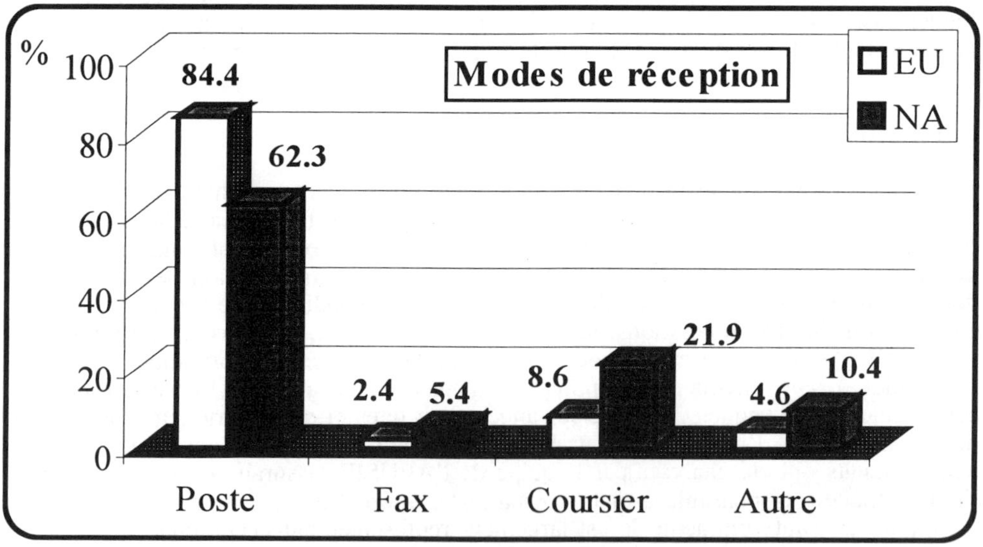

Figure 2 : Modes de réception des documents

Objectifs de l'étude, méthodologie

L'objectif de cette étude est d'évaluer et de comparer les services de fourniture de documents primaires sous quatre aspects essentiels:
- le mode de commande et de réception des documents,
- leurs délais d'obtention,
- le coût.

L'enquête se déroule sur une période de trois semaines: la première semaine chaque participant note toutes les commandes de photocopies effectuées et le mode de commande (fax, poste, en ligne...), pour chaque commande honorée, il note la date et les modalités de réception et ceci jusqu'à la fin des deux semaines suivantes. Les documents non arrivés à la fin de cette période sont considérés comme non reçus.

Un questionnaire a donc été élaboré pour y consigner toutes ces données auxquelles s'ajoutent des données concernant les participants: domaine d'activité, organisme public ou privé, taille de l'organisme, nombre annuel de photocopies demandées...

Résultats

L'étude a porté sur 16 pays en Europe, et l'Amérique du Nord (AN). Seules ont été prises en compte les demandes de photocopies, les demandes de prêt, livres en particulier, sont donc exclues.

Les documents commandés sont essentiellement des articles de périodiques puisqu'ils représentent 93,6% des demandes en Europe et 87,5% en AN; ils sont suivis par les brevets, moins nombreux en Europe qu'en AN.

Trois modes de commande dominent (cf figure 1): la commande en ligne (au cours de la recherche, par réseau de type ARTtel), le fax, et la poste, mais avec une très grande disparité suivant les pays: la commande en ligne est < 10% dans les pays scandinaves, > 75% en Autriche.

Le nombre de documents non reçus est fort élevé et que, plus grave, dans 50% des cas en EU (25% en AN) cette non-fourniture n'est accompagnée d'aucune explication. De plus, en AN, ce nombre est de 50% plus élevé qu'en Europe. A nos recherches d'explication, nos collègues américains ont répondu qu'ils commandaient beaucoup de documents sans savoir si le fournisseur les possède.

La poste reste le mode de réception très largement prédominant (cf figure 2). Les délais de livraison sont surprenants: 6,2 jours en Europe, 4,7 en AN. On est étonné par cette longueur, bien éloignée de ce qu'annoncent les grands fournisseurs de documents. Pourquoi, d'autre part, l'Europe est-elle nettement plus « lente » que l'AN? Faut-il incriminer la poste ou un manque de performance de la part de trop nombreux fournisseurs?

Un point intéressant est apporté par la confrontation délai / modes de commande et de réception: si l'on excepte le couple commande par fax livraison par coursier ou courrier spécial, nettement plus rapide, le mode de commande, fax, en ligne, poste, influe très peu sur le délai de fourniture: 6,4 jours, 6,4 jours, 7,1 jours.

Les données sur le coût ne peuvent être comparées entre Europe et AN: en effet, les américains ont modifié le questionnaire en demandant le coût réel des photocopies commandées, mais sans précision sur le nombre de pages, le nombre de copies... rendant ces données inexploitables. En Europe, 11,2% des documents sont obtenus gratuitement, 77,8% contre paiement: 83,7% à un prix standard, 12,5% à un prix réduit et 4,2% à un tarif élevé (envois en urgence...). Comparé à la moyenne générale, le secteur biomédical arrive en tête pour les prix forts (moyenne générale, 2,5%) comme pour les prix réduits (moyenne générale, 7,5%). Ceci pourrait, à notre avis, refléter les deux entités ayant contribué à cette enquête: Industrie pharmaceutique / bibliothèques universitaires.

La commande est prépayée (compte de dépôt, coupons) dans 46,7% des cas et post-payée (facture) dans 53,3% des cas. L'étude de l'influence du statut de l'organisme demandeur, montre que 69% des documents du secteur public sont post-payés, 65% de ceux du secteur privé étant prépayés. De plus, pour le secteur public, les coûts se décalent vers le bas (prix réduits ou gratuité).

Les fournisseurs sont extrêmement dispersés: 236 en Europe, 117 en AN, plus de 80% fournissant seulement de 1 à 5 documents tandis que 3 se détachent très fortement de la moyenne, la British Library, l'INIST (France) et le Karolinska Institute (Suède), et en AN, UMI.

Conclusion

Cette étude montre que « l'Europe du document » n'est pas encore faite ! Il existe une grande diversité de comportement, de politique, de coûts,... entre les pays.

Les « autoroutes de l'Information » sont encore très peu utilisés dans la fourniture des documents primaires, la poste la poste restant le moyen dominant. L'utilisation croissante d'Internet accompagnée des modifications éditoriales des éditeurs modifieront-elles les habitudes de commande des utilisateurs et permettront-elles de réduire les délais d'obtention des documents, délais encore très longs.

Il faut regretter les trop faibles effectifs de certains types de documents, par exemple brevets, normes, réglementations,.. ce qui ne permet pas de juger les performances des prestataires sur l'ensemble des documents qu'ils fournissent.

Les « autoroutes de l'Information » sont encore très peu utilisés dans la fourniture des documents primaires, la poste restant le moyen dominant. La croissance d'Internet accompagnée des modifications des politiques éditoriales des éditeurs modifieront-elles les habitudes des utilisateurs et permettront-elles de réduire les, encore très longs, délais d'obtention des documents?

La répétition de cette étude permettra de disposer de données quantitatives évolutives et ainsi participer à l'amélioration des services de fourniture des documents primaires.

THE COST OF DOCUMENT DELIVERY AND THE LIBRARY SERVICES PERFORMANCE

Giuseppe Merlo, Valentina Comba
UNIVERSITY OF TORINO, CENTRAL MEDICAL LIBRARY, TORINO, ITALY

Introduction

Cost-effective and timely document delivery is a major concern as many academic libraries face cuts in their budget for journals.

This study examines the performance of five commercial document suppliers and compares them with an Italian Interlibrary Loan service called GIDIF, RBM (which stands for Gruppo Italiano Documentalisti dell'Industria Farmaceutica e degli istituti di Ricerca BioMedica). GIDIF,RBM (henceforth Gidif) is an Union Catalogue of serials, which allows participating Libraries to receive copies of articles on an exchange basis. A sample of 29 requests for periodicals articles was sent both to commercial suppliers and to 17 Gidif Libraries at the same time. Data were collected on each supplier's ability to fill requests, costs and quality of the service.

Commercial suppliers

The following suppliers were selected among the most important ones, on the basis of their strong holdings in the field of Biomedicine and partly based on our precedent positive experience in their document delivery services:

- EBSCO Document Services, part of the EBSCO Information Services group (henceforth EBSCO);
- INIST Document Delivery Service (henceforth INIST);
- British Library Document Supply Centre (henceforth BLDSC) ;
- the Universitätsspital-Bibliothek of the University of Zurich (henceforth ZU100); the Internet Public Access Catalog (IPAC) of the DOBIS/LIBIS-network provides a catalogue for 41 local libraries which represent more than 100 libraries of the University of Zurich from every faculty, except for the School of Law,;
- ISI Document Solution (from now on ISI), a part of the Institute for Scientific Information.

Methodology

A two-month trial period, with a target sample of 30 requests for articles not held in Central Medical Library was defined. There was no filtering of the requests, which were sent alternately to each one on a rotational basis.

The authors co-ordinated the trial, assessing the suppliers' performance in the areas of: actual holdings; procedures to request and deliver; copy quality; cost per transaction (including copyright fee); time required to submit a request. A log sheet was designed to record such data.[1]

Results

Table 1 shows the results of this trial. (All currency exchange rates were calculated on 6/10/1998)

Table 1: Comparison of performance

SUPPLIER	Ebsco	Inist	British Library	Zu100	Isi	Gidif,Rbm
Time for delivering	12,6	10,5	7,3	12,6	17,6	11,1
mode (req)	3	3	3	1	3	1
mode (rec)	2	2	2	2	2	2
Pages for article	5,6	6,6	6,8	6	6,8	6,36
Hold	100%	100%	100%	100%	100%	86%
Qual. txt	1	1,16	1	1,2	1	1
Qual. graph.	1	1	1,33	1,4	1	1,2
Cost (Usd)	19,423	10,258	9,914	11,888	20,931	7,307
Time for requesting	2' 35"	2' 30"	1' 50"	5'	3' 40"	1' 30"
TOTAL cost per item (Usd)	20,187 Usd	11,115 Usd	10,542 Usd	13,775 Usd	22,056 Usd	7,787 Usd

Average delivery time ranged from 7.3 days for BLDSC to 17.6 days for ISI; this last collected the articles requested before sending them to Italy from the US.

Except for ZU100, all suppliers had the on-line request option (by e-mail, telnet or the web). ZU100 allows Swiss libraries to make on-line requests, but from abroad accepts only faxes ILL IFLA forms. Suppliers addressed all requests, although we did not carry out any beforehand control of the journals listed in their catalogues. All suppliers supplied documents of good to excellent quality, with few exceptions.

Suppliers had different basic fee for standard service:

- EBSCO applies a standard fee of 12.50 $, (copyright payment apart);
- ISI applies a standard fee of 10.95 $, (copyright payment apart);
- INIST applies a standard fee depending on the number of pages, (plus a standard copyright fee of 7 FF);

- BLDSC and ZU100 apply a standard fee depending on the number of pages, including the copyright fee.

INIST, BLDSC and ZU100 required customers to open a prepaid account, and purchase a minimum number of "Units" or "Coupon"; Ebsco asks the customer to open an account before ordering online.

The time required to submit the request differed, depending on the methods used and connection time: it ranged from 1 min. and 20", for a request to the BLDSC (ArtTel) via Telnet, to 7 min. and 30" for Zurich, time being needed to check, write, print and fax a request.

Performance analysis indicates BLDSC as the cheapest and fastest commercial supplier of documents, followed by INIST.

GIDIF,RBM INTERLIBRARY LOAN NETWORK

The GIDIF Union Catalogue was set up in 1984 to enable pharmaceutical companies, research institutes, hospital libraries and University libraries to exchange photocopies of articles for research purposes. The Italian copyright law allows this exchange of paper copies. Due to the important differences between these various libraries, the provision of copies is frequently imbalanced. Since it was first established, the number of corporate/pharmaceutical libraries has decreased and public/special libraries has increased. Forty-nine libraries were included in 1998.

As a partner of an Interlibrary Network such as Gidif implies that we have to fullfill requests from other Libraries. According to literature,[2,3] service costs have to be therefore calculated considering the number of articles received and sent.

In order to find out the actual cost for each item received through the Gidif service of document delivery, the following items have to be considered:

i) number of transactions per year;
ii) participation to costs of processing and updating of the Catalogue;
iii) paper, photocopying, stationary;
iv) mailing and fax;
v) personnel.

Table 2 shows the data collected for cost analysis. Statistical data on our article requests were calculated on the basis of past two years: in 1996 and 1997, our Central Library received an average of 596.5 articles, and supplied 909. Articles requested from other libraries are increasing by about 8%, and articles received are decreasing, by about 19%.

Table 2: GIDIF cost analysis/item

Components	Cost for Item
Maintenance	957 Itl
Paper	74 Itl
Copying, material	1,100 Itl
Mailing	1,219 Itl
Fax	305 Itl
Personnel	9,143 Itl
TOTAL Cost	12,798 Itl 7,307 Usd

Processing and printing of the Catalogue with a yearly update was performed by a private bibliographic agency, and costs were 570,697 ItL, [L. 957 per article]. We recorded an average of 7 pages per article requested from other libraries, corresponding to 74

ItL a page; stationary and copying processes had an average cost of 1,100 ItL. per item. Surface mail cost of 1,219 ItL per article; a standard request by fax, lasting 28" on average, had an actual cost of 305 ItL.

A mean of 10 minutes was required to fulfil requests. Part-time contracted employees were assigned to our Union Catalogue normal service; their cost for the university is 27,000,000 ItL gross a year.

GIDIF and commercial suppliers: a comparison

Requests collected at the reference desk were submitted to a commercial supplier -on a rotation basis- and to a Gidif Library -after checking journal holdings-, tracking performances. Data were collected and then compared, and results are shown in Table 1.

Out of 29 articles requested, commercial suppliers fullfilled 100% of our request, while Gidif Libraries only 86%, missing 4 items ; 6 of the 25 articles supplied by Gidif were received by fax (although not requested), and were not considered. Average time to fulfil normal Gidif Libraries requests was 11.1 days, ranking third in performance.

Text quality of the articles received through Gidif Libraries proved to be excellent, graphical quality (tables or pictures) almost excellent.

The major Gidif cost item was the time needed for fullfilling requests; personnel assigned to service in 1997 spent 152 hours of work. An average time for sending requests to Gidif Libraries was assumed 1 min. and 30", considering that self-access facilities in our Library are very good.

Gidif Libraries' average cost per item provided appears to be the lowest one, followed by BLDSC.

Conclusions

Our analysis indicates that Gidif offers actually the most cost-effective service of document delivery, and although four days slower than BLDSC, their average time per item received meets our customers' actual needs. However, the trend whereby private libraries are leaving the Gidif Catalogue is a serious problem, as it will cause increasing costs.

The Central Medical Library plans to continue the participation to Gidif, mainly because of the low-cost of ILL services if compared to commercial suppliers. Commercial suppliers have to remain for articles not owned by Gidif Libraries.

Gidif will remain convenient according to the title it has in its Catalogue. Current trends seeing private Libraries -mainly pharmaceutical companies or research documentation centres- leaving or freezing the service will lead to i) increasing costs for Catalogue updating and ii) increasing requests from outside for the remaining Libraries.

As a result of this work the Central Medical Library has defined performance indicators for Gidif document delivery service in order to improve the quality of the service, especially the speed and accuracy of data. Another result has been the definition of 'break even points' for the statement of convenience.

Articles supplied are actually almost twice the articles requested; if requests from Gidif Libraries are four times greater than our requests to Gidif Libraries, articles supplied by BLDSC or Inist - under 10 pages- will become cheaper.

References

[1] Sekerak RJ, Light JC, Wang H, Hall EF. A trial of three commercial document delivery suppliers with strong holdings in biomedicine. Med Ref Serv Q 1997;16(2):27-36
[2] Abbott C. Performance measurement in library and information services. London: Aslib, 1994
[3] Kurosman K, Durniak BA. Document delivery: a comparison of commercial document suppliers and interlibrary loan services. Coll Res Libr 1994;55(2):129-39

REMOTE ACCESS TO A LIBRARY AND INFORMATION RESOURCE FOR PRIMARY HEALTH CARE PROFESSIONALS

Andre Tomlin, Ian Owens, Marie Montague, Anne Brice
[1]CENTRE FOR EVIDENCE-BASED MENTAL HEALTH, DEPT. OF PSYCHIATRY, UNIVERSITY OF OXFORD, OXFORD, UK

The PRISE project

The Primary Care Sharing the Evidence (PRISE) Project lasted for 2 years, finishing in March 1998. It followed on from the Primary Healthcare Needs (PHIN) Project[1] that concluded that there were a number of areas where further research would be useful. PHIN highlighted the generation, communication and use of information by general practitioners (GPs), showing that one quarter of GPs had unmet information needs in their daily practice. This information was required for a range of primary health care activities. PRISE aimed to develop a pilot information service to test the requirements of primary care teams, in order to enable and support those who wish to find evidence that can support their provision of patient care.

Twelve general practices (8 general practices and 4 dental practices) in the local area (Oxfordshire, Berkshire, Buckinghamshire and Northamptonshire) were selected to take part in the PRISE project. The practices were a mixture of fundholding/non-fundholding, large/small, urban/rural and teaching/non-teaching. They all had to meet minimum technical set-up criteria before they were accepted to take part in the project. Each practice set up a stand-alone personal computer (PC) with a modem, which was connected to a telephone line and installed with dial-in software. This PC became the remote electronic link to a PC at the library end of the project that gave the remote user access to a range of general networked resources, including MEDLINE, The Cochrane Library, The Internet, and the local IHS (Institute of Health Sciences) Library catalogue.

PRISE OBJECTIVES

The main objectives of PRISE were to:

- Monitor the remote library connection
- Provide on-site training in the use of the library connection to the pilot sites
- Monitor use of the IHS Library and related services
- Produce guidelines to enable local information providers establish a similar service
- Produce a sample database of seminal primary care articles

Remote connections

Providing an electronic link meant that communications software was required. The PRISE team took the advice of a local consultant who advised that ReachOut software would suit their purposes. This software was installed on four PCs in the IHS Library; each connected via a modem to a telephone line. These four PCs sat in the library awaiting calls from the PRISE practices. When connected, users were given access to all of the resources available on the library network. There were some technical problems with ReachOut. It soon became clear that the software was slow to use and unreliable in the way that it was viewed from the practice end. Printing and downloading information at the practice end was difficult, and access was always limited to four simultaneous users due to the fact that there were only four PCs available in the library at any one time. The PRISE team decided to implement another software system to improve the link. The SHIVA software that was installed enabled the user to dial-in directly into the University network. Any database software required was installed at the practice end. This new system meant that downloading and printing became much easier, and that the link became considerably faster. However, SHIVA also presented the project team with problems. Two of the twelve practices involved in the project could not use the new link, because they did not have a good enough hardware/software set up in the practice to utilize the SHIVA software. The link also excluded a handful of resources which were only available on the library network, and not on the wider University network.

Once the link had been installed and tested a training program began. The program sought to teach all members of the practice team how to find high quality evidence to answer questions relevant to day-to-day practice in primary care. The program was broken down into five sessions:

- Orientation session
- Finding the Evidence Workshop
- Introduction to MEDLINE
- Developing MEDLINE search skills
- Finding biomedical information on the Internet

Training program

The training was supported with a training pack that was added to at each session. Training was also evaluated each time it took place, and in a follow up questionnaire. There were a number of problems that arose in relation to the training program. The PRISE team found it difficult to arrange times for training to take place, particularly as the sessions were aimed at the entire practice team. The main focus of the sessions were the key resources available on the PRISE link (MEDLINE, The Cochrane Library, Internet). This meant that specialist resources that may have been of greater use to some practice team members (CINAHL, Healthstar, Health-CD, Dental MEDLINE) were neglected. A number of practice team members also found it difficult to spare the time to follow up the training session with a reminder session, in order that they might develop and remember the skills taught.

The PRISE training program was generally well received, with 62% of total training sessions taking place. One of the twelve practices completed the entire program, but all twelve received at least one session. It was felt that evening training may have been a useful addition to the program, with a 5-7pm slot perhaps suiting more members of the practice team than the lunch time slot which was on offer. All trainers involved in the PRISE training agreed that a successful program would always be dependent on the trainer first spending a few weeks developing a good working relationship with the practice in question; attending practice meetings, and becoming a valued member of the general practice set up.

Evaluation
Formal evaluation of PRISE was extremely difficult. Three questionnaires were delivered over the course of the project, in different formats (postal, fax, telephone). The final questionnaire looked specifically at four areas:

- Practice profile
- PRISE costs
- Information seeking behavior & impact
- PRISE satisfaction

The questionnaires showed that the PRISE link was used by all professional groups involved in the project. MEDLINE came out on top as the most popular resource, with Internet usage increasing greatly over the course of the project. PRISE took up 5% of total library usage at the IHS Library. Practice members identified a lack of search skills among the majority of users, and also commented that restricted access to the PRISE link PC in the practice was a major barrier to use.

Best Answers
One of the original PRISE objectives was to produce a sample database of seminal primary care articles. This became known as Best Answers, and was beta-tested as part of the project. The database is currently being developed to be searchable by topic, drug, keyword etc. It will contain critically appraised structured abstracts, and will be made available in a variety of formats, all aimed at getting information to the clinician in less than 15 seconds.

PRISE findings

The PRISE project has shown that a dial-in link can be made to work, although standard equipment and good technical support are essential. However, dial-in access is now being superseded by Internet developments, and this is viewed by the project team as a far better future solution to the problem of providing remote access to an information service. This solution does still rely very heavily on the development of the NHSNet, which is slow to get into every practice.

Access to a link PC in the practice setting is of vital importance. The physical positioning of the PC and time of day when it is made available to various members of staff must be a priority in the set up specification. Users require tailored resources. Members of the primary health care teams do not generally have the time or inclination to perform lengthy literature searches. Appraised and abstracted material relevant to their questions is required.[2]

RECOMMENDATIONS FOR LIBRARY SERVICES FROM THE PROJECT INCLUDE:

- Library catalogue availability (do you want to make your catalogue available?) You might need Internet software to do this
- Commercial database availability
- What resources are required?
- Are they on the network/Internet?
- Can you afford access for your user community?

TECHNICAL ISSUES

- Do you have support for the technical set up (at both ends)?
- Are you aware of the NHSNet-type developments?

TRAINING AND SUPPORT

- What training have you planned?
- Where and when is this training taking place?
- Does this training match up with what your users want?

PUBLICITY AND PROMOTION OF SERVICE

- Do your users know about the whole of your library service?
- What do the users want?
- What are your group's information needs?
- What type of information do they need to answer their questions (guidelines, systematic reviews, RCTs etc)
- Where is the funding coming from?

Future developments

The PRISE project team are currently deciding how best to continue with the development of remote access to a library service for primary health care. The final PRISE workshop in early July 1998 will elicit recommendations from an invited audience as to the next steps, given the emergence of primary care groups and the continuing and increasing emphasis on primary care within the NHS.[3] Internet access is likely to provide users with the majority of resources required to continue the promotion and implementation of evidence-based general practice. Although the Internet was a useful resource at the beginning of the project, it is only now that it's potential impact has been realized. NHS Net developments across primary care will provide users with access to evidence relevant to their specialties. Library services will remain an important element in this process, particularly in training users how to find and appraise high quality evidence relevant to primary care. PRISE has identified a need for local information officers to support the new primary care groups, acting as roving information specialists around the local area, visiting the practice when their expertise is required. If primary health care information needs are to be met by librarians, we must adapt our services to reflect the Internet developments of recent years, provide our users with gateways to the evidence that they need, and then facilitate their learning in how to effectively use these resources.

References

[1] Palmer J, Simpson S. Primary healthcare information needs. Oxford: Health Care Libraries Unit, 1995
[2] McColl A, Smith H, White P, Field J. General practitioners' perceptions of the route to evidence based medicine: a questionnaire survey. BMJ 1998;316:361-365
[3] Department of Health. The new NHS: modern, dependable. London: The Stationery Office, 1997

INTERNET, INTRANET ET LE KIOSQUE ÉLECTRONIQUE

Moreno Curti, Andrea Gelmetti, Marco Rettani, Andrea Gorini, Cesare Carrà, Gabriella Gabutti, Andrea Zeccato, Carmine Tinelli, Catherine Klersy
DIRECTION SCIENTIFIQUE, IRCCS POLICLINICO SAN MATTEO, PAVIA, ITALY

Introduction

En 1995 un "Local Area Network" (LAN) a été instauré dans l'hôpital Policlinico San Matteo de Pavie. La Bibliothèque Scientifique a été une des premières unités reliées au LAN. Depuis, une série d'initiatives et de projets ont été lancés pour développer des services centralisés et utiliser le potentiel du réseau local, le but étant de dépasser les limites géographiques de l'hôpital et de distribuer l'information scientifique à tous les clients reliés au réseau. En effet l'hôpital a des charactéristiques architecturales et organisatives qui justifient de telles exigences: un développement horizontal, des unités se distribuant sur une surface étendue qui souvent est cause de problèmes de communication. La présence jusqu'en 1995 de 40 bibliothèques en est un signe éloquent.

Depuis, des services ont été activés, tel que la consultation de banques de données biomédicales à distance, la réalisation d'un site Web Intranet, la publication sur le net d'informations locales, telles que la production scientifique des chercheurs de l'hôpital, le calendrier des rencontres scientifiques, le catalogue collectif de revues biomédicales et d'autres encore. Tout a été réalisé afin d'éviter les déplacements du médecin/chercheur dans les différentes bibliothèques de l'hôpital, tout en lui permettant d'avoir à disposition, sur son propre lieu de travail, la plus grande quantité d'informations scientifiques et les intruments pour pouvoir récupérer celles qui ne sont pas immédiatement disponibles.

Le projet

Le projet initial, de ce qui représente le sujet de cette communication, n'incluait ni Internet ni ses revues électroniques. Il devait se baser uniquement sur le potentiel du réseau hospitalier (Intranet) et sur les ressources de la bibliothèque scientifique. Le kiosque électronique ne s'entendait que come expositeur électronique des revues auxquelles était abonnée la bibliothèque. Cette dernière, lors de l'arrivée de chaque nouveau fascicule des revues, sur papier, devait penser à passer au scanner les tables des matières et à les publier sur les pages web. De cette façon, tous les utilisateurs Intranet pouvaient les consulter d'où, comme et quand ils le désiraient et, comme devant l'expositeur d'un kiosque à journaux, commander à la bibliothèque les copies retenues importantes et/ou nécessaires à leur travail.

L'idée de faire convivre les informations dérivant d'Intranet avec celles d'Internet a été successive à la constatation, d'une part, de la disponibilité toujours plus grande d'informations bibliographiques directes sur Internet et d'autre part à la réalisation dans notre bibliothèque d'une cablage ISDN entre notre réseau Intranet et Internet. Le kiosque électronique initialement conçu devient quelque chose de plus grand et complexe et avec des limites moins nettes et difficilement identifiables. Il ne doit plus se réduire à la vision uniquement de ce qui est possédé par la bibliothèque, mais il peut aller récupérer le contenu de toutes les revues électroniques présentes sur Internet et, en particulier, avec des temps d'attente et de mise à jour rendus minimaux, le contenu des revues auxquelles nous sommes abonnés.

DES PROBLÈMES

Deux problèmes émergent de notre expérience:

- *la vitesse de connection* passe des 10 Mbps du réseau Intranet aux 64 Kbps de la connection Internet et représente donc un goulot et une limitation technique non négligeable. Cela est vrai en particulier lorsque plusieurs utilisateurs sont reliés au même moment (actuellement les utilisateurs Intranet sont environ 150!) ou bien quand il est nécessaire de transférer des documents de grandes dimensions (par exemple file full-text en format pdf);
- *la récupération d'informations scientifiques* sur Internet est en général gratuite jusqu'à la référence bibliographique, mais elle requiert ensuite un paiement pour l'accès et la récupération du document full-text. L'utilisateur individuel, souvent aux possibilités économiques limitées, peut en tous cas, voir les revues à disposition en format électronique, en parcourir les tables des matières et à travers une expansion de l'idée de "kiosque électronique", remplir la demande de copie de l'article scientifique d'intérêt et l'envoyer au service de documentation scientifique local.

REALISATION

Pour réaliser notre projet, tout en tenant compte des problèmes relevés, nous avons réalisé sur un serveur de la bibliothèque, un système de pages web qui fait un usage ample de "frames", c'est-à-dire de différentes fenêtres en format .html insérée dans une même page. Ces frames peuvent récupérer des informations de pages web situées sur des serveurs se trouvant même à des milliers de kilomètres de distance l'un de l'autre et les montrer sur un seul écran. Le kiosque électronique part, du point de vue opérationnel, d'une page web visible uniquement sur Intranet: celle-ci reporte la liste des revues nous intéressant, dont les tables des matières (tables of contents - TOC) sont consultables sur le réseau.

En sélectionant une quelconque de ces revues, on ouvre une liaison avec une autre page web composée de plusieurs cadres ou frames:

- dans *le premier frame* est reportée la liste des fascicules dont il est possible consulter la table des matières, à laquelle ils sont reliés par un link;

- *un deuxième frame*, rappelé à partir du premier, montre les TOC des revues. Les informations qui apparaissent dans cette fenêtre peuvent avoir une double origine: 1) pour les revues avec une propre version électronique, les TOC sont pris directement des pages web de la revue en question. Les éditeurs, en général, en permettent la visualisation gratuite, quelques fois incluant le résumé et occasionellement la version full-text de certains travaux. Pour augmenter la vitesse de visualisation qui généralement est lente à travers Internet, nous avons réalisé une sorte de mirroir des TOC d'intérêt, en les copiant sur notre serveur web; celui-ci, nous l'avons déjà dit, permet des temps de consultation et de réponse beaucoup plus rapides; 2) pour les revues n'ayant pas une propre version électronique, mais auxquelles nous sommes abonnés, et que nous retenons devoir diffuser rapidement, le TOC est publié sur Intranet après passage au scanner des pages des tables des mattières et inclusion comme images jpeg dans les frames leur étant réservés;

- *un troisième frame* contient un formulaire à remplir par l'utilisateur à distance, quand, après consultation des tables des matières, il trouve des informations bibliographiques sur des articles scientifiques l'intéressant et dont il désire lire le texte intégral. Le form est en réalité un formulaire en format web pour l'insertion de données dans une banque de données réalisée avec Microsof Access. Toutes les demandes de récupération de documentation scientifique sont donc archivées à l'intérieur de celle-ci. Le form contient deux types de champs: d'une part ceux qui sont nécessaires pour identifier le document scientifique à récupérer, et d'autre part ceux pour l'identification de l'utilisateur à qui faire parvenir ledit document. Quand le formulaire est correctement rempli, il suffit d'un 'click' sur un interrupteur électronique pour que la requête arrive à la bibliothèque à travers le réseau.

CHANGEMENT BIBLIOTHÉCAIRE?

Le personnel de la bibliothèque, à travers une interface web de consultation réservée, peut visualiser sur base journalière les nouvelles requêtes; il les analyse et par ses propres canaux de "document delivery", il les fait parvenir aux utilisateurs. C'est en effet la bibliothèque qui décide de la stratégie à appliquer pour récupérer le texte intégral, sur la base des revues pour lequelles il existe un abonnement, des revues full-text accessibles au moyen d'un mot clé, ou à travers des services de "document delivery" nationaux ou internationaux. L'interface de gestion réservée à la bibliothèque visualise aussi d'autres champs, tel que la date de requête de la part de l'utilisateur, la date d'activation de la recherche et celle d'évasion.

Le service offert ne veut absolument pas représenter une alternative aux banques de données biomédicales, mais bien les intégrer à travers une différente modalité d'interrogation: il ne répond pas aux exigences de celui qui fait une recherche par mots clé, mais comme je l'ai déjà dit, il veut remplacer l'expositeur du kiosque où l'utilisateur feuillette les tables des matières des fascicules les plus récents qui l'intéressent, recherche les nouveautés et enfin demande une copie des articles à lire. Contrairement à l'expositeur du kiosque traditionnel, le kiosque électronique peut être consulté 24 heures par jour et directement de l'ordinateur sur son propre bureau.

Lorsque dernièrement nous avons commencé à écrire la version définitive de ce travail, il est apparu qu'un projet, qui au moment de son activation (il y a 2 ans environ) apparaissait innovateur, est à ce jour dépassé sous certains aspects: la plupart des éditeurs internationaux, pas exemple, a réalisé, ou est en train de réaliser, des systèmes payants pour la consultation de leurs propres revues online, avec la possibilité de liaison en temps réel et la disponibilité d'informations extrêmement à jour. Ceci permet d'éviter les retards liés à la réalisation sur papier du document et à sa distribution.

Malgré tout cela, nous sommes convaincus que quelque chose d'innovatif soit resté: il suffit de penser à la possibilité de consulter les tables des matières des revues auxquelles l'Institut n'est pas abonné mais pour lesquelles il est possible eventuellement de demander la copie des articles retenus intéressants; la possibilité de consulter les tables des matières passées au scanner des revues non encore disponibles sur Internet; la possibilité d'utiliser le serveur local, lequel se comportant en mirroir, permet une utilisation des informations avec des temps bien plus rapides que ceux d'Internet; la possibilité de se servir du système sans même se rendre à la bibliothèque, mais en utilisant les services que la bibliothèque peut fournir. La bibliothèque d'autre part devient ainsi un intermédiaire fonctionnel entre utilisateur et revue. Elle vient en effet à connaissance des exigences de ses propres médecins/chercheurs, elle fait une évaluation de leurs requêtes et elle résoud leur problèmes en les libérant ainsi de charges qui ne sont pas de leur compétence, telles que abonnements, récupération de documents et/ou leur paiement. La liaison aux revues électroniques full-text qui devrait sous de nombreux aspects rendre invisible la bibliothèque à l'utilisateur, représente elle aussi un des points à la charge de la bibliothèque. Les problèmes technologiques permettant (ceux de vitesse d'accès et de transfert des données sur Internet seront tôt ou tard dépassés), la bibliothèque choisira et prendra en charge les abonnements avec leurs mots-clé; mais l'accès au texte intégral des revues électroniques sera fait par l'utilisateur final, grâce au travail, à ce point invisible, de la bibliothèque.

EXPANDING LIBRARY SERVICES TO MEDICAL STAFF AND STUDENTS AT SMALL AND REMOTE HOSPITALS

Ragnhild E. Lande
UNIVERSITY LIBRARY OF TRONDHEIM, TRONDHEIM, NORWAY

Introduction

Norway is a sparsely populated country, with only 4 million inhabitants. This creates complex administrative problems, not least within our health service. More than 100 hospitals of various sizes and degrees of specialisation are scattered widely over the country. The world's northernmost hospital at Spitsbergen, at the same latitude as the northern part of Greenland, is one of them with only 2-3 physicians and patients of all shapes and sizes. Here you see a picture from Longyearbyen at Spitsbergen. The yellow building is the hospital, the brown one the University Centre, and there is a reindeer in the foreground, one of the inhabitants in Longyearbyen.Here you see the hospital from the outside, and from the inside, with an isbear waiting for consultation.

Administratively Norway is divided into 18 counties which are responsible for the administration of the hospitals. In addition five health regions have been introduced, each covering three or four counties. Recently the administration has been instructed to further closer cooperation within the health regions, and political, medical and other committees have been established for this purpose.

The project

BACKGROUND

My project study is limited to Health Region 4. This region covers the three counties in central Norway, with Trondheim and its University Hospital in the middle. There are eight somatic hospitals in Region 4. The University Hospital in Trondheim functions both as central hospital for the Region for patients with special needs, who cannot be treated by the other hospitals, as well as local hospital for Trondheim and its neighbouring municipalities. At present the hospital has some 1000 beds.

The Norwegian University of Science and Technology in Trondheim has 600 medical students, and this is to be increased by 30% within a few years. The curriculum is now based on problem-based learning with six years of pre-clinical and clinical studies totally integrated. This means that students have to meet with patients nearly "all the time". Many patients at the University Hospital are not "ordinary" patients, since they have been transferred from the district hospitals where they cannot be treated because their illnesses are rare. This creates a problem for medical education, because there are not enough patients for all students, and the patients they see are often not suitable for studying common problems and diseases. A result is that students have to go to other hospitals in the Health Region for part of their studies.

There is a close relation between problem-based learning and library services. In periods when students are beeing trained in clinical practice in smaller hospitals, they will need continous access to adequate library and information services. In clinical practice it is important to have easy access to relevant and updated information. In addition to the usual problem of having adequate funds, the smaller hospitals face difficulties in recruiting and keeping qualified specialists. In Norway we have a shortage of health professionals, and specialists prefer to work in the professional and scientific environment of larger hospitals, with daily challenges, better facilities and infrastructure.

These were some of the reasons why the University and the hospital authorities in Trondheim initiated a project that would make the Medical Library and Information Centre of the University Hospital into a resource centre for all hospitals in Region 4.A resource centre would secure easy and speedy access to information sources and relevant literature for staff and students working at any hospital in the Region. As well as securing better service for staff and students, efficient cooperation within the Region will result in better utilisation of the resources provided for the libraries.

AIMS AND OBJECTIVES

What are the dimensions of the project? How many users will there be totally? How many persons are involved in library services today? What is the budget for the libraries? What can the libraries do better in the future if they cooperate?

The Medical Library and Information Centre at the University Hospital is part of the main university library (NTNU Library). It serves all occupational groups and students working in the Hospital, approximately 3000 people. Health professionals outside the hospital can also use the library. The other seven hospitals in the Health Region employ 2800 professionals, consisting of 450 physicians, 1900 nurses and 350 others. This gives a total of nearly 6000 library users in Region 4.

The literature budget at the University Hospital is about USD 400 000, coming partly from the University and partly from the Hospital. 15 librarians work in the Medical Library and Information Centre, and the management is done by NTNU Library. Nearly all district hospitals have a medical library with a librarian. In only two hospitals these librarians are fully-trained and work full-time. The medical libraries at the district hospitals have a total budget for literature of USD 340 000.

Discussions with heads of departments at these hospitals, focused on several cooperative areas, which can be grouped in three sections: (1) the digital library, (2) other cooperation areas, for example acquisition and cataloguing, and (3) patient information (which will be included in other projects).

THE DIGITAL LIBRARY

All hospitals in Norway have the same problem. For security reasons their data networks are closed. As in many other countries the authorities do not allow free access to Internet from in-house hospital networks. On the other hand, a personal computer with connection to Internet is often placed in the medical library. Some hospitals have their library catalogues, MEDLINE and the Cochrane database on CD-ROM, running in their local hospital network.

The Norwegian National Health Network is a high priority national initiative. The main objective is to ensure the implementation and use of information and communication technology that enables the healthcare service to fulfil its common needs and objectives for efficient and secure information management, collaboration and development. The local networks will be linked to the Health Region networks, and the five regional networks will be linked into a national network. There will be one national link to the Internet, to secure the technical, organisational and ethical aspects.

For the regional network in Health Region 4 we are planning a digital library, providing:

- Bibliographic databases
- The national library system, BIBSYS
- The library catalogues
- Full text journals
- Multimedia textbooks and teaching files
- Digitised textbooks
- Physician and hospital directories

These sources will be available to all. A national pilot project has just started at the University Hospital in Trondheim. This will test a secure Internet connection from the closed hospital network. We feel that this is the first step in the process of setting up our digital library for the eight hospitals in Health Region 4.

OTHER POTENTIAL COOPERATION AREAS WILL BE:

Acquisition: If the small hospital libraries become a part of the Medical Library and Information Centre, the main library can buy their books and journals with advantageous price reductions. We estimate the reduction to be between 10-20%.

Cataloguing: Today nearly all hospitals have a small in-house library system. The Medical Library and Information Centre uses BIBSYS, the national library system for academic and research libraries in Norway. BIBSYS is a system with nearly the same modules and routines as PICA in The Netherlands. If the small hospitals use the same system, they will save registration time. Larger libraries buy and catalogue the same documents. The hospitals will thus have access to each others‘ catalogues, and it will be possible to order books and litterature for all users in a health region.

Periodicals: It is a long way to a complete digital library. Economic, technical and practical problems have to be solved before we can have all journals in electronic form. In the meantime printed journals will play an important role in the daily work for health professionals and students. Closer cooperation between hospitals in the Health Region will offer better service to all and save money.

Consultation: The librarians in the Medical Library and Information Centre have experience from a large, active library, and are able to solve difficult information questions. They are updated through courses and conferences, and from experience through in-house educational programmes. They can advise and teach library staff in the smaller hospitals, and give information about books, journals and electronic material. They know what staff and students need for updating in their professional field, and can make guidelines for the holdings in the smaller libraries.

User education and courses: The Medical Library and Information Centre is currently running many courses for professionals and students in the health sector. For example, in information retrieval using different electronic interfaces, various databases and the Internet. At present all the courses are being held at the University Hospital. It would be cheaper and more convenient for users if these courses could be held locally.

The aim for the future must be to offer maximum user education in electronic form when it is convenient for each user and that can be made available on the local network.

Quality control: Using the Medical Library and Information Centre as resource library, will enhance the quality of service to students and staff in all hospitals in the Region.

Outcome

The first part of the project study is finished. The recommendations are now forwarded to the authorities. We are confident that this project that will expand library services to medical staff and students in our region has shown considerable advantages that can be measured in financial and qualitative terms.

PANORAMA DES RESSOURCES DOCUMENTAIRES HOSPITALIÈRES FRANÇAISES SUR INTERNET

Hélène Breul, Laurence Boué, Armelle Martin
CENTRE DE DOCUMENTATION MÉDICO-PHARMACEUTIQUE AP-HP/PCH-AGAM, PARIS, FRANCE.

Abstract

Recently, many web sites have been developed on the Internet network by institutions, companies, individuals and state organisations. The world of health care has followed this development and has witnessed a real proliferation of information targeted at the various members of this sector (doctors, pharmacists, etc...).

Searching information requires new tools to facilitate the selection of those web sites best adapted to the needs of the users. We have therefore deemed it necessary to establish an evaluation structure for use by documentalists and librarians. For the health care field, we suggest that we undertake an evaluation of the resources available on the Internet sites for French hospitals and that we present an overview of these sites in 1998.

The first stage of our study was to make an inventory of all the Internet sites established by French hospitals and health care units by using search engines as well as the list created by the web site of the University Hospital of Rouen. All of these selected sites were then subjected to an evaluation.

The evaluation filter, created in conjunction with the ADBS (Association des professionnels de l'information et de la documentation), was devised to be applicable to all Internet sites, regardless of their speciality. It is therefore not designed to evaluate the intrinsic scientific quality of the information presented by the sites but rather to estimate the relevance of the organisation and the services proposed. The criteria used may be divided into two categories: criteria judging the formal presentation of the site (access, structure and design) and criteria listing the content of the sites (authors, bases of validation, information layouts, audience, documentary products, access to primary documents, multilingualism).

The analysis and the comments on the results allow us to make an estimation of what is being produced on the Internet in the health care sector and to define the important criteria for making a better selection of resources available.

*AP-HP: Assistance Publique - Hôpitaux de Paris
*PCH-AGAM: Pharmacie Centrale des Hôpitaux - Agence Générale des Approvisionnements Médicaux

Introduction

L'objectif de ce travail était de présenter un « état des lieux » des ressources hospitalières françaises sur Internet. Une grille d'évaluation a été élaborée en collaboration avec l'ADBS (Association des professionnels de l'information et de la documentation) et appliquée aux sites Web hospitaliers ou hospitalo-universitaires. Les sites ont été recensés à partir de la liste des centres de santé du site Web du Centre Hospitalo-Universitaire de Rouen (http://www.chu-rouen.fr) et de différents moteurs de recherche (Nomade, Yahoo et CarrefourNet).

Nous avons visité 68 sites Web hospitaliers ou hospitalo-universitaires en 1998. Parmi ceux-ci, 50% environ sont bien développés et présentent plusieurs niveaux de hiérarchie. En revanche, 10% des sites ont au moins une partie importante en construction.

Résultats obtenus pour les critères les plus significatifs de la grille d'évaluation

CRITÈRES QUALITATIFS

- Critères d'accès: peu de sites sont multilingues et le plus souvent il s'agit d'une version bilingue anglaise. Nous avons trouvé un site comprenant une version russe et un site en version français-allemand-espagnol.
- Organisation du site Web: la plupart des sites remplissent le critère de bonne navigabilité et présentent un plan du site, par contre le moteur de recherche ou la rubrique «Quoi de neuf» sont souvent absents. Quand ils existent, les liens hypertextes externes sont satisfaisants et renvoient sur les sites les plus représentatifs et/ou spécifiques. La majorité des sites affichent le logo de l'institution qui est indispensable car il permet de toujours localiser le site pendant la recherche.
- Critères de validation: l'identité du Webmaster est souvent mentionné mais il y a beaucoup d'articles qui ne sont pas signés ce qui pose un problème pour la validité des informations. Seuls 10% des sites mentionnent l'existence d'un comité de rédaction.
- Coordonnées du site: l'e-mail du Webmaster n'y est pas systématiquement précisé.
- Critères de dates: seuls 36% des sites visités précisent leur date de mise à jour qui est un critère majeur pour la validité et la fraîcheur de l'information.

CRITÈRES DESCRIPTIFS

- Nature des informations: les images sont très présentes sur les sites et parfois en taille réduite, ce qui accélère l'affichage de l'écran et sa visualisation. Les cartes ou graphiques complètent le texte dans environ 50% des sites.
- Audience: ces sites visent principalement le grand public et secondairement les médecins et étudiants. Seuls 15% d'entre eux nous ont semblés intéressants pour les professionnels de l'information car ils proposent des ressources documentaires (catalogues, renvois vers des banques de données, textes législatifs, etc...).
- Critères d'interactivité: les différents modes d'interactivité propre à l'Internet (listes de discussion, «FAQ» etc..) sont peu développés.
- Produits documentaires: en général, ils ne sont pas présents dans les sites recensés. On retrouve le plus souvent les bibliographies liées aux services médicaux, les annonces de congrès et des listes de sources d'informations, le plus souvent des liens hypertextes vers d'autres sites ou des banques de données.

COMMENTAIRES SUR LES RÉSULTATS

Quels sont les critères importants dont les résultats sont satisfaisants?
Tous les critères d'organisation des sites sont assez bien respectés: bonne présentation, repérage facile dans le site ce qui incite à la visite. En ce qui concerne l'audience, l'information aux patients est privilégiée car ce sont les usagers de l'hôpital. L'information aux médecins est développée à part par d'autres médecins ou par des services médicaux particuliers.

Quelles sont les améliorations indispensables?
Il nous paraît vraiment nécessaire d'avoir une version anglaise des sites pour permettre une meilleure ouverture internationale. Pour faciliter la recherche et accéder plus rapidement à l'information pertinente, il est indispensable de proposer un moteur de recherche. Une rubrique «Quoi de neuf» est aussi un avantage supplémentaire pour les sites souvent visités.

Mentionner systématiquement les divers auteurs, la date de mise à jour et la présence d'un comité de rédaction permettrait d'améliorer la validation des informations et leur utilisation. Il faudrait augmenter le nombre de listes ou forums de discussions à l'intérieur des sites mêmes car ils sont presque inexistants, ce qui conduit à des échanges limités. De plus l'existence de tels outils dynamisent le site.

Sauf exception, le professionnel de l'information en milieu hospitalo-universitaire est encore peu impliqué dans la création ou l'évolution des sites Web. La bibliothèque médicale n'est presque jamais nommée dans ces sites alors qu'elle est indispensable aux personnels de santé, elle ne fait donc pas l'objet d'un développement spécifique. Il est souvent impossible de connaître le fonds documentaire possédé car peu de catalogues sont disponibles sur les sites Web.

Spécificités des sites Web hospitaliers

Nous avons distingué six différents groupes d'informations proposés: l'information sur l'hôpital, l'information aux patients, l'information médicale ou scientifique aux médecins, l'information sur la formation et l'enseignement, l'information juridique et l'information par accès Intranet.

INFORMATION SUR L'HÔPITAL

On retrouve souvent une présentation générale de l'hôpital, son historique, les différents plans (du site hospitalier même et plans d'accès), la liste des services médicaux et le plateau technique, les pôles d'activités, les services administratifs et les organigrammes, le bilan d'activité, l'annuaire Internet des différents acteurs de l'hôpital et les photos de l'établissement, du personnel et de l'équipement.

Ponctuellement, il est possible de prendre des rendez-vous par e-mail, de remplir une fiche d'admission pour l'hospitalisation ou d'avoir des informations sur la disponibilité des lits. On retrouve parfois le sommaire ou le texte intégral du bulletin publié par l'hôpital.

INFORMATION AUX PATIENTS

Le patient peut retrouver sur les sites Web les livrets d'accueil et toutes les informations pratiques liées aux consultations et à l'hospitalisation (horaires, noms des médecins, pièces à fournir). Il peut aussi y remplir le questionnaire de satisfaction de l'établissement. Un site propose aussi d'écrire à un patient hospitalisé par e-mail. Les sites Web hospitaliers offrent beaucoup d'informations concernant les pathologies, leurs traitements et les adresses des associations de malades. Plus rarement, il est possible au patient de poser des questions au médecin.

INFORMATION MÉDICALE

Elle concerne les pathologies, les traitements, les techniques, la recherche. Le médecin peut aussi s'inscrire à différents congrès et a la possibilité de répondre parfois aux appels à communications. Les sites Web proposent de nombreux liens hypertextes vers des sites Web médicaux généraux ou spécifiques, vers des revues scientifiques en texte intégral sur abonnement, vers les sites d'accès gratuits à MEDLINE. Ponctuellement, les médecins peuvent aussi publier leurs travaux sur Internet. Quand les services médicaux ont développé une partie propre dans le Web hospitalier, ils insèrent leur bibliographie d'articles publiés et référencés dans MEDLINE.

INFORMATION SUR LA FORMATION ET L'ENSEIGNEMENT

Tout ce qui concerne les inscriptions, les programmes d'enseignement, les coûts et les offres d'emplois est souvent mentionné sur le site. Parfois, il existe des possibilités de téléenseignement pour l'étudiant et quelques occasions de déposer son Curriculum Vitae. Un site permet le télédéchargement de polycopiés de faculté, un autre présente et critique des CD-ROMs interactifs.

INFORMATION JURIDIQUE

De nombreux textes juridiques sont présents sur ces sites, notamment pour le patient la charte du patient hospitalisé, la protection juridique du patient, le don d'organes, l'accès au dossier médical et administratif. Pour le médecin, on retrouve les textes concernant la carte professionnelle de santé. Un site a développé un catalogue des textes législatifs dans le domaine de la santé avec recherche par matière ou chronologiquement. Un autre site donne des informations sur la législation spécifique à l'hospitalisation psychiatrique.

INFORMATION PAR INTRANET ET/OU PAR ACCÈS RÉSERVÉ (AUX MÉDECINS)

Cet accès est parfois mentionné et propose ponctuellement la possibilité de discuter des dossiers médicaux difficiles avec des experts internationaux, d'interroger MEDLINE ou Cancerlit et de visualiser les résultats de laboratoire. Il nous a été impossible d'accéder à ces informations et donc de les présenter plus précisément. L'Assistance Publique - Hôpitaux de Paris a développé son propre réseau Intranet accessible à l 'ensemble du personnel hospitalier (annuaire, liens externes, banques de données...).

Conclusion générale

L'utilisation d'une grille d'évaluation nous a permis de définir des critères indispensables à une meilleure sélection des ressources hospitalières sur Internet et de mieux connaître le développement et l'apport de l'Internet à l'hôpital.

Nous voulons souligner la faible participation des Centres de Documentation dans les sites Web hospitaliers français. Il est vrai que le contexte hospitalier actuel n'est pas toujours favorable aux professionnels de l'information et de la documentation. Malgré de réelles avancées, leurs fonctions sont encore mal reconnues et ils ne bénéficient d'aucun statut au sein de la Fonction Publique Hospitalière.

Pourtant dans le domaine médical français, il existe un site de référence (http://www.chu-rouen.fr), et d'autres sites Web innovants sont de plus en plus présents sur Internet.

L'Assistance Publique - Hôpitaux de Paris quant à elle, a mis en place un Comité d'Orientation du Web (COWEB), qui a émis des recommandations incluant notamment le respect d'un certain nombre de critères de qualité.

Bibliographie

Régie régionale de Montréal-Centre. Grille d'analyse des sites Web. Montréal, 1997. <URL: http://www.rrsss06.gouv.qc.ca/publications/grille.html>

Centrale Santé. Critères de qualité de l'information médicale sur Internet. Démarche de Net Scoring. Paris, 1997. <URL:http://www.apuis.com/santé/fqualic0.htm>

Joly Monique et al. Evaluation de l'information présente sur Internet. Lyon, 1998. <URL: http://www.insa-lyon.fr/Departements/DocInsa/Fristi/fristi36.html>

GRILLE D'EVALUATION DES SITES INTERNET

(appliquée à 68 sites WEB hospitaliers)

CRITERES QUALITATIFS

	Oui	Non
Accès :	%	
Référencé par un moteur de recherche	100	0
Statistiques d'utilisation	15	85
Multilinguisme	18	82
Organisation :		
Page d'aide	0	100
Repérage dans le site (aide à la navigabilité)	85	15
Plan du site	85	15
Moteur de recherche	12	88
Pertinence des liens hypertextes	67	33
Rubrique "Quoi de neuf"	16	84
Logo sur toutes les pages	78	22
Validation :		
Identité des auteurs/rédacteurs	40	60
Comité de rédaction	10	90
Site institutionnel	69	31
Site référencé dans d'autres sites	100	0
Coordonnées :		
Adresse E-mail	63	37
Adresse courrier	40	60
Téléphone	33	67
Fax	25	75
Dates :		
Date de création	19	81
Date de mise à jour	36	64

GRILLE D'EVALUATION DES SITES INTERNET

(appliquée à 68 sites WEB hospitaliers)

CRITERES DESCRIPTIFS

	Oui	Non
Nature des informations :	%	
Statistiques	34	66
Textes	91	9
Images	88	12
Documents animés	19	81
Documents sonores	1	99
Cartes, plans, graphiques...	46	54
Audience :		
Etudiants	42	58
Experts, spécialistes	51	49
Grand public	88	12
Professionnels de l'information	15	85
Interactivité		
Liste de discussion	7	93
"Chats"	10	90
FAQ (frequently asked questions)	9	91
Produits documentaires	%	
Bases de données	3	97
Bibliographies	10	90
Revue de presse	3	97
Revue de sommaires	3	97
Dossiers documentaires	1	99
Index de mots-clés	1	99
Catalogues en ligne	4	96
Littérature grise	6	94
Congrès (abstracts, proceedings...)	7	93
Agenda (congrès, salons...)	21	79
Répertoire de sources d'informations	19	81

SUPPORT FOR INFORMATION SEEKING ON THE MEDICAL LIBRARY WEB

Anamarija Rozic-Hristovski, Ljupco Todorovski, Dimitar Hristovski
CENTRAL MEDICAL LIBRARY, LJUBLJANA, SLOVENIA

Introduction

Advances in information technology offer many opportunities for improving the access to local resources as well as delivery of information from external resources. The common goal of all medical libraries is to provide access as efficiently as possible to the information resources needed in the work of their users. It can be approached by creating library web sites by offering users better access to information and services.[1] The Central Medical Library (CMK) of the Faculty of Medicine in Ljubljana, Slovenia challenged by growth of information resources in medicine and increasing users' computer literacy decided to built its own web site with embedded search engine.

Web site design

CMK web site aim is to serve as a library guide to its resources and services. It has a menu/hypertext link structure with two frames displaying the current menu and active text, where information screens and hypertext links allow cross-menu navigation. The menu structure is limited to three levels, so that users have a limited number of layers to penetrate before reaching the information pages. Besides, some hot links are established to enable fast access to the most important items. The web pages are embedded in uniform graphic design. Every page offers interactivity via e-mail. Text version is prepared to overcome communication delays. Users can choose between Slovene and English version of the web pages. The main menu offers access to eight sub-menus, among them services, information resources and Internet resources.

Search engine implementation

Browsing web pages can be an effective method of information-seeking in a situation where the need of information seeker is not very well defined. But it is often much less effective and efficient in case where this need can be expressed by a small number of relatively precise terms. This is the reason why we incorporated a search engine in the CMK web site.

As a search engine we used *Harvest*[2] customised to our needs. Harvest is an integrated set of tools to gather, extract, organise, search, cache, and replicate relevant information across the Internet. We used two of the several Harvest subsystems: the *Gatherer* and the *Broker*. The Gatherer subsystem collects indexing information from the resources available at provider sites. The Broker subsystem retrieves indexing information from the Gatherer, indexes the collected information, and provides a WWW query interface to it. We indexed the whole Faculty of Medicine WWW site and also the first web pages of the cites listed in the "Internet resources" section of the CMK web site. We customised the Harvest search form and the results page to suit our needs.

Evaluation

Nine month after CMK web site is operating we noticed an increasing interest among the Slovene biomedical community and from abroad. The users accessed CMK home page 6805 times. They put special attention to the Internet resources, which were browsed 2725 times.

Conclusions

Information resources accessible using the WWW excite users' interest also in Slovenia. CMK home page access statistics shows that web pages facilitate active dissemination of information and enable interactivity using search engine and e-mail. In the future, we plan to improve the capabilities for searching CMK web pages and to conduct user evaluation of the system.

References

[1] Biddiscombe R, Knowles K, Upton I, Wilson K. Developing a web library guide for an academic library: problems, solutions and future possibilities. Program 1997;31:59-73

[2] Bowman CM, Danzig PB, Hardy DR, Manber U, and Schwartz MF. The Harvest information discovery and access system. In: Proceedings of the 2nd International WWW Conference: Mosaic and the Web; 1994 Oct; Chicago, Illinois. p. 763-71

SUPPORTING FAMILY CARERS WITH TELEMATIC INTERVENTIONS - THE ACTION-PROJECT

Olof Sundin, Harriet Berthold
BORAS UNIVERSITY COLLEGE OF HEALTH SCIENCES, BORAS, SWEDEN

Introduction

ACTION is a 36-month nursing-led European project, involving England, Northern Ireland, the Republic of Ireland, Portugal, and Sweden. The project started in January, 1997 and is to be completed in December, 1999. The project is funded through the Fourth Framework Telematics Programme for the Disabled and Elderly.

The primary aim of the project is to maintain the autonomy, independence, and quality of life for frail old and disabled people, as well as their family carers by opening new information channels into their homes - channels involving the application of new information and communication technology.

Research design

The ACTION-project is divided into four phases. The first phase, carried out during 1997, studied the health care systems of the different countries, the users' needs and priorities, and the technical specifications necessary. Data in the user needs' study came from focus groups of family carers and another 451 family carers who completed questionnaires in the five participating countries. In the second, and current, phase of the project different information programmes are being created and put together in an overall software architecture. In the third and fourth phase the service architecture will be tested and demonstrated in the countries involved.

Results

The user needs and priority study revealed that television is an important part of the daily life of old people.[1] The informants made statements such as "A television is often a life line to people who can't get out." Data from the questionnaire indicated that an average of 82% of all informants had "a lot" or "quite a lot" of experience using television. An average of 70% of all informants also indicated that they had "a lot" or "quite a lot" of experience using a remote control. On the other hand an average of 87% of the family carers stated that they had no experience using a PC.

The family carers would, however, be happy to use new technology if they believed it would be beneficial to them and easy to understand.

The ACTION-system is based on familiar technology such as the end-user's own TV, a computer, and a remote control for navigation. The text-based information resources are delivered through a web-based Intranet system using ISDN2B and are information programmes including skills training in daily life, financial information, long term planning, respite care, emergency situations and coping instruments. Oral communication is supported by a high quality videoconference system that links the family carer to different health providers as well as to other family carers through ISDN6B.

Discussion

The user-friendliness of an information service directed at old people is crucial for its adoption. According to Rogers[2] an innovation that is compatible with the user's life situation is more likely to be used. The study shows that TV plays an important role in an older person's life and the ACTION-system is therefore built around this familiar technology.

Through the support of new communication technology, oral information has the potential of playing an important role for the health consumer even from distance. The ACTION-system integrates both text-based and oral information, through one information and communication channel.

References

[1] Rogers E. Diffusion of innovations. New York: Free Press, 1995

[2] Sundin O. Diffusion of telematics. In: Berthold H (ed.) D 04.1. Users needs and priorities (p. 46-53). Research report, European Commission DGXIII Telematics Applications Programme, Disabled and Elderly Sector, 1997

Chapter 13: THE (MEDICAL) LIBRARY PROFESSION

Editorial introduction

Changing needs of library users and changing roles of librarians have their consequences for the medical library professions. Linda Smith of the Graduate School of Library and Information Science of the University of Illinois at Urbana-Champaign, draws our attention to the issues in library education. In this paper she makes a plea for more collaboration, also across national boundaries. Alison Hicks reports on distance learning for librarians as part of their training in teaching evidence based medicine, which is a very good example of using modern methods in education to adapt to new challenges for medical librarianship.

Professional associations have a responsibility and therefore an important role to play in further education and developments in librarianship. One way of showing their involvement in and adaptation to modern technology is how they are presented and what they publish on the Web. A valuable inventory with comments is presented by Vanna Pistotti and Manuela Colombi. The papers from Spain and Hungary discuss the importance of public relations for the medical library in order to achieve its aims and goals of better usage of available information sources and optimal use of library services. The importance of attending medical meetings and taking part in the scientific discussion and information exchange is underlined by Marta Jordà-Olives from Spain.

EDUCATION FOR HEALTH SCIENCES LIBRARIANS: PAST, PRESENT AND FUTURE POSSIBILITIES

Linda C. Smith
GRADUATE SCHOOL OF LIBRARY AND INFORMATION SCIENCE, UNIVERSITY OF ILLINOIS AT URBANA-CHAMPAIGN, CHAPAIGN ILLINOIS, USA

Introduction

The Medical Library Association (MLA) celebrates its centennial in 1998, so health sciences librarianship has been recognized as a distinct area of specialization in North America for 100 years. Course work in health sciences librarianship has been offered as part of a degree program in several schools of library (and information) science (LIS) since 1939, when Thomas P. Fleming first taught a course at Columbia University School of Library Service. MLA has been influential through its credentialing and continuing education (CE) programs over several decades[1] and its two recent policy documents on education and research.[2,3] The National Library of Medicine (NLM) has also played an important role in furthering education through its post-master's internships (since 1957), its support for educational programs through grant funds, the 1995 recommendations of its Planning Panel on the Education and Training of Health Sciences Librarians,[4] and the subsequent award of seven planning grants.[5] This paper considers the past, present and future possibilities of education for health sciences librarians from a North American perspective, but with the recognition that technologies for distance learning may enable more global collaboration.

Aspects of educational programs and experiences

Rather than present a chronology of how education for health sciences librarians has developed over the past 100 years, this paper briefly reviews changes in the following aspects of educational programs and experiences: purpose, method, location, scheduling, participants, and content. The discussion highlights the potential impact of distance learning, drawing on the author's experience with the LEEP3 program, a distance enrollment option for the M.S. degree offered by the Graduate School of Library and Information Science at the University of Illinois at Urbana-Champaign (http://leep.lis.uiuc.edu). LEEP3 allows students in locations ranging from Alaska to the Virgin Islands to earn a degree with limited time spent on campus in the midwestern state of Illinois. Teachers and students collaborate through a variety of technologies supporting asynchronous and synchronous communication. Although some LEEP3 students currently work in health sciences libraries, in-depth specialization is not yet supported by course work available through the program.

PURPOSE

The purpose of pursuing an educational program may be to earn a degree, to gain experience under the guidance of more experienced professionals through an internship or residency, or to develop new knowledge and skills through continuing education. Independent study is also a part of the lifelong learning recognized as a responsibility of the health sciences librarian. In the U.S. and Canada the master's is the first professional degree. Only 56 institutions currently offer an accredited degree and even fewer offer advanced certificates or doctoral-level study, meaning that many geographic regions are unserved. While most degree programs include a practicum or field work in which a student can gain experience in a health sciences library, post-master's internship or residency programs exist in only a few academic health sciences libraries. CE opportunities are much more numerous, because there is a wider variety of providers. Technology-mediated distance learning makes degree programs available to more people and also increases the potential number of participants in CE offerings.

METHOD

Educational methods vary depending on the purpose of study and the content to be learned. Formal degree study has traditionally involved a professor lecturing to a group of students who in turn are responsible for completing readings and writing papers or taking exams covering the course material. Lectures are now being supplemented or replaced with more active learning strategies. Internships and residencies involve learning by observing and doing, though they may also include some more formal instruction. Independent reading of the professional literature is one important means of continuing education. Teleconferences broadcast to multiple sites now provide an alternative to CE workshops or short courses involving face-to-face interchange between instructors and students. Structured interaction with peers is another form of continuing education, including such options as the journal club for discussing selected professional literature (with electronic journal clubs as an alternative to face-to-face discussion) and peer-assisted learning in which a librarian spends time "shadowing" a colleague at another institution.

LOCATION

While independent study can take place anywhere and in-service training can be planned for any place of employment, other educational opportunities have focused on face-to-face communication in set locations, whether the college classroom or the conference hotel meeting room. Teleconferences expand the number of people who can participate in educational programs from many downlink sites. Delivery of instruction via the Internet has extended learning opportunities to any desktop computer capable of connecting to the Internet.

SCHEDULING

Such educational activities as the college class, journal club discussion, or CE workshop typically take place at set times. While the Internet supports synchronous communication through such technologies as RealAudio broadcasts and text chat, computer conferencing tools that support asynchronous communication allow individuals to participate in discussions and review course materials at times that are convenient for them.

PARTICIPANTS

Participants in the educational process include students, teachers, and organizations sponsoring educational programs. For face-to-face educational offerings, students and teachers must be in the same place at the same time. Although LIS schools often draw on adjunct faculty (practicing health sciences librarians) to teach courses, such individuals come from a limited geographic area. Local and regional CE workshops also often depend on local presenters. Through technology-mediated options such as the Internet, students may be in multiple sites and guest speakers or instructors from various locations can share their expertise. Organizations sponsoring educational programs include universities, professional associations, and (in the U.S.) the National Library of Medicine and the National Network of Libraries of Medicine. Although these organizations function largely independently, there is increasing interest in forging partnerships to meet educational needs in innovative ways.

CONTENT

Design of educational programs is aided by efforts undertaken to identify content needed to practice a particular specialty. MLA's Platform for Change[2] defines seven areas of knowledge and skills for the health sciences librarian: health sciences environment and information policies; management of information services; health sciences information services; health sciences resource management; information systems and technology; instructional support systems; and research, analysis, and interpretation. Giuse and colleagues[6] have developed an even more exhaustive knowledge and skill taxonomy including such categories as medical informatics, management/personnel, and marketing.

Conclusion

The brief outline of aspects of educational programs and experiences demonstrates that many options are potentially available for degree-oriented and continuing education. Challenges to those concerned with the development of educational programs include insuring quality and fostering collaboration. In 1963 Meyerhoff observed that "over and over again, medical librarians have demonstrated their appreciation of further study and their willingness to engage in it. The problem here is not to stimulate interest, but to channel it into the most fruitful course".[7] This involves taking best advantage of independent study vs. collaborative learning, asynchronous vs. synchronous interaction, and face-to-face vs. technology-mediated instruction by determining which means are most effective in achieving desired educational outcomes.

While lifelong learning remains an individual responsibility, many organizations have an interest in creating educational offerings. To avoid unnecessary duplication, coordination and collaboration are desirable. As MacKenzie and Greenes observe, "the WWW signals a potential shift from independent, entrepreneur-driven development of isolated curricula to a new era in which faculty collaborate to share educational resources".[8] Extending this effort across national boundaries poses additional challenges of addressing multi-cultural and multi-lingual concerns.[9]

Acknowledgment

Preparation of this paper was supported in part by NIH Grant no. 1 T15 LM 07098-01 from the National Library of Medicine. The views expressed are solely those of the author and do not represent the official view of the National Library of Medicine.

References

[1] Roper FW. MLA's professional development program: how we took control of our future. Bull Med Libr Assoc 1998;86:211-6

[2] Medical Library Association. Platform for change: the educational policy statement of the Medical Library Association. Chicago: The Association, 1991 (http://www.mlanet.org/education/pfcindex.html)

[3] Medical Library Association. Using scientific evidence to improve information practice: the research policy statement of the Medical Library Association. Chicago: The Association, 1995 (http://www.mlanet.org/research/science1.html)

[4] National Library of Medicine. Report of the Planning Panel on the Education and Training of Health Sciences Librarians. Bethesda (MD): National Institutes of Health, National Library of Medicine, 1995 (http://www.nlm.nih.gov/ep/rfa_libr_training/title.html)

[5] Johnson FE (ed). Symposium: NLM planning grants for the education and training of health sciences librarians. Bull Med Libr Assoc 1996;84:513-68

[6] Giuse NB, Huber JT, Kafantaris SR, Giuse DA, Miller MD, Giles DE Jr, Miller RA, Stead WW. Preparing librarians to meet the challenges of today's health care environment. J Am Med Inf Assoc 1997;4:57-67

[7] Meyerhoff E. Continuing education of medical librarians: evaluation of the Association's past performance and suggestions for the future. Bull Med Libr Assoc 1963;51:376-83

[8] MacKenzie JD, Greenes RA. The World Wide Web: redefining medical education. JAMA 1997;278:1785-6

[9] Aronson B, Comba V. Multi-cultural and multi-lingual dimensions for the education of the European medical librarian. In: Bakker S, Cleland MC (eds). Information transfer: new age - new ways. Dordrecht: Kluwer, 1993:103-6

BECOMING ADEPT: TEACHING EVIDENCE BASED MEDICINE TO LIBRARIANS USING DISTANCE LEARNING

Alison Hicks
INFORMATION RESOURCES, SCHOOL OF HEALTH AND RELATED RESEARCH, UNIVERSITY OF SHEFFIELD, SHEFFIELD, UK

Background

Evidence based medicine has brought new challenges and opportunities[1-3] for librarians and information professionals but the ability to respond is limited by the need to develop additional skills and techniques whilst working in a busy setting. The ADEPT (Applying Diagnosis, Etiology, Prognosis and Therapy filters) programme was an intensive training course aiming to equip librarians for new and extended roles. Commissioned by the South Thames Library and Information Service, ADEPT was designed by Andrew Booth of the School of Health and Related Research (ScHARR) at the University of Sheffield. Alison Hicks joined ScHARR during the project and contributed to the writing of materials and the evaluation of the programme. ADEPT, delivered using a mix of workshops and distance learning, draws on a number of influences. The content of the programme is influenced by the research conducted at McMaster University, Canada,[4] on search techniques for specific types of study design. The format of the programme takes a lead from techniques used to teach evidence based medicine.

Structure and delivery

The structure of ADEPT is summarised in Table 1.
Units 1 through 5 followed the same structure: learning objectives; introduction; search strategies & filters; worked example; exercises; take home messages; summary; recommended reading. Participants were given one month to read units and complete exercises for return to ScHARR. Completed exercises were subject to review by the ADEPT trainers; a model answer was constructed and disseminated with detailed feedback.

Experience within the South Thames region has shown that, even within a relatively compact region, librarians are reluctant to spend much time away from their libraries, or travelling to training venues. This situation was further complicated by the fact that the trainers were based in Sheffield and were unable to travel the long distance on a regular basis to run the whole programme in the form of workshops. The ADEPT team were required to develop a programme which would reach as large an audience as possible but would also provide participants with intensive support.

The practical nature of the skills required a hands on approach and it was important that participants be able to sustain their skills in the workplace. These considerations led to the decision to use a blend of workshops and distance learning modules.

To deliver the training in an innovative fashion, it was decided to make use of techniques used in teaching evidence based medicine. In particular, the ADEPT team used the following: problem-based scenarios as the basis for small group work; the See-one, Do-one, Teach-one methods of progressive learning; the use of small group teaching; and the use of educational prescriptions to determine the content of the final workshop.

Table 1. Structure of ADEPT

UNIT	SUBJECT AREA	FORMAT	MONTH (1997)
1	Searching for therapy studies	Workshop	March/April
2	Searching for diagnosis studies	Workshop	March/April
3	Searching for systematic reviews	Distance learning	April/May
4	Searching for prognosis studies - Searching for aetiology studies	Distance learning	July
5	Searching for economic evaluations - Searching for guidelines	Distance learning	September
Final	Adapting ADEPT: getting knowledge into practice	Workshop	October

Evaluating ADEPT

As ADEPT was a pilot programme, it was important to collect a variety of evaluative data. The following evaluations were conducted: evaluations of individual units; evaluation of the concluding workshop; evaluation of the distance learning component; and a six-month follow-up evaluation.

UNIT EVALUATIONS

An evaluation form was included in each unit to assess the level of participants' familiarity with MEDLINE, the level of difficulty of the unit and whether or not the learning objectives had been met. In general, those at beginner or intermediate level found the units more difficult than those at advanced or expert level. The area causing most difficulty for all participants was the characteristics of the various study types, the area where participants are less likely to have prior knowledge. Participants were most confident with the searching techniques for the various study designs.

EVALUATION OF FINAL WORKSHOP

A short questionnaire was used to evaluate participants' satisfaction with the content and delivery of the workshop. Participants graded various aspects of the workshop using a Likert scale. This quantitative analysis was supplemented by qualitative questions where participants were asked to comment on the workshop content. It was clear from the evaluations received that participants appreciated a workshop environment to consolidate on skills learned through distance learning and welcomed the opportunity to work within a group.

EVALUATION OF DISTANCE LEARNING COMPONENT

Participants also evaluated the distance learning component of ADEPT (Units 3, 4 and 5) giving details of which units had been completed and, where relevant, reasons for non-completion. Of 33 evaluations, 9 respondents had completed and returned all three units, 11 had completed and returned two of the units and 2 had completed and returned one unit. Other respondents were able to read and complete the units but were unable to return the exercises to ScHARR by the deadline. A number of reasons were given for non-completion: pressures of day-to-day work; domestic circumstances; involvement in other courses; and involvement in exceptional project-based activities. Reasons relating to the programme itself included too much reading material; too little turnaround time between units and the level of difficulty.

It is obvious from the evaluations that distance learning can be a very isolating experience. The ADEPT course could be improved by actively promoting a learning community encouraging participants to keep in contact between workshops. It would be beneficial to offer a formal support service to help with any problems encountered. Several participants felt that the amount of time taken to complete units was too great and the time allowed between units was too short. The materials could be improved by adhering more closely to a distance learning style;[5] evaluations of earlier units showed that participants preferred shorter units. The mixed ability of the participants also proved problematic as the materials were aimed at intermediate level and above.

The introductory and closing workshops were well received and it has become clear from evaluations that a course delivered solely by distance learning would have been less popular. Participants were pleased with the extent of practical work; the units are based on a great deal of hands-on work thus encouraging learning by doing. The participating librarians were able to develop skills which are relevant to their work and several have since had the opportunity to put those skills into practice. The scope and coverage of the course was also well received; the main study types associated with EBM are covered and several participants have since used the course materials.

6-MONTH FOLLOW-UP EVALUATION

Six months after the completion of the course, a short questionnaire was sent to all participants to evaluate how they had used the skills and materials from ADEPT. 13 evaluations were received and of these, 11 have referred to the ADEPT materials since completing the course. The most common uses of the materials were to develop search strategies (9 respondents) and teaching/training purposes (9 responses). The materials have also been used to define literature search questions and to cascade skills to library colleagues. Several respondents suggested a quick reference guide summarising the main points of ADEPT; other suggestions included an index to the materials, the creation of "support teams" and the possibility of a refresher course.

What next..?

The ADEPT trainers are applying the lessons learned to develop the materials for other training programmes and to build on their existing knowledge of distance learning. For example, the materials are being adapted for a training programme for health librarians within the Trent region in the UK. PRECEPT (Programme for Encouraging Clinically Effective Practice in Trent) runs from March 1998 to December 1998, and consists of three stages: Sources of clinical effectiveness (one day workshop); Tips and tricks of using MEDLINE (half-day workshop); and Using methodological filters (four half-day workshops). Having learned from ADEPT, the final stage of PRECEPT, on methodological filters, is offered to a maximum of 12 participants who have identified this as a training need.

ADEPT, though by no means a finished product, represents an innovative attempt to address an immediate learning deficit and in this sense may be viewed as a success. All involved recognise its experimental nature and its impact to date is largely due to the commitment of the participating librarians. Both the participants and course providers have gained useful skills. The extensive feedback and evaluation mechanisms have contributed to the team's knowledge base and the team is confident that colleagues will be able to enhance and refine the ADEPT model.

References

[1] Batstone G & Edwards M. Professional roles in promoting evidence based practice. Br J Health Care Management 1996;2:144-147

[2] Haines M. Evidence based practice: new opportunities for librarians. Health Libr Rev 1994;11:221-225

[3] McCarthy LH. Evidence based medicine: an opportunity for health sciences librarians. Med Ref Serv Q 1996;15(4):63-71

[4] Haynes RB, Wilczynski N, McKibbon KA et al. Developing optimal search strategies for detecting clinically sound studies in MEDLINE. J Am Med Info Assoc 1994;1:447-458

[5] Rowntree D. Teaching through self-instruction: how to develop open learning materials. London: Kogan Page, 1990

THE INFORMATION PROFESSIONAL ASSOCIATIONS ON THE WEB: IDENTIFICATION AND QUALITY

Vanna Pistotti, Manuela Colombi
[1]ISTITUTO DI RICERCHE FARMACOLOGICHE 'MARIO NEGRI'; [2]SCHERING-PLOUGH SPA, DOCUMENTATION SERVICE AND LIBRARY, SEGRATE, MILANO, ITALY

Introduction

The professional isolation felt before Internet entered our daily work is now completeley overcome through the easy contact created from the net both among the members of the same association and associations sharing similar interest.
All this thanks to the web sites: But which are the most usefull sites for the professional and managerial evolution of the librarian/information officers? How to recognize their soundness? Which guidelines should be considered if one of us gets the opportunity to create a web site?

Aim of this poster presentation was to evaluate which information professional organizations are on the Internet and to assess and compare the contents of their web sites.

Material and methods

Our starting point was to choose the web site of the Italian Librarians' Association which we knew had a wide and updated list of professional associations worldwide. We immediately perceived the lack of a criterion for the evaluation of the sites of said associations. Thus, they being very numerous, we decided to choose eleven among them (see Table 1), considering their country of origin, their notoriety, and their historical and cultural value. We analyzed the single web sites keeping the following parameters in mind: graphics, language, speed of loading, the presence of the members' list, information on how to subscribe, information about the activities performed, special services for members, link to opac, publishers, libraries, database producers, and professional associations, presence of advertisements, availability of search engines.

Results and general considerations

In globally evaluating all those sites, and considering both the content and the appearance of the single webs, the first favourable impression arises from those sites demonstrating to have a permanent editorial board and not a simple though appreciable voluntary one. Here we find AIB, MLA, SLA, and, though not made clear, ASLIB and DGB.

The second characteristic, though apparently superficial, concerns the graphics of the site from the viewpoint of both iconography and colour. This aspect is very important when uploading the site and for the empathetic approach. Among the best EAHIL, GIDIF-RBM, ABF, SLA.

Another consideration concerns the presentation of the association itself: who they are, who they represent, which are their aims, information for aspiring members. This information is present even if not always immediate.

The fourth judgement was based on the various services offered to the association members. MLA, IFLA, DGB are the best, offering even employment opportunities. AIB, MLA, EAHIL offer a discussion list.

The fifth aspect considered was the presence of links with other associations, opac, libraries, publishers and database producers. The best are MLA and AIB, good GIDIF-RBM and ABF.

The last aspect considered is the site updating, which turns out to be quite timely for all the associations examined, except for GIDIF-RBM, ASLIB, and EUSIDIC. In this last the most timely updating may probably emerge in the section open to association members, only. It is a certainty that their 1996 homepage does not provide a good impression.

Following our observations, there is no operative standard for the creation of a web page well representing an association. Sure, the page shall be quickly loaded and provided with a pleasant, not excessively coloured and image-rich graphics. Its content should be well indexed at least at homepage level in order to allow a quick link with the desired sections. The introduction of services for members is a very important aspect even in view of the recruitment of new members. Worth mentioning - if subdivided into categories - is the presence of links with publishers, associations, and libraries. As to products, an excellent example is provided from the buyers' guide by the Medical Library Association.

Last but not least: the site updating is extremly important granting seriousness and continuity to the existence of the site itself.

Table 1: Eleven web sites included in comparative evaluation

ACRONYMS, NAMES, and URLS OF THE ASSOCIATIONS		
ABF	Association des Bibliothécaires Français	www.abf.asso.fr
AIB	Associazione Italiana Biblioteche	www. aib.it
ASLIB	Association for Information Management	www.aslib.co.uk
DGD	Deutsche Gesellschaft für Dokumentation	www.darmstadt.gmd.de/DGD
EAHIL	European Association for Health Information and Libraries	www.ub.ntnu.no/eahil/
EBLIDA	European Bureau of Library Information and Documentation Associations	www.kaapeli.fi/~eblida
EUSIDIC	European Association of Information Services	www.vito.be/eusidic
GIDIF-RBM	Gruppo Italiano Documentalisti Industria Farmaceutica e Istituti Ricerca Biomedica	www.gidif-rbm.it
IFLA	International Federation of Library Associations and Institutions	www.ifla.org ifla.inist.fr (european mirror)
MLA	Medical Library Association	www.mlanet.org
SLA	Special Libraries Association	www.sla.orgu

PRACTICE OF COLLEGIALITY: MISSION AND GOALS

Márta Virágos
CENTRAL LIBRARY, MEDICAL UNIVERSITY OF DEBRECEN, DEBRECEN, HUNGARY

Introduction

The Hungarian academic library profession experiences exciting times, because of not just the speed of change, but also by the recognition that significant contributions to progress within the academic community can be made. The bottom line for a library is the effectiveness of its service to its users.

Core skills for the academic librarian of today and the foreseeable future are: educational credibility, user education, IT-related skills and management skills.

Educational credibility

It is vital for librarians to gain credibility in an educational role. This represents the key to their effective integration into the academic community. The perception of academic staff can be reinforced or altered by, e.g., participating in official bodies or presenting papers at influential meetings.

User education

The librarian of today should develop a range of methods to train students in the skills of self-reliance. This is particularly important given the shift from teaching to learning, the high profile of transferable skills and the increasingly electronic environment. These changes have profound implications for librarians as trainers as well as for the student body. Library media professionals have worked hard to move from teaching isolated "library skills" to teaching integrated information skills.

Effective integration of information skills has two requirements:

- to be directly related to the contents area curriculum and to classroom assignments, and
- to be tied together in a logical and systematic information process model.

IT-related skills

It is information technology which generates the most vigorous debate in relation to the changing role of the librarian. Technological advances continue to ask questions of the supports services including the library. Library services - whether converged or not - are examining their policies on the balance between collection development and accessing information electronically.

IT-related competencies: tailored navigational support implies that the librarian keeps up-to-date with subject-based knowledge and accompanying IT-developments, and has an advisory role in guiding users through the maze of electronic sources and formats. Trainee librarians of today have to know how to use the machine, and how to interrogate the system through the machine, but the important thing is which information is useful to the individual being helped.

IT related infrastructure: the academic librarian of this decade and beyond has to possess a portfolio of IT-related skills in order to complement and support the navigational skills. Such skills help staff to manage the information more widely and, transfer these skills to the users as appropriate.

Management skills

External developments should be ensured for the advancement of library services. The staff who are required to adopt the skills and techniques of sound management practice will depend largely on the ethos, organisation and structure of the service. There are a number of factors suggesting that managerial responsibilities need to be more widely adopted. These include:
- the breakdown of hierarchical staffing structure
- increasingly participative decision-making
- greater emphasis on teamwork
- the need for flexibility in working arrangements
- the devolution of responsibilities and budgets

ATTENDING MEDICAL CONFERENCES AS A MARKETING STRATEGY FOR PROMOTING ONLINE SERVICES

Marta Jordà-Olives
HOSPITALS VALL D'HEBRON, RESEARCH AGENCY, BARCELONA, SPAIN

Introduction

The amount of information generated in the biomedical field is growing too fast to be easily embraced by potential users. To better reach end users, biomedical information providers have always been pioneers in using technological advances to make information more accessible.

We, as information professionals play (or should play) an active role in these developments because, as technology evolves, we must adapt our work strategies and routines to the new information requirements. And, as we have always done, we have to help users in the formulation of their demands in order to supply them not only with the information they request but also with the information they really want.[1] On the other hand, the new technologies have heavily affected people's information seeking behaviour. CD-ROMs have introduced the possibility of end-user searching, which on our part implied the organisation of specific training sessions. The most widely used database in CD-ROM format was (and still is) MEDLINE, which enjoys a privileged position as part of a non-profit organisation. A strong marketing strategy, which includes the awarding of grants and extensive training programs around the world, has made MEDLINE the most visible database in the biomedical field.

Now, with the widespread influence of the Internet on information retrieval, what will happen to the existing electronic and hard-copy information services? Will more time be allocated to information seeking, or will there be a knock-on effect with other sources/systems being displaced? What of the future of the commercial online hosts?[2] What is our role as information providers who work in the online environment? Should we give the users exactly what they ask for? Or should we keep working to satisfy their presumed information needs?

An emerging role in our everyday tasks involves the knowledge and application of marketing strategies to better reach our users and provide them with the best available answers to their explicit or implicit information demands. As new technologies evolve, we need to adapt our strategies to the new information requirements.

In this paper, I will focus on a specific aspect of our work: The Online Services. I will try to explain how the new information technologies, together with the MEDLINE phenomenon, seriously affect the result of the information retrieval process and I will suggest another way of marketing online services.

The MEDLINE phenomenon

As we all know, accessing bibliographical databases by means of telematic processes made us indispensable intermediaries between the physician and the literature retrieval. At that time, we believed that marketing our service would be difficult because we had to convince people to move from their old searching habits to the faster and more reliable ones. We also tried (and succeeded in) moving them from the "serendipity" habit to the "subject-oriented" searching system. We did this by a practical demonstration which showed the good results obtained with a ten or fifteen minute literature search. These results were retrieved from several databases. MEDLINE, EMBASE, PASCAL and others were constantly used to give the best and most relevant results possible.

But with the introduction of CD-ROM technology, MEDLINE is now the most widely used database in the Biomedical environment and the attitude has become: "if it's not in MEDLINE it is not worth knowing about". Thus, the success of MEDLINE has led to deficiencies in decision-making processes because online searches have gradually declined, while MEDLINE on CD-ROM has become the only database used, or even known about. Moreover, end-user access to MEDLINE on CD-ROM has lead to less refined searches. Despite all our user training efforts, searches are not well prepared and the capabilities of the database are not fully used. As a result, search strategy is very often inadequate and errors due to incorrect use, or lack of use, of the thesaurus are frequent.[3]

The new technologies' effect

The advances in information technologies do not take into account the complexities of the perception of information needs. We are witnessing the entrance of millions of end-users into the market in a relatively short time, many of them having more knowledge of certain information systems than do some information professionals. "The fact that the Internet offers much that is free will also play an important role in the end-user (...) with cheap or seemingly free online access another potential barrier has been demolished".[2] Also, "with the increasing availability of a range of web versions of commercial databases, many librarians are now faced with problems in justifying subscriptions to traditional Online Services. In particular, small medical libraries are faced with justifying expenditure on locally networked versions of MEDLINE when the database may be accessed freely via Internet".[4]

Another undesired effect of accessing information through the Internet is the difficulty in using search engines. On their part, traditional online hosts are announcing continuous changes in their products or adapting them to the new market. A good example is The new services and features introduced by Dialog Corporation (http://www.dialog.com).

Marketing Online Services

User studies are the first stage of marketing. The word "marketing" is sometimes associated with "manipulation" but this is not necessarily true. According to Webster's Encyclopaedic Unabridged Dictionary of the English Language marketing is defined as "the total of activities by which transfer of title or possession of goods from seller to buyer is effected, including advertising, shipping, storing and selling".

This is almost exactly what we do in our libraries: acquire information (shipping), catalogue and store it (storing), disseminate this information by means of OPACs or databases (advertising) and finally, provide the information according to our user's demands (selling). Following this concept we can state that marketing is the set of techniques concerned with matching products and services with needs, as well as improving communication with actual and potential users. McClure and Samuels[5] say that "libraries must carefully study what market exists for their services and what these services should be (...). To develop a marketing strategy, libraries must devote far more time to assessing community and potential information demands" because librarians tend to think that their product is so good that there is no need to advertise it, however "the information professional is the intermediary between the producer of recorded knowledge and the consumer of recorded knowledge".[6]

Going to the clients

One of the first steps of marketing is targeting the audience. My contribution to this topic is to address the users by working on a common project with them and submitting the results to medical congresses. "Professional congresses provide a forum for the exchange of professional news and ideas. Library congresses are useful for our profession but do not go beyond this. Thus, if we wish to communicate the contents and the use of certain information sources (and to increase the use of our services), we need to approach the potential user of this information and express ourselves through the same channels."[3] With this in mind, and always in collaboration with medical professionals, I began to participate in medical congresses and clinical sessions. Following the same methodology in each case (database reviews for specific fields) the results have sometimes been surprising for me and always unexpected for the doctors. Through their own experience they have had the opportunity to discover database options: the use and differences between thesauri, searchable fields, etc. They have also seen that MEDLINE is just another database among many others on the market, and that the others may meet their needs equally well or even better, depending on the search required. This result may seem obvious to us, but the advantage of the experience is that it provides us with scientific data to buck up our arguments and, moreover, it allows us to convey our knowledge through medical information channels. The immediate effect of this work in our case has been a renewed increase in use of the online service, which, complemented by the MEDLINE database accessible through the internal hospital network, has led to a more rational use of information sources, at least in the fields studied so far.

Conclusion

To keep marketing our services we have to experiment with different ways to approach our users. We, as information professionals should be present in their scientific meetings and in their electronic discussion lists to be ready to answer their information demands, since our job directly affects their work.

References

[1] Hoffman D. News and views from online world: optimism reigned among speakers, exhibitors... and most attendees (Online Inc.'s Online World Conference & Expo). Information Today 1997;14(4):14
[2] Nicholas D, Fenton D. The Internet and the changing information environment. Managing Information 1997;4:30-32
[3] Jordà-Olives M. From user training to medical conferences: Two ways for us... EAHIL Newsletter 1997;40:11
[4] Anagnostelis B, Cooke A. Evaluation criteria for different versions of the same database - a comparison of MEDLINE services available via the world wide web. (http://omni.ac.uk/agec/iolim97) donwloaded on:12/12/97; originally presented at Online Information 97. London 9-11 Dec. 1997
[5] McClure Ch, Samuels A (eds). Strategies for library administration: concepts and approaches. Libraries Unlimited 1982, p.391
[6] Oldmann C. Marketing library and information services: The strengths and weaknesses of a marketing approach. Eur J Marketing 1977;11:460-474

PUBLIC RELATION MANAGEMENT IN MEDICAL LIBRARIES IN HUNGARY

Lívia Vasas, Imola Jehoda
CENTRAL LIBRARY OF THE SEMMELWEIS UNIVERSITY OF MEDICINE, BUDAPEST, HUNGARY

PR and quality assurance in our library

Regarding Public Relations we can find numerous kinds of definition for it. "Public Relations" is defined as an attempt to influence public opinion by conveying information that benefits the (library) through a variety of techniques that will result in favourable publicity. We can say it very simply, "do your best and speak about it" in order to have good relation with those who could help in doing better services.

We should take into consideration that everything we are doing is for the sake of Quality Assurance. If one visits the library then wants as good services as possible and he must receive the proper information to his questions. If the library was not able to help, it is natural to give good and useful advice to the visitors. The PR activities help us in maintaining the high level of quality in our services.

The role of PR in ordinary life of libraries

Naturally, we have no time to deal with all the aspects of our topics, so we concentrate on some very important tasks we are doing all the time as a part of our work, hoping to do the best. This is a very important factor of our success! Doing our job well, every member of the library staff must think about Public Relations as a part of her/his daily routine!

Some years ago we hardly knew anything about PR but we have done something similar to it. We thought that to be polite was important for only those who were dealing with the "customers" or "visitors" in the library. At the moment the new financial and economic circumstances require more and other type of activities than being polite!

The libraries are very important segments of PR activities of publishers and database distributors. Opening new gates to the market, they want to influence our decision on buying new information technology to shape and improve our help-desk services. This is the first case (passive side) of PR in the library and we learn from them. The other case is, when after getting this information and the ways of knowledge we pass these new sources to our users, sponsors, visitors by promoting us! This is the active side of public relations work.

Characterising the present situation

In Hungary the economic and cultural systems have changed and are changing even today. The aims of these are to get closer to the European higher education standards. Instead of the small universities the government support the establishing of so called "classical" large universities with more faculties. This tendency can be traced in the health services as well as.

There are new financial facilities for the libraries but they have to fight for every penny. Libraries receive money from different budgets but they need to apply for money to different foundations. They helped us in buying new technologies, subscribing new periodicals that we could not afford. Nowadays, they limited their sponsorship, so we have to make money to maintain these services.

Planning

The Senate of the universities and the management in the hospitals make long-run and short-run activity plans. Regarding Public Relations the management generally makes yearly plans. The plans for the "Public Relations" work is completely different in case of the university libraries and the hospitals.
- Libraries must make a list on the new publications, events and special occasions for promoting the library.
- After summarising the goals we must characterise how we would want to achieve our targets, know how much this would cost, how much money we have, how we could get additional money.
- Deadlines and agenda must be determined according to the proper tasks. Confusion makes bigger harm than doing nothing!
- We dedicate the tasks to one or two persons who take the responsibility for this job.

Goals

It serves the better understanding to regard visitors as customers. The management has to organise this "business", because everything must be kept in one hand. The management knows competitive products and the services, prices and the payable segments of the market. Value added services must be introduced. Practically the customers take the new acquisitions for granted but they would like to have more additional information as well. The value added services are good opportunities to ask for extra money.

There are more than a dozen tenders in a year to get money from. The library management must work out a schedule of allocating and spending money. This work helps us in getting additional financial sources. The results of a harmonised and economical financial policy increase the reputation of a library and the reliability of the management. The better the reputation is the bigger amount of money one can get.

Librarians always could give new ideas to customers. Customers highly appreciate our help given to their new ideas. If they have good opinion of our services that also encourage us in giving new ideas in the future.

PR tools & devices

Most of the PR devices are well known among the librarians. The Media for example can destroy our work or multiply even the smallest result within some minutes. There is nothing more important than having good relations with the Media. One or two librarians from the staff should write articles about our work and services. We should inform the televisions and the radios on the happenings that could be widely interesting.

The management of the library has to organise open days, exhibitions, scientific conferences, special courses etc. in order to invite more and more people to take part in these events. We have to seize special events and anniversaries to establish any program that increase the reputation of the library. Every visit in the library is a very good opportunity to give better inspect not only into the document but the life of our library as well.

Naturally the staff must collect all information and opinions from the customer that could be very useful for the future. This inside communication could improve our services. The staff could correct the insufficiencies instantly and react properly. The image of the library is one of the basic element that must be also kept in sight. Sometimes the library has grants and donations from contributors free of charge but the library also supports organisations and institutes or anybody else as goodwill services. We have a special information group to serve those who want to know more about the library, about the collection of the books as well as our value added services. Last we should mention the representation of the interest in Public Administration. We usually invite some decision maker into the library from the Ministries.

PR in practice

From time to time - at least quarterly - we have to review the realisation of our PR plan. We have to look for the heel of Achilles that will help us in getting over the problems. After this analysis we have to settle down the new idea (if it is necessary) the new tasks and goals that must be achieved. We have to examine the new circumstances as well the possibilities with their financial backgrounds. The new stand of points must be worked out as well. These will serve the basis to do well in the new run. Carrying out needs consistency and flexibility as well. After doing the tasks one by one we have to go back to the beginning but at higher level to start again with analysis.

Last but not least

As you can see the practices of PR in our library's life. It is impossible to survive this new situation without doing public relations. You could see how Public Relations got their positions in the daily routine, how they became basic principals of our work. We cannot get result by doing PR as campaign once or twice for some days per year!

Training and workshops on this topic are more than useful for every library that wants to get over the difficulties that were brought up by the social changes and the lack of money. I am sure, we can declare there is no professionalism without doing public relations.

We hope to achieve this goal by doing PR very consistently. Nowadays we are organising a training on the specialities of PR for the medical libraries. We would like to help them this way hoping the common co-ordinated work is much more productive and the success will became permanent and long-lasting!

Bibliography

Annual report of 1997 Semmelweis University of Medicine Central Library. Budapest, 1998

Bussey HJ. Public relations vs. marketing: The information professional's role as mediator. Spec Libr 1991;82:154-158

St Clair G. Marketing and promotion in today's special library. Aslib Proc 1990;42:213-217

Zimmermann ME. Public relations at SLA: An introduction article to a special issue. Spec Libr 1991;82:151-153

Chapter 14: HISTORY

Editorial introduction

The last chapter of these proceedings is devoted to historical aspects: not only the history of medicine as subject of library studies and activities, including the historical medical collection of the library, but also the history of medical librarianship.

The papers of Maria Francesca Ribes Cot, Heidi Seger, Clarissa Szabo and Rosella Aprea differ greatly in subject and angle of view on the subject. They have in common, though, the call for interest in history and the importance of history towards a better understanding of the present. Librarians have a special role in conserving the past, especially the information sources that have build up to the knowledge base of a profession. This special role of librarians is very well presented by Guus Mathijsen (p. 146). Although he claims that the medical library profession is in a better position, because of the support of the US Medical Library Association and the NLM, it is still very important to *all* European medical librarians to contribute to the professional heritage, not only of their own profession but also of nurses and other health professionals (see also the paper of Linda Parr p. 181).

THE HISTORY OF MEDICAL LIBRARIES: A BIBLIOGRAPHICAL CONTRIBUTION

Maria Francesca Ribes Cot, M.C. Jara Mirones, V.M. Cuñat Ciscar
[1 2]Hospital Universitario Marques de Valdecilla, Library; [3]Universidad de Cantabria, Dept de Historia Moderna y Contemporanea, Santander, Spain

Introduction

To judge from published articles, studies and communications presented at scientific meetings by medical librarians, the history of medical libraries does not appear to be a priority for these professionals more especially corcerned about areas such as the applications of new technologies, integrated information systems, user training, quality control and so on. Nevertheless, the study of the historical forerunners of modern health science libraries is an excellent example of historical development, from the general libraries of classical times, through the personal libraries of the Middle Ages, wich still exist in modern times, up to the libraries belonging to scientific institutions of the 17th, 18th and 19th centuries. This is of great interest because it allows us to analyse the development shown by medical libraries, from and element of personal learning, to a key service in the clinical decision making process of medical staff.

A review of the literature on the subject, provides numerous articles on present day medical libraries.

Results

The bibliographic search carried out through these systems gives access to a large amount of published work on history of medical libraries in the contemporany period, specially on North American libraries, with the Bulletin of Medical Libraries Association as the main source. However, the bibliography obtained on the subject prior to the 20th century is scarce (tables I-II) and difficult to obtain, acces being mainly through references given by other authors. Figure 1 shows the number of publications relating to different historical periods. Figure 2 shows percentages of articles found in the North American literature and the rest of the world.

Sources and methodology

Automated bibliographic searches: ON-LINE: Eric, LISA, Dissertation, EMBASE; CD-ROM: MEDLINE, Indice Medico Español and Rebius.

Several search profiles were implemented, using natural language and documentary language where possible. Key words used to prepare searches belong to the areas of medical libraries and biomedical information services, with no chronological lines from classical times up to the 20th century. The most frequert concepts were: medical libraries, history, hospital libraries, libraries, librarians, library association, etc.

Specialized bibliographies

Specialist journals, indexed and non-indexed in the data-bases

Medical libraries in Europe and North America were consulted for information on published work relating to the history of medical libraries in their countries.

Through Internet information on the subject was requested from the following groups: Library History Round Table, Wellcome Institute, British Library, Library Today, New York Academy of Medicine, National Library of Medicine (U.S.A.), Library Association Group of History and automated catalogues of medical and non-medical libraries were interrogated via Internet.

Discussion

North American medical library groups were founded in 1898 and this long-standing, tradition probably explains the large number of studies on the history of libraries carried out in the USA, as compared to Europe where the creation on health, science library groups is much more recent. In England the medical library group was set up in the sixties, and in Germany in 1973 [in the Netherlands in 1953]. It was not until the eighties that library associations were established in other countries such as Spain, Portugal and Italy (1991), culminating with the formation in 1986 of the European Association of Health Libraries, EAHIL.

The work of the European associations of medical libraries has been an extremely positive contribution, helping membres to work more efficiently in multiple aspects. The EAHIL would be an excellent forum for discussion and a stimulus for the study of the history of European medical libraries. This would surely be worth the effort, since the key to the future of on libraries lies is the study of their origins. It would be a nice project, let's go ahead with it.

Bibliography

BOOKS

ALCOLEA S. La Biblioteca de la Universitat de Barcelona. Barcelona: Pub. de la Universitat, 1994

ANNAN GL. Handbook of Medical Library Practice. Third ed. Chicago: Medical Library Association, 1970

AVELAR SOARES ME, RODRIGUES MABM. Les fonds anciens des imprimes de la Bibliotheque de la Faculte de Medicine de L'Universite de Porto. Les medicins-auteurs portugais. En: Medical Libraries: Cooperation and new technologies. North Holland: Amsterdam, 1985:445-4447

BONNETT P, FORRESTER WH, JOSE RH. The British Medical Association's Nuffield Library. Past, Present and Future. Health Inform Libr 1990;1: 53-59

BURKE RA. Culture and communication through the ages. Chicago: dePaul University, 1953

CASTIGLIONI A. Historia de la Medicina. Barcelona: Salvat, 1941.
CHESNEY AM. The Johns Hopkins Hospital and the Johns Hopkins University School of Medicine. A Chronicle. Vol. I Early Years 1867-1893. Baltimore: The Johns Hopkins Press, 1943
DE LA CAMARA JP. Fisonomia y vida del hospital moderno americano: estampas de un viaje de estudio. Madrid: Ministerio de Trabajo. Instituto Nacional de Previsión, 1948
DOE J (ed). A handbook of medical library practice. Chicago: Medical Library Association, 1943
DOE J, MARSHALL LM (eds). A handbook of medical library practice. 2d. ed. Chicago: Medical Library Association, 1956
DOYLE G. The provision of medical information in a Dublin Medical School in the 19th century. En: Health Information: New Possibilities. Dordrecht: Kluwer Academic Publishers, 1995:205-207
ELMER P. The library of Dr. John Webster: The making of a seventeenth-century radical. London: Wellcome Institute for the History of medicine, 1986
GROEN FK. Sir Willian Osler and Medical Libraries. En: Health Information: New Possibilities. Dordrecht: Kluwer Academic Publishers, 1995:200-204
GUTHRIE D. Historia de la Medicina. Barcelona: Salvat Ed., 1947
INVERT J. Histoire des Hôpiteaux en France. Toulouse: Ediciones Privat, 1982
IORI R. The medical knowledge in Reggio Emilia through the period of activity of the University of Medicine (1571-1772). En: Medical Libraries: Cooperation and new technologies. North Holland: Amsterdam, 1986:463-4o
JOHNSON ED. A History in the Western World. New York: Scarecrow Press, 1965
OLIVER MUÑOZ MV. La Biblioteca del Colegio Maximo de San Pablo de Lima (1568-1767): Analisis Bibliograficos y Socioculturales. (Tesis Doctoral). Madrid: Universidad Complutense, 1989
PARSONS EA. The Alexandrian Library: Glory of the helenic word. New York: Elsevier Press, 1952
PEKKARINEN P, TOIVARI S. On the origin and early development of medical libraries and transfer of medical information: an essay on ancient medical texts En: Information transfer: New age-new ways. Dordrecht: Kluwer Academic Publihers, 1992:369-372
PISHA LJ. Library Collections at Harvard, Yale and Brown from 1780's to the 1860's (Dissertation) Columbia University 1991
PONS ALOS V. Archivo del Hospital "Major de Pobres" de Xàtiva: Catálogo y Estudio. Valencia: Generalitat Valenciana. Conselleria de Cultura Educacio i Ciencia. Diputacions d'Alacant, Castelló i València, 1987
POSTELL WD. Development of Medical Literature. New Orleans: Luisiana State University, School of Medicine, 1943
RODRIGUEZ ALVAREZ R. La Biblioteca de la Universidad de Oviedo (1765-1934). (Tesis doctoral). Oviedo: Universidad de Oviedo, 1992
ROJO VEGA A. Ciencia y Cultura en Valladolid. Estudio de las bibliotecas privadas de los siglos XVI y XVII. Valladolid: Universidad de Valladolid. Ediciones del Seminario de Historia de la Medicina, 1985
SEBASTIANI B, SALVATORI G. The pre-Salernitan period, the codices and the italian libraries: A page in the history of medicine. En: Health Information: New Possibilities. Dordrecht: Kluwer Academic Publishers, 1995:197-199
SILLERO SARASUA MP. La Biblioteca de Philipp Hauser. Análisis Bibliometico e Inventario. (Tesis Doctoral). Sevilla: Universidad de Sevilla, 1992

SERIALS

BALLARD JF. The past history of the Medical Library Association. Bull Med Libr Assoc. 1948;36:227-241
BIRCHETTE KP. The History of Medical Libraries from 2000 B.C. to 1900 A.C. Bull Med Libr Assoc 1973;6:302-308
BRAUDE RM, WOOD SJ. On the origin of a species : evolution of health sciences librarianship. Bull Med Libr Assoc 1997;85:1-10
BRODMAN H. Education and attitudes of early medical librarians to their work: a discussion based on the oral history project of the medical library association. J Libr Hist 1980;15:167-182
COLAIANNI LA. The vision thing. Bull Med Libr Assoc 1992;80:1-8
CULP RW. The Mount Sinai Hoispital Library, 1883 to 1970. Bull Med Libr Assoc 1972;60:471-480
CUSHING H. The doctor and his books. Am J Surg 1928;4:100-110
DEBAKEY M. The National Library of Medicine evolution of a premier information center. JAMA 1991;266:1252-1258
DURAN CAÑAMERAS F. La Biblioteca de la Facultad de Medicina de Barcelona (Historia). Anales de Medicina y Cirugía. 1947:256-265

GARCIA A. Tres bibliotecas de médicos valencianos, renacentistras (Luis Alcañiz, Pere Pintor y Pere Martí). Asclepio. 1974-5;XXVI-XXVII:527-546

GARCIA BALLESTER L. Tres bibliotecas médicas en la Valencia del siglo XV. Asclepio. 1966-67;XVIII-XIX:383-406

GARRISON CHJ. How to Use Package Libraries in the Building Program. The Modern Hospital 1930;34:49-52

GROEN FK. Three who made an association; I. Sir Williams Osler. 1849-1919. II. George Milbry Gould, 1848-1922. III. Margaret Ridley Charlton, 1858-1931 and the founding of Medical Library Association, Philadelphia, 1898. Bull Med Libr Assoc 1996;84:311-319

HELWIG D. Ancient medical library being resurrected in Egipt. Can Med Assoc J 1989;140:452-453

HOLLMAN E. Sir Willians Osler and Harvey Cushing. Two great personalities and medical bibliophiles. Stanford Med Bull 1961;19:173-185

HOLLEY EG. The past as prologue: The work of the library historian. J Libr Hist 1977;12:110-127

HOW Hospital Libraries are Growing in England. The Modern Hospital 1932:63

HUNTINGTON AT. The Association of Medical Librarians; past, present and future. Med Libr Hist J 1907;5:111-123

JONES P. What the Librarian Can and Should Mean to the Hospital. The Modern Hospital. 1931;37:53-56

KRONICK DA. A lending library for medical students in the eigteenth century. Bull Med Libr Assoc 1989;77:69-70

LITTGER KW. Dr. Johann Scheifler (1612-1671) and his library. A prosopographic study. Sudhoffs Arch Z Wissenschaftsgesch 1990;74:75-103

SPIVAK CD. The medical Libraries of United States. Med Libr 1898;1(suppl):1-14

WIDDES JDH. Medical Libraries in the Republic of Ireland. Libri 1954;3:81-87

Figure 1. Number of publications relating to different historical periods

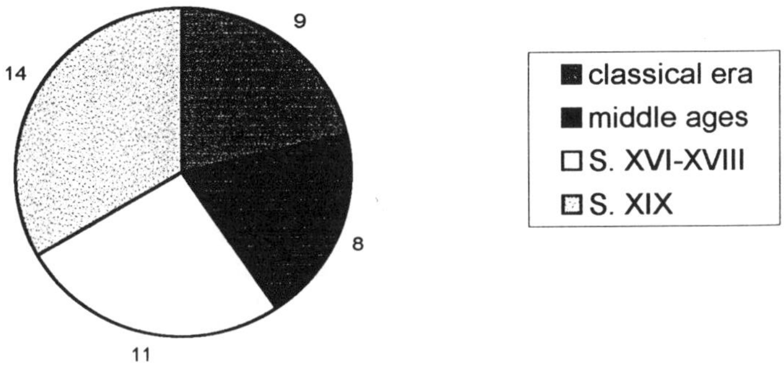

Figure 2. Number of articles/Countries

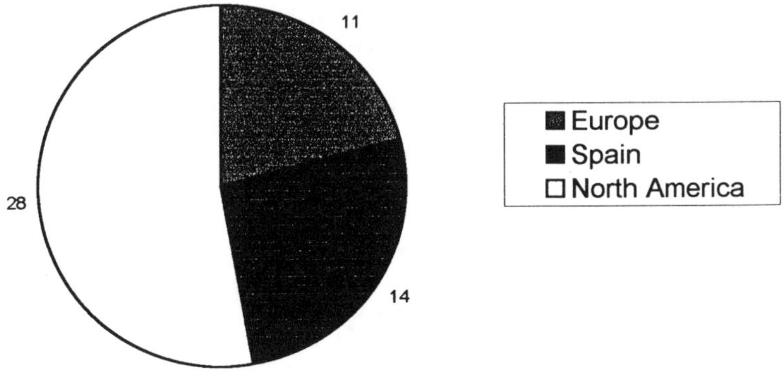

LES BIBLIOTHÈQUES DES INSTITUTS D'HISTOIRE DE LA MÉDECINE EN SUISSE / MEDICAL HISTORY LIBRARIES IN SWITZERLAND

Heidi Seger, Gertraud Gamper, Pia Burkhalter, Danièle Calinon, Brigitte Clerc
ZURICH; BERNE; LAUSANNE; GENEVA, SWITZERLAND

Zurich

La Bibliothèque de l'Institut d'histoire de la médecine a été inaugurée en 1951 lors de la création d'un institut et d'une chaire d'histoire de la médecine à l'Université de Zurich. Depuis de nombreuses années déjà, le médecin zurichois Gustav Adolf Wehrli (1888-1949) avait enseigné l'histoire de la médecine comme privat-docent. La Bibliothèque comprend actuellement env. 160'000 titres (monographies, tirés-à-part, thèses, périodiques et documentation diverse). Une collection de manuscrits, des lettres autographes de médecins et d'importantes documentations biographiques et iconographiques complètent les fonds. La littérature scientifique comprend des titres de presque tous les temps et toutes les régions et couvre une multitude d'aspects des disciplines médicales. Depuis 1994 les nouvelles acquisitions sont annoncées dans le catalogue informatisé du réseau DOBIS/LIBIS des bibliothèques des instituts universitaires. Des pourparlers pour un nouveau système (Aleph) sont en cours; il est prévu qu'il entrera en fonction en 1998/99. DOBIS/LIBIS est accessible par Internet à l'adresse de l'Université: http://www.unizh.ch/. La Bibliothèque participe au prê interbibliothèques au niveau suisse et étranger.

ADRESSE Bibliothek, Medizinhistorisches Institut und Museum (directeur: Prof. Beat Rüttimann), Universität Zürich, Rämistr. 71, CH-8006 Zürich, <http://www.mhiz.unizh.ch>

Responsable de la Bibliothèque: Heidi Seger; e-mail: hseger@mhiz.unzh.ch

Berne

La bibliothèque à été fondée en 1963 par Erich Hintzsche (1900-1975), professeur d'anatomie à l'Université de Berne. Il a légué sa bibliothèque privée ainsi que sa collection d'instruments scientifiques au Canton de Berne, à condition que sa donation soit maintenue en bon état et augmentée et qu'elle soit mise à la disposition de la recherche. Jusqu'à sa mort, il s'occupait personellement de la bibliothèque. Après la création de la chaire d'histoire de la médecine, la première titulaire, le professeur Esther Fischer-Homberger prit la responsabilité de la bibliothèque, qui changea de nom en s'appelant désormais "Institut d'histoire de la médecine". Depuis 1985, le professeur Urs Boschung est le directeur de l'institut.

Ouverte au public, la bibliothèque contient environ 35'000 monographies, de la littérature originale aussi bien que de la littérature secondaire, ensuite des tirés à part, des illustrations, des correspondances, des fonds d'archives et des manuscrits.
Ce sont les publications biographiques et les publications concernant la vie et l'oeuvre d'Albert de Haller, ainsi que la médecine du XVIII siècle, des manuels de diverses matières médicales, l'histoire de la psychiatrie, l'histoire de la pharmacie, et le thème "femmes et médecine" qui forment les domaines de collection privilégiés.

ADRESSE

Institut d'histoire de la médecine / Université de Berne. Bibliothèque, Bühlstrasse 26, CH-3012 Bern, Tél.: +41 31 631.8486 - Fax: +41 31 631.8491
<http://www.ana.unibe.ch/MHIUB/mhiub.htm>
e-mail: pia.burkhalter@mhi.unibe.ch

Lausanne et Genève

L'Institut romand d'histoire de la médecine et de la santé comprend deux sites complémentaires, Lausanne et Genève, et deux bibliothèques qui se développent selon leurs spécificités. Tous les ouvrages sont annoncés dans le catalogue informatisé VTLS comportant 2 millions de notices provenant d'environ 100 bibliothèques de recherche et de références situées dans les cantons suisses de langue française et italienne. Ce catalogue est accessible à l'adresse: http://www.rero.ch

L'Institut universitaire de la médecine et de la santé publique de Lausanne a été fondé en 1989, il est dirigé par le professeur Vincent Barras.

La bibliothèque renferme environ 10.000 ouvrages, les plus anciens datant du 16e siècle. Les centres d'intérêt comportent: histoire de la médecine et des neurosciences, médecine antique, histoire des hôpitaux, histoire de la médecine en Suisse et plus spécialement dans le canton de Vaud et à Lausanne, anthropologie et philosophie de la médecine, éthique. Elle possède aussi une collection de 30 périodiques, la plupart depuis les premiers numéros, et une collection de tirés-à-part et de dossiers biographiques.

Fondée en 1992, la bibliothèque de Genève est reliée à deux institutions: l'Institut Louis-Jeantet d'histoire de la médecine, dirigé par le professeur Bernardino Fantini, et l'Unité de recherche et d'enseignement en bioéthique, dirigée par le professeur Alex Mauron. Elle comprend environ 10.000 ouvrages. Les fonds anciens datent pour la plus grande partie du XIXe et du début du XXe siècle et concernent surtout la pathologie, l'anatomie, la physiologie, la biologie, la médecine légale et la psychiatrie, les maladies infectieuses et les médecines parallèles. Ils comprennent également des tirés-à-part et des thèses de professeurs et de médecins genevois. La littérature secondaire est centrée sur l'histoire de la santé publique, l'histoire des maladies infectieuses, la philosophie de la médecine, l' histoire des aspects scientifiques de la médecine, la bioéthique, l'histoire médicale genevoise.

Responsables des bibliothèques
Lausanne: Danièle Calinon, e-mail: Daniele.Calinon@inst.hospvd.ch
Genève: Brigitte Clerc, e-mail: brigitte.clerc@medecine.unige.ch

Summary

Medical History is taught at the Universities of Zuerich, Berne, Lausanne and Geneva. The Medical History Library of Basel is in the process of being reorganized. The four chairs are combined with academic research institutes and important specialised libraries.

ANALYSIS OF THE LIFE WORK AND LIBRARY BEQUEST OF TIBOR GYÕRY A HUNGARIAN MEDICAL HISTORIAN

Clarissa Szabo-Balogh, Laszlo Molnar, Piroska Prepok
CENTRAL LIBRARY OF THE SEMMELWEIS UNIVERSITY OF MEDICINE, BUDAPEST, HUNGARY

Summary

In 1998, it is the sixtieth anniversary of Tibor Györy's death. Tibor Györy (1869-1938), physician, historian of medicine is even now not yet acknowledged. Our poster will demonstrate stations of Györy's life, our information sheets show the results of our investigations. We are employed at the Semmelweis University of Medicine. Our University is bearing the name of Ignac Semmelweis from the year 1969. It was Tibor Györy, who made the name of Semmelweis internationally known.
He left his book collection of 2211 documents, his archival material by will to the library of the medical faculty.
On the presented poster photos were to be seen of the life of Tibor Györy, the exhibition of medical history in 1898. We show the international congress of medical history in September 1929 in Budapest on several photos.
In information sheets we analyze in detail the historical work of Tibor Györy, his archival and library bequest.

References

[1] Györy Tibor. In: Biographia az Állatorvostudományi Egyetem elhunyt tanárainak és elõadóinak életrajza. szerk. Kovács Gyula, Fehér György. Bp. 1967. Mezõgazdasági Könyvkiadó, 54-56
[2] Györy Tibor: Különfélék. Tünõdés. Népegészségügy 1934;15:1009-10
[3] Györy Tibor: Orvosi szaklapjaink történetébõl. Népegészségügy 1934;15:954-59
[4] Schultheisz Emil: Györy Tibor 1869-1938. Orvosi Hetilap 1964;105:751-2
[5] Szállási Árpád: Emlékezés egy kiváló orvostörténészre. Orvosi Hetilap 1979;120:346-8
[6] Vámossy Zoltán: Györy Tibor 1869-1938. Orvosi Hetilap 1938;82:1

SEXUALLY TRANSMITTED DISEASES: TRAVELLING THROUGH SPACE AND TIME

Rossella Aprea, Jeanette Gaido, Pietro Puddu
ISTITUTO DERMOPATICO DELL'IMMACOLATA (IRCCS), SCIENTIFIC LIBRARY, ROME, ITALY

Introduction and methodology

In this report we present an historical review on the evolution of STDs in different regions of the world to highlight the most characteristic factors involved in the propagation and/or the fall of STDs during the centuries and all over the world. We selected a certain number of articles as a result of a bibliographic research on MEDLINE database (January 1966 - September 1997), using the keywords "sexually transmitted diseases" and "genitourinary diseases" crossed with "history of medicine", from the ancient times to 20th century. One hundred and four articles were found pertinent for this study. The number of publications concerning STDs in the pre-Aids and Aids-era were not numerically different. During the period 1966-1984 (still pre Aids-era) of the 58 publications selected, 40 (68,96%) were found in north-east European journals (mostly from Russia, Germany and Poland) and these publications analyzed exclusively the history of STDs in each individual country. On the contrary, during the Aids-era, there has been a considerable increase of publications in American and Western European journals, which examined the evolution of STDs not only in their own countries, but in Africa and Asia as well. Only 33 articles [1-33] of original 104 were further selected and analyzed for their completeness and possibility to best describe the historical and geographical situation of STDs in the various regions of the world.

Historical periods of STDs

We have identified 5 significant historical periods concerning the evolution of STDs:
1) Before Christ: Gonorrhea and sexual and social behavior among the Greeks, Egyptians and Asiatics;[5,21,28]

2) After Christ until 1492: Modest information concerning prevention and therapies;[3,5,7,11,22]

3) 1493-1800: The spread of syphilis after the return of Colombo from Spain;[2,6-9,11-15,17,18,20,22,30]

4) 1801-1980: The progressive fall of syphilis and other STDs for the identification of the microorganism responsible for sexual infections, for numerous and strict preventive measures focused on the control and the regulation of prostitution and for new diagnostic and therapeutical forms;[1,3,6-17,19,22,23,29,30]

5) from 1981 on, AIDS era: a new disease, an old problem for similarities with syphilis in forms of transmission (i.e. sexual contact, blood transfusion, from mother to the fetus during pregnancy), and in terms of social isolation and moral condemnation.[3,6,10,12,26,27]

STDs today: a global problem

From this analysis STDs do not result only a biological entity, but a group of diseases that are rooted and engaged on certain attitudes, values and beliefs and that all this factors are strongly associated with the historical periods of the world (i.e. social conditions, environmental phenomena, wars, industrialization) more than on geographical location.[27,34,35]

Everywhere the history of STDs shows a sheer pendular movement. Phases of major spread of STDs have as a consequence severe control of sexual habits. This severe control brings to phases of less spread of STDs with a result of progressive higher sexual permissiveness, opening a new epidemiological and sociocultural cycle.[22] Nowadays the knowledge and the awareness of the risks connected with sexual contacts are essential for everyone to avoid infection, not only for some social categories as homosexuals, prostitutes and drugs addicts. Also the situation concerning the forms of prevention has deeply changed, because the factors involved in the increasing incidence of STD are multiple and variable. Changing social, economical, cultural and biological factors (i.e. sex tourism, high urbanization, drug addiction, life style, teenager sex) plays more and more a decisive role in the spreading of STDs. For this reason, all these factors, alone and combined, should not be underestimated in the formulation of "new forms" of prevention and control of STDs.[27]

References

1 Hübschmann K. History of Dermatology and Venereology from 1848 to the end of 1944 in Prague, Czechoslovakia. Int J Dermatol 1982;21:356-360

2 Waugh MA. Venereal diseases in sixteenth century in England. Med Hist 1973;7:192-9

3 Ziperman HH. A medical history of the Panama Canal. Surg Gynecol Obstet 1973;137:104-14

4 King A. Venereology - a backward look. Br J Vener Dis 1972;48:412-5

5 Morton RS. Sexual attitudes, preferences and infections in Ancient Egypt. Genitourin Med 1995;71:180-6

6 Pellow D. STDs and AIDS in Ghana. Genitourin Med 1994;70:418-23

7 De Silva PA, Gomez MG. The history of venereal disease and yaws (parangi) in Sri Lanka (Ceylon). Genitourin Med 1994;70:349-54

8 Weindling P. Sexually transmitted diseases between imperial and Nazi Germany. Genitourin Med 1994;70:284-9

9 Fyrand O, Granholt A. The history of venereology in Norway. Genitourin Med 1994;70:215-7

10 Tibbits D. Safer sex now and then. Med J Aust 1994;161:83-84,86-7

11 Lyons M. Sexually transmitted diseases in the history of Uganda. Genitourin Med 1994;70:138-45

12 MacDougall H. Sexually transmitted diseases in Canada, 1800-1992. Genitourin Med 1994;70:56-63

13 Hall LA. "The Cinderella of medicine": sexually transmitted diseases in Britain in the nineteenth and twentieth centuries. Genitourin Med 1993;69:314-9

14 Dikotter F. Sexually transmitted diseases in modern China: a historical survey. Genitourin Med 1993;69:341-5

15 Cronberg S. The rise and fall of sexually transmitted diseases in Sweden. Genitourin Med 1993;69:184-6

16 Conde-Glez CJ, Calderon E, Juarez-Figueroa L, Hernandez-Avila M. Historical account of venereal diseases in Mexico. Genitourin Med 1993;69:462-6

17 Mattelaer JJ. History of venereal disease [French]. Acta Urol Bel 1993;61:19-28

[18] Bamber SD, Hewison KJ. Underwood PJ. A history of sexually transmitted diseases in Thailand: policy and politics. Genitourin Med 1993;69:148-57
[19] Davidson R. Measuring "the social evil": the incidence of venereal disease in interwar Scotland. Med Hist 1993;37:167-86
[20] Arnold D. Sexually transmitted diseases in nineteenth and twentieth century in India. Genitourin Med 1993;69:3-8
[21] Morton RS. Sexual attitudes, preferences and infections in Ancient Greece: has antiquity anything useful for us today? Genitourin Med 1991;67:59-66
[22] Remotti G. Sexually transmitted diseases: yesterday and today [Italian]. Ann Ostet Ginecol Med Perinat 1989;110:273-82
[23] Fee E. Sin vs. science: venereal disease in Baltimore in the twentieth century. J Hist Med Allied Sci 1988;43:141-64
[24] Adler MW. The terrible peril: A historical perspective on the venereal diseases. Br Med J 1980;281:206-11
[25] Janier M, Saada V. From venereology to sexually transmitted diseases. Ann Dermatol Venereol 1989;116:957-64
[26] Cater W Jr. Acquired immunodeficiency syndrome, sexually transmitted diseases and epidemiology. Past lessons, present knowledge and future opportunities. Am J Epidemiol 1990;131:749-58
[27] Darrow WW. Health education and promotion for STD prevention: lessons for the next millennium. Genitourin Med 1997;73:88-94
[28] Bafverstedt B. Dermatological and venereal diseases told about in the Bible [Swedish]. Lakartidningen 1971;68:3793-802
[29] Auvin M. The beginning of venereal disease control in the USSR (V.M. Bronner, 1876-1938) [Russian]. Vestn Dermatol Venerol 1971;45(5):54-8
[30] Schoenfeld J. History of venereal diseases [Germany]. Offentl Gesundheitswes 1982;44:660-3
[31] Roberts A. The pox and the people: a history of venereal diseases and sexual attitudes. Nurs Times 1982;78:1177-85
[32] Handsfield HH. Sex, science and society. A look at sexually transmitted diseases. Postgrad Med 1997;101:268-73,277-8
[33] Zone RM. Venereal diseases: a historical perspective. J Tenn Med Assoc 1991;84:451-3
[34] Schoefeld CBS. Sexually transmitted diseases. Edinburgh: Longman, 1972
[35] Brandt AM. No magic bullet. A social history of venereal disease in United States since 1880. New York-Oxford: Oxford University Press, 1987

AUTHOR INDEX

Appendix: LIST OF SIGs AND CECs

Special Interest Groups	contacts
Academic Medical Libraries	Rikie Deurenberg
Editors of Medical Library Journals/Newsletters	Suzanne Bakker
Clinical Librarians	Suzanne Bakker
Database Producers	Rüdiger Schneemann
Nursing and Allied Health Libraries	Patrica Flor
Pharmaceutical Libraries	Vincent Maes
Problem-based Learning	Fons van den Eeckhout, Ingegerd Rabow
Veterinary Libraries	Gerdien de Jonge
WHO Documentation Centres	Arne Jakobsson

Continuing Education Courses	course leaders
Quality management	Carl Gustav Johanssen
User education	Jean Yeoh
Editors' workshop	Shane Godbolt, Penny Bonnett, Suzanne Bakker
Cochrane Library	Julie Glanville
Medical information on the web	Lisa Blankenship, Lynn Fox
Medical Subject Headings	Marie Monik, Gun Brit Knutssøn
Internet sources	Paul Nieuwenhuysen
Public health information sources	Anke Scheiber
Serveurs Web	Corinne Verry
Copyright	Charles Oppenheim
Medical information databases	Christine Wickman